THE GENETICS OF CANCER

CANCER BIOLOGY AND MEDICINE

Series Editors M.J. Waring and B.A.J. Ponder

THE GENETICS OF CANCER

Edited by

B.A.J. Ponder

Professor of Human Cancer Genetics
University of Cambridge
UK

and

M.J. Waring

Reader in Chemotherapy
University of Cambridge
UK

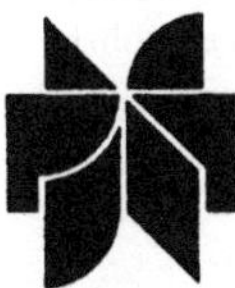

SPRINGER SCIENCE+BUSINESS MEDIA, B.V.

A catalogue record for this book is available from the British Library

Library of Congress Cataloging in Publication Data

The genetics of cancer / edited by B.A.J. Ponder and M.J. Waring.
p. cm. -- (Cancer biology and medicine ; CABM 04)
Includes bibliographical references and index.
ISBN 978-0-7923-8886-9 ISBN 978-94-011-0677-1 (eBook)
DOI 10.1007/978-94-011-0677-1
1. Cancer--Genetic aspects. I. Ponder, B. A. J. (Bruce A. J.), 1944- . II. Waring, Michael J. III. Series.
[DNLM: 1. Neoplasms--genetics. W1 CA673L v.4 1995 / QZ 202 G33193 1995]
RC268.4.G459 1995
616.99'4042--dc20
DNLM/DLC
for Library of Congress 95-31821
CIP

Copyright

Typeset by EXPO Holdings, Malaysia

Contents

List of Contributors

N.E. CAPORASO
Genetic Epidemiology Branch
National Cancer Institute
National Institutes of Health
EPN 439
Rockville
MD 20892
USA

T.A. DRAGANI
Division of Experimental
Oncology A
Istituto Nazionale Tumori
Via G. Venezian 1
I-20133 Milan
Italy

D. ECCLES
Wessex Clinical Genetics Service
Level G
Princess Anne Hospital
Southampton
SO16 5YA
UK

R.A. EELES
Institute of Cancer Research and
Royal Marsden Hospital
Downs Road
Sutton
Surrey
SM2 5PT
UK

L.R. FERGUSON
Cancer Research Laboratory
University of Auckland Medical
School
Private Bag 92019
Auckland
New Zealand

M. GOULD
Department of Human Oncology
University of Wisconsin-Madison
K4/332 Clinical Science Center
600 Highland Avenue
Madison
WI 53792
USA

P. GRUSS
Department of Molecular Cell
Biology
Max Planck Institute for Biophysical
Chemistry
Am Fassberg
D-37018 Göttingen
Germany

M. HALL
Cancer Research Campaign
Mammalian Cell DNA Repair Group
Department of Zoology
University of Cambridge
Cambridge
CB2 3EJ
UK

R. HOULSTON
Section of Epidemiology
Institute of Cancer 2
Research
Sutton
Surrey SM2 5NG
UK

R.T. JOHNSON
Cancer Research Campaign
Mammalian Cell DNA Repair Group
Department of Zoology
University of Cambridge
Cambridge
CB2 3EJ
UK

P.G. NORRIS
Department of Dermatology
Addenbrooke's NHS Trust
Hills Road
Cambridge
CB2 2QQ
UK

M.A. PIEROTTI
Division of Experimental
Oncology A
Istituto Nazionale Tumori
Via G. Venezian 1
I-20133 Milan
Italy

J.D. POTTER
Cancer Prevention Research Program
Fred Hutchinson Cancer Research
Center
1124 Columbia, MP 702
Seattle, WA 98104
USA

S.S. RICH
Bowman Gray School of Medicine
Wake Forest University
Medical Center Blvd.
Winston-Salem, NC 27157-1063
USA

T.A. SELLERS
Division of Epidemiology
University of Minnesota
School of Public Health, Suite 300
1300 South Second Street
Minneapolis
MN 55454-1015
USA

C.M. STEEL
School of Biological and Medical
Sciences
University of St. Andrews
Bute Medical Building
St. Andrews
Fife KY16 9TS
UK

E.T. STUART
Department of Molecular Cell Biology
Max Planck Institute for Biophysical
Chemistry
Am Fassberg
D-37018 Göttingen
Germany

Preface

Families in which there seems to be inheritance of cancer have been recognized for almost 200 years. Only in the past decade, however, have molecular genetics and epidemiology combined to define the role of inheritance in cancer more clearly and to identify some of the genes involved.

Using cancer-prone families, the causative genes can be tracked down by genetic linkage and positional cloning. Several of these genes have subsequently proved to play critical roles in normal growth and development. There are also implications for the families themselves as regards genetic testing, with its attendant dilemmas if it is not clear that useful action will result.

The chapters in this volume illustrate what has already been achieved, but also look critically at the future directions of this research and its potential clinical application.

1
Breast cancer genetics

D. Eccles and R. Houlston

INTRODUCTION

The observation that some families have an excess of breast cancers, not readily accounted for by chance, is not new. Breast cancer families have been recognized since Ancient Roman times[1]. One of the earliest and most striking published reports was by a French physician, Paul Broca, who in 1866 reported a four-generation family where breast cancer had affected ten out of twenty-four women[2]. It is only in the last 10 years, however, that significant advances have led to a better understanding of familial clustering of this disease.

Systematic epidemiological studies of familial risks have shown an increased risk of breast cancer in the relatives of breast cancer patients. Results from segregation analyses of pedigrees have suggested that, whilst the majority of breast cancer cases are sporadic, around 5–10% of cases can be attributed to a highly penetrant gene which is dominantly inherited. Molecular genetic studies have directly implicated some specific loci predisposing to breast cancer.

The aim of this chapter is to review the evidence supporting a role for genetic factors in breast cancer aetiology and to discuss the value of such information in clinical practice.

GENETIC EPIDEMIOLOGY OF BREAST CANCER

Case-control and cohort studies of familial breast cancer risks

Case-control and cohort studies of the familial risks of breast cancer have been published by a number of workers[3–9]. All have demonstrated a significant familial risk of around two-fold. Of the published studies, the largest by far is that based on the Cancer and Steroid Hormone (CASH) Study conducted by the Centres for Disease Control[10]. This study is based on the family histories of 4730 confirmed cases of breast cancer, diagnosed between the ages of 20 and 54, and 4688 matched controls. Since this is to date the largest and most detailed population-based study of familial breast cancer, it will be referred to extensively.

A number of features of the familial breast cancer risk suggest that a proportion of breast cancers can be attributed to the inheritance of a highly penetrant gene, with the proportion of genetic cases being greatest at younger ages. Firstly, familial breast cancer risk is strongly age dependent. For example, in the CASH study, the risk in relatives was 5-fold greater if the case was diagnosed before the patient was 40 years old compared with less than 2-fold if diagnosed after age 50. Secondly, the risk of breast cancer is greater in women with two or more affected first-degree relatives than in women with only one affected relative, and thirdly, familial risks are greater in relatives of bilateral metachronous cases than in relatives of unilateral cases.

Segregation studies of breast cancer

Possible genetic models of familial breast cancer have been formally tested using segregation analysis by a number of workers[10–13]. All have found support for the inheritance of a dominant gene underlying the familial aggregation of breast cancer. Those studies based upon high-risk families, i.e. those selected for multiply affected relatives, are fundamentally less satisfactory than those based upon unselected series of patients. This is because of the problem of ascertainment correction and because the genetic basis of breast cancer in selected families may not necessarily reflect the familial aggregation of breast cancer observed in the general population.

In the analysis of the CASH dataset, the best fitting model for the familial aggregation of breast cancer was an autosomal dominant gene with a population frequency of 0.0033, such that the cumulative risk of breast cancer is 38% by age 50 and 67% by age 70 in gene carriers, compared with 1.5% and 5% respectively in non-carriers. Under this dominant model, the proportion of breast cancer cases attributable to the deleterious gene falls from approximately 35% among cases of breast cancer diagnosed below age 30 to 1% in cases diagnosed after age 80.

A number of epidemiological studies have demonstrated a higher risk of breast cancer in sisters of affected cases than in mothers. If real, this is a feature of familial breast cancer unaccounted for by a dominant model and could reflect either the presence of recessive genes predisposing to breast cancer or the effect of common sibling environment. Alternatively, it could be a reflection of the

Table 1.1 Genetic risks in breast cancer*

Risk category	*Risk relative to population*
First-degree relative of patient over 55 years at diagnosis	× 1.6
First-degree relative of patient under 55 years at diagnosis	× 2.3
First-degree relative of patient under 45 years at diagnosis	× 3.8
First-degree relative of patient with bilateral breast cancer	× 6.4

* Based on Houlston *et al.*, 1992[18]

temporal trend of increasing breast cancer incidence which has also been observed in familial breast cancer[14].

Relationship of familial breast cancer to other cancers

A striking feature of familial breast cancer is the association of familial breast cancer with other cancers. There are many anecdotal reports of families with multiple cases of early-onset breast cancer and ovarian cancer which are consistent with the inheritance of a dominant gene with pleiotropic effects[15]. This association is supported by epidemiological studies of breast and ovarian cancer which have found that the risk of ovarian cancer increased by 1.3–1.7-fold in relatives of breast cancer patients and vice versa[16].

The other cancer type for which a familial association with breast cancer is well established is childhood bone and soft-tissue sarcomas. This association undoubtedly reflects in part the contribution of the Li-Fraumeni syndrome to the overall total burden of breast cancer risk.

The evidence for an association between breast and other cancers is more tenuous. There is some evidence from both case reports of high-risk families and epidemiological studies for an association between breast and prostatic cancer[9,17,18]. The risk of prostatic cancer in relatives of breast cancer patients has been variously reported as increased between 2.2- and 3-fold. However, Peto and co-workers (unpublished data), in a large cohort study, found a relative risk of only 1.1, giving less support for such an association. Taken together, all studies would be compatible with an increased risk of around 1.3-fold. An association has also been reported between breast and uterine cancer by Anderson *et al.*[8], and Tulinius *et al.*[9]. Schildkraut *et al.*[16], however, found a significant correlation between cancers of the ovary and breast, but no significant association was observed between endometrial and either ovarian or breast cancer. Other associations have been reported between breast cancer and cancers of the lung[8] and thyroid[19,20]. It is noteworthy that an association between thyroid cancer and breast cancer exists as a feature of Cowden syndrome.

BREAST CANCER GENES

There are a number of rare genetic conditions with distinct phenotypes which are associated with an increase in the risk for breast cancer (e.g. Cowden disease and Peutz–Jeghes syndrome). These conditions are clinically and genetically distinct from the hereditary breast and breast/ovarian cancer families, in which there is no consistently recognizable phenotype which will distinguish gene carriers from non-carriers in a family before the onset of malignant disease. The high incidence of sporadic breast cancer in the population and the lack of a recognizable carrier phenotype complicates linkage studies. The emergence of the polymerase chain reaction as a simple but powerful laboratory tool has considerably increased the amount of family material for linkage studies because pathology material from deceased family members can now be utilized. There are at least four dominantly inherited genes predisposing to breast cancer; three have been located (BRCA1 on chromosome 17q12-21, BRCA2 on chromosome 13q12-13 and p53 on chromosome 17p13.1). However, clearly these do not account for all familial breast cancer.

The biology of sporadic and familial breast cancers is similar in that they both involve the accumulation of mutations in genes which are involved in regulating cellular growth and differentiation. Studying the molecular events in sporadic tumours may provide clues about possible sites of heritable predisposing mutations. Conversely, knowledge about inherited genes predisposing to cancer gives insight into the mechanism of sporadic cancers of the same type.

Cytogenetic and molecular studies in breast cancer

A number of lines of evidence point towards the existence of genes whose products negatively regulate cell proliferation. Studies of a number of rare cancers suggest that, in certain families, the predisposing genes might act recessively at the cellular level[21]. Formal statistical analysis of data from retinoblastoma cases led Knudson to propose his two-hit hypothesis of tumorigenesis[22]. Knudson calculated that the pattern of familial versus sporadic retinoblastoma cases was best accounted for by two separate events. In familial cases, the first hit is inherited (i.e. transmitted via the germ line and present in every cell), and only a single somatic (acquired) hit in any cell is necessary for the malignant phenotype to emerge. In sporadic cases, both hits must be acquired in the same cell for the malignant phenotype to develop (Figure 1.1).

Proof of this hypothesis followed characterization of the retinoblastoma gene on chromosome 13q14 in 1987[23]. Furthermore, it was shown that the introduction of a normally functioning (wild type) retinoblastoma gene into a malignant cell line could suppress the malignant phenotype[24]. Genes with this property are termed tumour suppressor genes or anti-oncogenes. One property of this class of cancer-predisposing gene which makes them candidates for hereditary types of cancer is that, although inherited in an autosomal dominant fashion, their action at the cellular level is recessive. That is, the inactivation of one copy of the gene does not alter the phenotype of the cell until the second copy is altered. However, some tumour suppressor genes can cause a change in cellular behaviour even though a mutation affects only a single copy of the gene. One example of such a gene is p53 which is located on the short arm of chromosome 17. Mutations leading to the production of a protein which is able to bind and change the conformation of the wild-type protein can effectiveley inactivate all normally functioning p53[25].

When a tumour suppressor gene has undergone a mutation, there is a variety of ways in which the function of the wild-type copy can be lost. This will frequently appear as reduction of a heterozygous locus to homo- or hemizygosity (loss of heterozygosity) in a comparison of constitutional DNA with tumour DNA using markers in the vicinity of a putative tumour suppressor gene. This feature is a hallmark of tumour suppressor genes. Of course, a proportion of tumours will undergo point mutations in both copies of the gene and this would not then be detected as loss of heterozygosity. However, if there are some regions where loss of heterozygosity is detected frequently in a large enough

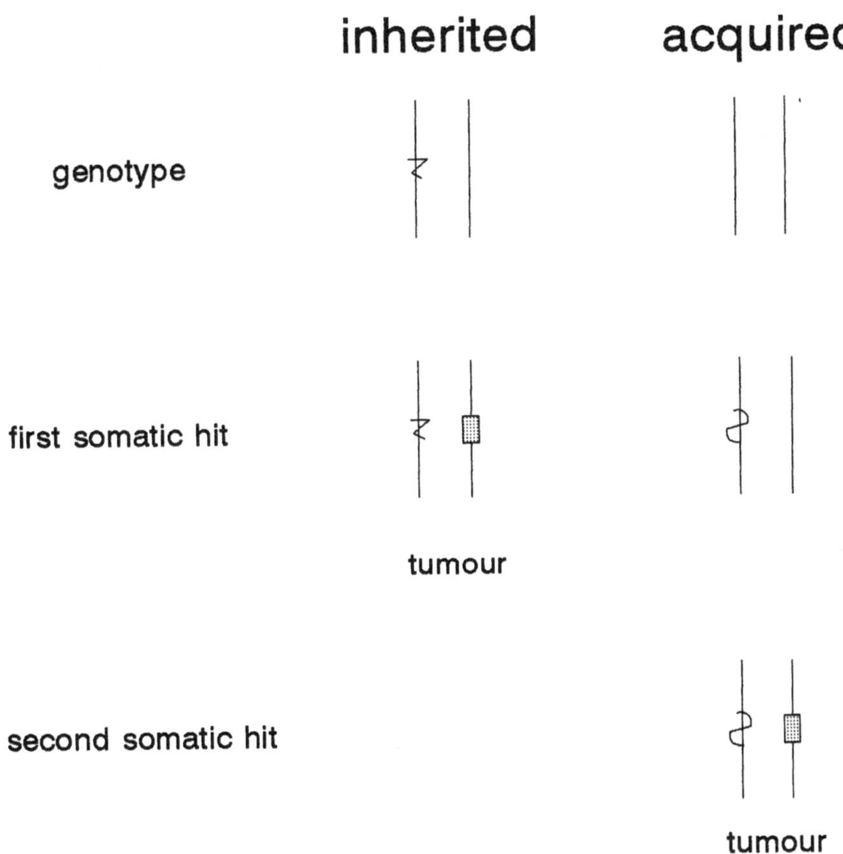

Figure 1.1 Development of tumour in inherited and acquired cancer

group of sporadic tumours, there are grounds for suspecting the presence in these regions of a tumour suppressor gene.

The supply of sporadic tumour tissue and paired constitutional DNA samples is potentially more plentiful than the supply of DNA samples from members of cancer families suitable for linkage studies. The molecular genetic events involved in the multistep process of carcinogenesis involve different combinations of oncogene activation and loss of function in tumour suppressor genes (Figure 1.2) and are broadly speaking the same in both familial and sporadic tumorigenesis and so information about the molecular events involved in sporadic tumour development may give some clues as to candidate loci for familial cases.

Initial cytogenetic studies on sporadic human breast tumours highlighted a range of non-random abnormalities involving chromosomes 1, 3, 6, 11, 13, 16, 17 and 18 (reviewed in Reference 26). Some of these changes are associated with oncogene activation and some with loss of tumour suppressor function. These

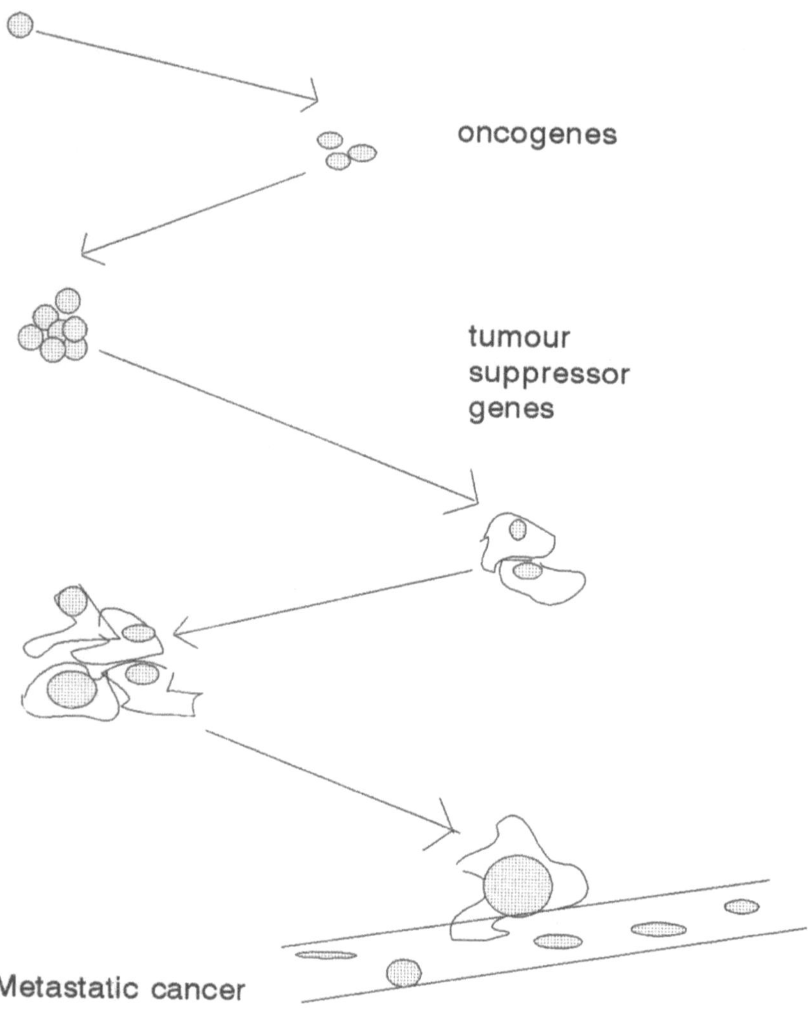

Figure 1.2 Multistep process of carcinogenesis

cytogenetic studies were limited, however, by technical constraints. Studies with highly polymorphic markers have confirmed these initial cytogenetic findings[27–30] with loss of heterozygosity frequently observed on chromosomes 1p, 3p, 11p, 16q, 13q, 17p, 17q and 18q.

Linkage analysis

Sporadic tumour studies provide candidate regions for linkage studies in breast cancer families. These candidate regions have been largely disappointing to date. Thus for example, chromosomes 11p, 13q and 18q, the locations respectively of the tumour suppressor genes, Wilms tumour gene, Rb gene and DCC gene, have not been shown to be implicated in familial breast cancer by linkage studies. There are a number of well-recognized problems associated with searching for breast cancer genes in families, even where there are quite good candidate regions and plentiful markers for carrying out linkage studies. Firstly, there are a number of different loci which account for breast cancer in families but where there are not necessarily features which will distinguish the disease pattern caused by one gene from the disease pattern caused by another. That is, the families are clinically homogeneous and so would be analysed as one group, although one or more genes are involved thus reducing the overall evidence of linkage (locus heterogeneity). Secondly, the presence of sporadic breast cancers (phenocopies) within a family can lead to inappropriate assignation of genotype on the basis of phenotype. Thus, it might be assumed that all women in the family with breast cancer were gene carriers; whereas, in reality, there will be the additional risk of sporadic breast cancer in any family member, just as in the population from which the pedigree is drawn.

The first convincing report of linkage in breast cancer families was published by Hall *et al.* in 1990[31]. Linkage was demonstrated to a polymorphic (VNTR) marker on chromosome 17q21 defined by the probe CMM86. Twenty-three extended families with 146 breast cancer cases were analysed in a number of different ways. When families were ranked according to the mean age of onset of breast cancer and LOD scores compared, not all the families showed evidence of linkage to chromosome 17q21. In the majority of families where the mean age of onset was 45 years or less, there was strong evidence of linkage to D17S74 (defined by probe CMM86) with a maximum LOD score of +5.74 at a recombination fraction of less than 10%. (This corresponds to odds of almost 1 000 000:1 in favour of linkage to this locus.) However, LOD scores for families with a later age at onset were mostly negative, with some sufficiently negative to exclude linkage to this locus completely. This suggested the involvement of more than one locus in predisposition in different families.

Following this first report, evidence of linkage of breast and ovarian cancer to the same locus was published by Narod *et al.*[32]. This group had used 5 breast and ovarian cancer families and found evidence of linkage to D17S74 in 3 families and evidence against linkage in 2 of the families. The maximum LOD score for the linked families was +3.03 at a recombination frequency of 10%. One family alone had a maximum LOD score of +2.72 at 7% recombination. The breast cancer gene at this locus is now referred to as BRCAI[33].

These initial reports led to the formation of an international consortium involved in linkage analysis in breast cancer. The results of pooled data on 214 families narrowed the interval in which BRCA1 must lie as well as defining more precisely the extent of heterogeneity and the penetrance of the BRCA1 gene[34]. The BRCA1 gene is described more fully in the next section of this chapter. The cloning of BRCA1 was reported 4 years after the original linkage[35].

Work on the hereditary non-polyposis colorectal cancer (HNPCC) syndrome demonstrated linkage to chromosome 2p markers in two very large kindreds. The main risk for those carrying the deleterious gene in these families is for colorectal cancer. However, an increased risk at other sites is recognized, including breast cancer[36]. The risks for breast cancer associated with this locus are, however, less clear than in site-specific breast and breast/ovarian cancer families. The hMSH2 gene on chromosome 2 has now been cloned[37,38] and shown to code for a DNA repair protein. More recently, another gene, hMLH2, on chromosome 3p, also coding for a mismatch repair protein, has been isolated[39]. Like proto-oncogenes and the tumour suppressor genes, mutations in this type of gene are likely to be implicated in a wide range of cancers[40]. This type of gene is dealt with in more detail in the chapter on colon cancer genetics.

The BRCA1 gene and breast/ovarian cancer families

The BRCA1 gene lies on chromosome 17 at approximately band q12-q21. Many of the candidate genes within the 1.5Mb region, defined by the work of the breast cancer linkage consortium[34], were sequenced and excluded before the gene was cloned[35]. With knowledge of the sequence of the gene, genetically predisposed individuals can be clearly defined and some of the bewildering questions about why some gene carriers defined by linkage do not seem to develop disease, and why some families show such a remarkably different pattern of cancers from others, can perhaps start to be answered.

What is already apparent from the published consortium data[34] is that families with ovarian cancer (at least two cases) as well as breast cancer have a high *a priori* chance of being linked to BRCA1 (over 90%). In contrast, those families with breast cancer only (even in families where the mean age at onset was under 45 years) had a much lower chance of being linked to BRCAI (67% for breast cancer families with a mean age at onset under 45 years of age but only 45% for all breast cancer families).

Examination of these data also allowed Easton *et al.*[41] to predict rough estimates of the cancer-specific risks, i.e. the age-specific penetrances of BRCA1 for breast and ovarian cancer: these were estimated for breast cancer as 49% by age 50 and 71% by age 70 and for ovarian cancer as 16% by age 50 and 42% by age 70. These figures are based on the assumption of homogeneous risk for breast and ovarian cancer across all linked families. This is unlikely to be the case given clinical observations of the widely different patterns of disease in families, some families with no cases of ovarian cancer and some with apparently only ovarian cancer. Easton *et al.*[41] proposed a model with two different susceptibility alleles at BRCA1, i.e. allelic heterogeneity, and calculated the risks by age 70 years for breast and ovarian cancer for the less common allele to be 71% and 87% respectively and for the more common allele the estimated risks are 86% and 18% respectively.

Resolution of these uncertainties about allelic heterogeneity, genetic heterogeneity and the effects of modifying genes may be possible now that the BRCA1 gene has been identified and direct mutation analysis is possible. This development is eagerly awaited and it is hoped that it will give some clues as to potentially useful intervention strategies in gene carriers: for example, the evaluation of screening techniques, the assessment of potential chemopreventive agents (e.g. tamoxifen), reduction in risk through lifestyle changes and interventions, such as prophylactic surgery. Eventually gene therapy may be possible; and all of these approaches might be applied more generally to sporadic breast cancer patients.

The Li Fraumeni syndrome and the p53 gene

The p53 protein was initially identified as a 53-kDa nuclear phosphoprotein which binds to the large T (transforming) antigen of the small DNA tumour virus SV40[42]. The gene encoding p53 is located on the short arm of chromosome 17[43]. Initially, p53 was thought to be a proto-oncogene because its transfection could render cells tumorigenic[44]. However, it was subsequently shown that all the p53 transfects used had been mutant and that a mutation in the p53 gene was essential for it to have transforming potential[45].

In 1989, an excess of lung, bone and lymphoid tumours were noted in mice transgenic for mutant p53[46]. A year later, two independent research groups showed inherited p53 mutations segregated with cancers in families with the Li Fraumeni cancer family syndrome[47,48]. The Li Fraumeni cancer family syndrome[49] comprises, classically, breast cancer in young women and childhood soft tissue sarcomas in association with a wide variety of other tumours, such as leukaemia, adrenocortical carcinoma and CNS tumours. About 50% of families with the classical pattern of disease have now been shown to have detectable germ-line mutations in the p53 gene (Reference 50 and Eeles, personal communication). There are, however, many families which do not conform to the classical pattern but which are somewhat similar. Rather less than 50% of these families have a detectable mutation in the coding region of the p53 gene, but other genes which control p53 activity may be implicated in some. Germ-line p53 mutations seem to be uncommon in individuals with a family history of breast cancer alone[51,52], with isolated very young age at onset of breast cancer[53,54] or bilateral breast cancer[55], or in isolated cases with tumours otherwise associated with the Li Fraumeni syndrome[56]. Multiple primary tumours in children and young adults may, however, be reasonable grounds for testing for p53 mutation in the germ-line[57].

Somatic mutations in the p53 gene are extremely common in the cells of sporadic cancers. The normal function of the p53 gene is becoming clearer. The working model is that, under normal circumstances, p53 is intimately involved in controlling the rate of cellular replication. When DNA replicates, occasional infidelities occur which need to be corrected before the cell divides. If this correction does not occur, the errors will be perpetuated in subsequent generations derived from the newly synthesized DNA; and, if the error happens to affect an oncogene or a tumour suppressor gene, this will contribute to future malignant transformation. p53 helps to ensure that this corrective repair is carried out. When the level of wild-type p53 in the cell rises above a certain critical level, the cell cycle is arrested at G1, allowing time for repair proteins to splice out the miscopied DNA and for a correct copy to be synthesized. The p53 levels then fall and mitosis can proceed[58]. If repair fails to occur, p53 drives the cell towards programmed cell death or apoptosis.

In individuals with an inherited mutant p53 gene, there is clearly much scope for a wide variety of tumours to arise when a mutation happens to knock out the function of the remaining wild-type p53 gene.

The problem with the clinical management of this type of cancer syndrome is the diversity of possible tumours which can arise. To date, there is no satisfactory screening test for many of these tumours. Current recommendations in the UK suggest an initial full clinical history and examination, urinalysis, full blood count and film, an ultrasound scan of the abdomen and an MRI scan of the head for children. The same test but without the MRI scan and with particular reference to examination of the breasts in females are recommended for adults[59]. Thereafter, because of the diversity of possible tumour sites, it is recommended that the individual and their General Practitioner are fully aware of the need for full evaluation if any untoward symptoms are noted. Open access to a hospital physician can be reassuring. One of the major difficulties in counselling such a family is the lack of accurate figures for risks in gene carriers for all of the possible tumours and the lack of reliable screening tools. Given the way in which it is proposed that p53 works in the cell, individuals with germ-line p53 mutations may be more sensitive to the mutagenic effects of X-rays. In addition, breast cancers in p53 mutation carriers tend to arise in much younger women (under 30 years) when mammography is less informative because of the greater gland density. There is an argument for avoiding mammography as a screening technique and properly evaluating other modalities, such as ultrasound scanning and magnetic resonance imaging.

Ataxia telangiectasia and risk of breast cancer

Ataxia telangiectasia is an autosomal recessive syndrome of progressive cerebellar ataxia and oculocutaneous telangiectasia in conjunction with immunological defects[60]. Affected individuals demonstrate an exquisite sensitivity to ionizing radiation and have about a 100-fold greater risk of developing cancer, especially lymphomas and lymphocytic leukaemia[61]. In addition to the increased risk of cancer seen in homozygotes, it is now well established that relatives of patients with ataxia telangiectasia show an excess risk of cancers, and of breast cancer in particular[62–68]. Although based on relatively young cases, the available data suggest that the risk of breast cancer in AT heterozygotes is not age dependent. Furthermore, the increased risk of breast cancer may be related to a history of exposure to ionizing radiation[67]. Combining the published studies, Easton[69] estimated that the risk of breast cancer in heterozygotes was increased 7.8-fold with 95% confidence intervals of 5.5 and 11.9. Although these risks are smaller than those conferred by either BRCA1 or p53 mutations, they are nevertheless of significance since the frequency of gene carriers for ataxia has been estimated as up to 1% of the population[67].

The overall impact of AT on the total burden of breast cancer is currently unknown; since the gene has not been cloned and there are no reliable tests for heterozygotes, neither the risk of breast cancer in heterozygotes nor the frequency of the AT gene mutations in the general population can be established with certainty. However, assuming the frequency lies between 0.2 and 0.5% and the risk associated with heterozygosity is between 5 and 8, Easton *et al.*[41] concluded that between 2 and 7% of breast cancer cases might be attributable to the AT gene. The gene for most complementation groups of AT maps to 11q22-23[70,71] but Wooster *et al.* were unable to demonstrate linkage to 11q22-23 in breast cancer families unlinked to 17q[72].

Other syndromes predisposing to breast cancer

Peutz–Jeghers syndrome

Peutz–Jeghers syndrome is a dominant disorder characterized by the association of melanin pigmentation on the lips, perioral region, buccal mucosa, hands, arms and feet, and gastrointestinal polyposis[73]. The cutaneous pigmentation is present in 95% of cases; it is present in early childhood but tends to fade by the middle of the third decade[74]. Multiple hamartomatous polyposis occurs throughout the entire gastrointestinal tract but is most prolific in the small bowel. Adenomatous change may occur within these polyps and a 13-fold increase in risk of gastrointestianal malignancies has been reported[75]. Patients with Peutz–Jeghers syndrome also have an increased risk of breast, uterus, pancreas, gonadal sex cord and sertoli cell tumours[76,77]. Many of these tumours occur at an early age and it has been estimated that 48% of affected individuals will die of cancer by age 57[75]. The syndrome is rare and the overall contribution to breast cancer risk must be very small.

Cowden syndrome

Cowden syndrome, an autosomal dominant genodermatosis of multiple hamartomas involving all 3 germ layers, is associated with an increase in breast cancer risk and with thyroid tumours[78–83]. Multiple trichilemommas occur, especially on the face, and facial papules, verrucous skin lesions and mucosal papules occur in more than 80% of cases[84,85]. Lipomas are common and polyps of the gastrointestinal tract have been found in 40–60% of cases[86,87]. Approximately one half of women affected suffer from fibrocystic disease of the breasts, and virginal breast hypertrophy may develop. Other phenotypic features include macrocephaly, kyphoscoliosis, pectus excavatum, vitiligo, and pit-like keratotic lesions of the palms and soles. Thyroid abnormalities (malignant tumour, adenomatous goitre and hyper- or hypothyroidism) and a variety of benign tumours of muscular and neural origin have been described in association with this disease.

The incidence of breast cancer is possibly 50% in female gene carriers. Those affected with breast cancer are young, typically premenopausal and the breast cancer is bilateral in a third of cases. Thyroid cancer has been described in 10% of cases and there may be an increased risk of other cancers (colon, uterus and bladder)[88]. Considerable intrafamilial variation is seen in Cowden syndrome which may be a consequence of the action of modifying genes or genetic heterogeneity.

The contribution of Cowden syndrome to breast cancer risk is likely to be small; however, this will only be fully defined with the identification of the location of the susceptibility gene(s).

Currently, the location of the susceptibility gene(s) for Cowden syndrome is unknown. Cytogenetic studies have been uninformative. No mutations were found in RAS, HER2/neu or pS2 genes in one patient[89]. A study of the tumour suppressor gene, p53, in one patient with multiple tumours and multiple trichilemommas of the scalp found a c/t mutation in exon 8 of the p53 gene[90]. However, no defects in exons 1–11 were found in a patient with Cowden syndrome and Lhermitte–Duclos disease[91].

Male breast cancer

As well as the increased risk of breast cancer in female relatives of breast cancer patients, male relatives also show an increased risk[92]. The pattern of increased risk is entirely compatible with an underlying genetic predisposition.

So far, there is no evidence for linkage to BRCA1[93] and there have been no reports of an underlying p53 mutation in any male breast cancer families. Male breast cancer is more common in men with Kleinfelter syndrome and other conditions with a relative androgen deficiency. Recently, there have been two reports of male breast cancer in three men from two families where partial androgen insensitivity was associated with a mutation in the DNA-binding domain of the androgen receptor gene (Xq11.2-q12)[94,95]. There were, however, no cases of females with breast cancer in these families. Furthermore, there is no suggestion in published pedigrees of X-linked transmission of a major gene for breast cancer. BRCA2, recently identified on chromosome 13q, is implicated in families with male breast cancer cases[107].

INTERACTION OF GENETIC AND ENVIRONMENTAL FACTORS

A number of environmental factors have been shown to alter the risks of breast cancer. These include exposure to both exogenous and endogenous oestrogens, diet, body mass index and height (reviewed in Reference 96). The impact of these factors is generally small and the findings from some studies have been inconsistent. Given that some individuals may be genetically predisposed to breast cancer, it is clearly important to understand the possible modifying effect that environmental factors may have on this genetic risk.

Adjustment for other known risk factors for breast cancer, such as parity and age of menarche, has generally been shown to have little effect on the familial relative risk, implying that the known hormonal risk factors act independently of genetic predisposition, and perhaps a significant genetic risk outweighs any environmental risk factors, However, a cohort study of women aged between 55 and 69 years reported by Sellers *et al.*[97] provides some evidence of interactions between familial and other factors. It was found that the effects of waist–hip ratio, parity and age at first birth on breast cancer risk were most pronounced among women with a family history of breast cancer. It is clearly of relevance that this study was conducted on older women where the genetic effect on breast cancer risk will be weaker.

The much lower risk of breast cancer in males, and the reduction in risk with an artificially early menopause[98] and a late menarche, point to oestrogens as likely promoters of breast cancer. However, oestrogens are unlikely to be involved in initiation of the mutations involved in breast carcinogenesis[99]. The effects of exogenous and endogenous oestrogens have been difficult to measure with certainty and a number of studies examining the effects of oral contraceptive use and hormone replacement therapy have given conflicting results. There is likely to be a lag period of 15–20 years between administration of a promoting agent and the onset of cancer. Since oral contraceptive use has only been common since the 1970s, it is probably still too soon to draw any firm conclusions from the available data on breast cancer incidence and oral contraceptive use. This may explain why published studies sometimes give conflicting results[100]. As far as hormone replacement therapy is concerned, the increase in risk becomes apparent after prolonged usage (more than 10 years), and it is not at all clear that a family history of breast cancer confers any significant additional increase in risk (References 101 and 102 and V. Blair, personal communication).

In practice, however, it is still difficult to recommend long-term oral contraceptive use or long-term hormone replacement therapy in a woman with a strong family history of breast cancer unless there are exceptionally good reasons to do so.

Radiation does cause some increase in breast cancer incidence[103], especially perhaps in those with an increased sensitivity (e.g. AT heterozygotes). These effects are relatively weak, and it is difficult to control for other factors, including genetic predisposition, in large population studies where the relevant data are often not available.

There are no really satisfactory studies which examine the interactions between the environmental risk factors identified through epidemiological studies and genetic predisposition to breast cancer. In the last few years, the genes responsible for at least some of these familial breast cancers are starting to emerge and studies which look at risk factors in clearly genetically predisposed individuals should become possible[14]. Undoubtedly, as our ability to recognize those at the highest genetic risk (i.e. those known to carry a predisposing mutant gene) becomes a reality, these types of studies must become a priority with a major thrust towards identifying factors, for example lifestyle changes (e.g. reduction of fat in the diet), new types of contraceptive agents[104] and potential chemopreventive agents (e.g. tamoxifen), which could delay the onset of disease or prevent it altogether.

ESTIMATION OF BREAST CANCER RISK IN CLINICAL PRACTICE

It is clear from the preceding sections of this chapter that family history offers an opportunity to identify those at a high genetic risk of breast cancer who may benefit from targeted screening, prevention strategies or prophylactic surgery. Furthermore, there is now considerable demand from women with a family history of breast cancer for their risk to be defined.

For some women, even without formal analysis of their pedigree, it is clear that the familial aggregation of breast and or ovarian cancer in their family is compatible with the inheritance of a dominant gene. Some families may have a phenotype diagnostic of one of the cancer family syndromes. However, in clinical practice, these possibilities are the exception rather than the rule and formal techniques of determining risk have to be applied.

Empirical risks, such as those shown in Table 1.1, can be used in clinical practice for counselling. However, every family history is unique and, in many circumstances, an empirical risk may be non-specific or unavailable. In contrast, where the mode of inheritance is inferred, a risk can be calculated for any pedigree structure. Using estimates of the probability of inheriting a deleterious gene for breast cancer and the age-specific penetrance enables the genetic component of risk at different ages to be calculated for relatives. With an early age of diagnosis, the genetic risk of cancer is high. Figure 1.3 shows the probability of being a gene carrier for breast cancer for cases diagnosed at different ages. With increasing age at diagnosis, the risk diminishes. This information can then be used to identify more precisely those family members who are at high risk and estimate the chance that a dominant gene is responsible for any family aggrega-

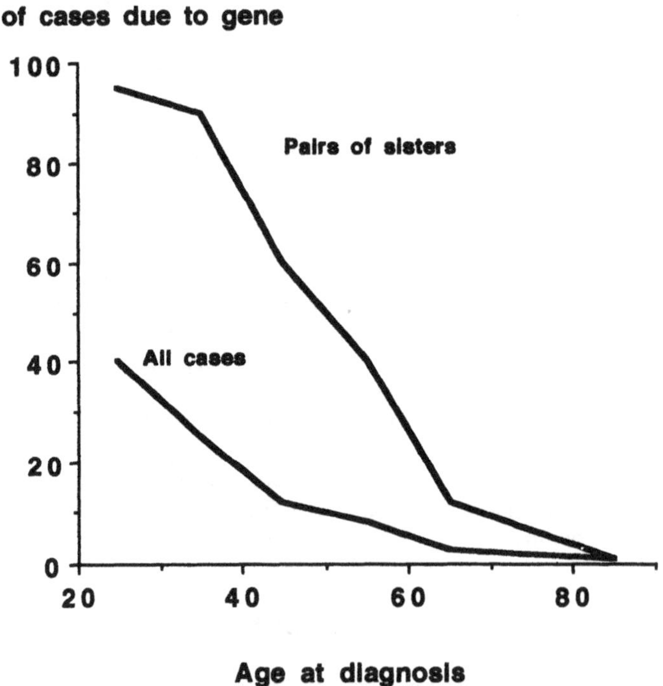

Figure 1.3 Probability of being a gene carrier for breast cancer (based upon the CASH segregation model of breast cancer[6]). The probability of carrying the deleterious gene is high at a young age of diagnosis but rapidly diminishes. Furthermore, the probability of being a gene carrier is higher where two sisters are diagnosed with breast cancer at the same age. Adapted from Reference 106

tion of breast cancer. The risk of breast cancer for a consultand is given by the likelihood of the pedigree with the consultand included divided by the likelihood of the pedigree with the consultand omitted. However, for all but the simplest of the pedigrees, such risk calculations will be complex and are best carried out within computer programs, such as MENDEL, devised by Lange *et al.*[105].

As previously discussed, inherited breast cancer is determined by a number of genes conferring a range of penetrances. The precise estimate of risk will depend upon the underlying basis of familial breast cancer in the consultand's family. However, in the absence of linkage, risk estimates based on segregation models can provide a basis for genetic counselling in families with multiple cases of breast cancer.

Pending molecular testing for the genes predisposing to breast cancer (imminent for BRCAI), presymptomatic testing largely resides in testing for linkage to BRCAI on chromosome 17q12-21. Probabilities of a consultand being a gene carrier are derived by combining the prior probability of breast cancer only families and breast/ovarian cancer families showing linkage to chromosome 17q with the LOD score obtained in the family of the consultand seeking counselling.

CONCLUDING REMARKS

Although much progress has been made in characterizing breast cancer genes, there are still many questions to be answered. Clearly, a number of different breast cancer susceptibility genes exist. The frequency and age-specific penetrance and phenotypic features associated with each locus will take many years to unravel. The interactions between environmental factors and these breast cancer susceptibility genes have yet to be explored, and this will be an important step towards developing potential preventive strategies. Because sporadic breast cancer is probably biologically the same disease as familial breast cancer, understanding the genes implicated in familial breast cancer may ultimately lead to a more general application of preventive measures within the general population. This in turn may reduce the high incidence of breast cancer in the Western world.

References

1. Steel CM, Clayton J, Thompson A. Genetic aspects of breast cancer. Br Med Bull. 1991;47(2):504–18.
2. Broca P (1866). Trait des tumeurs. Des tumeurs en general. Vol 1. Paris: Anselin, Becket et Labe.
3. Brinton LA, Hoover R, Frauneni JF Jr. Interaction of familial and hormonal risk factors for breast cancer. J Natl Cancer Inst. 1982;69:817–22.
4. Adami HO, Hansen J, Jung B, Rimsten A. Familiality in breast cancer: a case control study in a Swedish population. Br J Cancer. 1980;42:71–7.
5. Negri E, La Vecchia C, Bruzzi P *et al.* Risk factors for breast cancer: pooled results from three Italian case-control studies. Am J Epidemiol. 1988;128:1207–15.
6. Claus EB, Risch N, Thompson WD. Using age of onset to distinguish between symptoms of breast cancer. Ann Hum Genet. 1990;54:169–77.
7. Claus EB, Risch N, Thompson W. Age as an indicator of familial risk of breast cancer. Am J Epidemiol. 1990;131:961–72.

8. Anderson K, Easton DF, Mathews FE, Peto J. Cancer morbidity in the first degree relatives of young breast cancer patients. Br J Cancer. 1992;66:599–602.
9. Tulinius H, Egilsson V, Olafsdottin GH, Sigvaldon H. Risk of prostate, ovarian and endometrial cancer among selectives of women with breast cancer. Br Med J. 1992;305:855–7.
10. Claus EB, Risch N, Thompson D. Genetic analysis of breast cancer in the cancer and steroid hormone study. Am J Hum Genet. 1991;48:232–41.
11. Williams WR, Anderson DE. Genetic epidemiology of breast cancer: segregation analysis of 200 Danish pedigrees. Genet Epidemiol. 1984;1:7–20.
12. Iselius L, Slack J, Littler M, Morton N. Genetic epidemiology of breast cancer in Britain. Ann Hum Genet. 1991;55(2):151–9.
13. Newman B, Austin M, Lee M, King M-C. Inheritance of human breast cancer: evidence for autosomal dominant transmission in high risk families. Proc Natl Acad Sci USA. 1988;85:3044–8.
14. Narod SA, Lynch H, Conway T, Watson P, Fenteum J, Lenoir G. Increasing incidence of breast cancer in a family with BRCAI mutation. Lancet. 1993;341:1101–2.
15. Lynch HT, Harris RE, Guirgis HA *et al.* Familial association of breast/ovarian carcinoma. Cancer 1978;41:1543–9.
16. Schildkraut JM, Risch N, Thompson WD. Evaluating genetic association among ovarian, breast and endometrial cancer: evidence for a breast/ovarian cancer relationship. Am J Hum Genet. 1989;45:521–9.
17. Cannon L, Bishop DT, Skolnick M, Hunt S, Lyon JL, Smart CR. Genetic epidemiology of prostate cancer in the Utah Mormon genealogy. Cancer Surveys. 1982;1:47–69.
18. Houlston RS, McCarter E, Parbhoo S, Scurr J, Slack J. Family history and risk of breast cancer. J Med Genet. 1992;29:154–7.
19. Ron E, Kleinerman RA, Li Volsi VA, Fraumeni JF Jr. Familial non-medullary thyroid cancer. Oncology. 1991;48:309–11.
20. Goldgar DE, Easton DF, Cannon-Albright L, Skolnick MH. A systematic population-based assessment of cancer risk in first degree relatives of cancer probands. JNCI. 1994; 86:1600–8.
21. De Mars R. In: 23rd annual symposium on fundamental cancer research 1969. Baltimore: Williams and Wilkins;1970:105–6.
22. Knudson A. Mutation and cancer: statistical study of retinoblastoma. Proc Natl Acad Sci USA. 1971;68(4):820–3.
23. Lee WH, Bookstein R, Hong F, Young LJ, Shaw JY, Lee EYHP. Human retinoblastoma susceptibility gene – cloning, identification and sequence. Science. 1987;235:1394–9.
24. Huang HS, Yee J, Shew J *et al.* Suppression of the neoplastic phenotype by replacement of the RB gene in human cancer cells. Science. 1988;242:1563–6.
25. Srivastava S, Wang S, Tong Y, Pirollo K, Chang E. Several p53 proteins detected in cancer prone families with Li-Fraumeni syndrome exhibit transdominant effects on the biochemical properties of the wild-type p53. Oncogene. 1993;8 (9):2449–56.
26. Tripathy D, Benz CC. Activated oncogenes and putative tumour suppressor genes involved in human breast cancers. Cancer Treatment Res. 1992;63:15–60.
27. Devilee P, Van den Broek M, Kuipers-Dijkshoorn *et al.* At least four different chromosomal regions are involved in loss of heterozygosity in human breast carcinoma. Genomics. 1989;5:554–60.
28. Sato T, Tanigami A, Yamakawa K *et al.* Allelotype of breast cancer: cumulative allele losses promote tumour progression in primary breast cancer. Cancer Res. 1990;50:7184–9.
29. Cropp CS, Lidereau R, Campbell G, Champene M. Loss of heterozygosity on chromosome 17 and 18 in breast carcinoma: two additional regions identified. Proc Natl Acad Sci USA. 1990;87:7737–41.
30. Callahan R, Cropp C, Merlo GR *et al.* Somatic mutations and human breast cancer. A status report. Cancer. 1992;69 (6 Suppl):1582–8.
31. Hall JM, Lee MK, Newman B *et al.* Linkage of early-onset familial breast cancer to chromosome 17q21. Science. 1990;250:1684–9.
32. Narod SA, Lynch H, Feunteun J *et al.* Familial breast–ovarian cancer locus on chromosome 17q12-23. Lancet. 1991;338:82–83.
33. Solomon E, Ledbetter DH. Report of the committee on the genetic constitution of chromosome 17. Cytogenet Cell Genet. 1991;58:686–738.

34. Easton DF, Bishop DT, Ford D, Crockford GP and the Breast Cancer Linkage Consortium. Genetic linkage analysis in familial breast and ovarian cancer: results from 214 families. Am J Hum Genet. 1993;52(4):678–701.
35. Miki Y, Swensen J, Shattuck-Eidens D *et al.* A strong candidate for the breast and ovarian cancer susceptibility gene BRCAI. Science. 1994;266:66–71.
36. Peltomaki P, Aaltonen LA, Sistonen P *et al.* Genetic mapping of a locus predisposing to human colorectal cancer. Science. 1993;260:810–12.
37. Fishel R, Lescoe M, Rao M *et al.* The human mutator gene homolog HMSH2 and its association with hereditary nonpolyposis colon cancer. Cell. 1993;75:1027–38.
38. Leach FS, Nicolaides NC, Papadopoulos N, *et al.* Mutations of a mutS homolog in hereditary nonpolyposis colorectal cancer. Cell. 1993;75:1215–25.
39. Bronner C, Baker S, Morrison P, *et al.* Mutations in the DNA mismatch homologue hMLH1 is associated with hereditary non-polyposis colon cancer. Nature (London). 1994;368:258–61.
40. Wooster R, Cleton-Jansen A-M, Collins N *et al.* Instability of short tandem repeats (microsatellites) in human cancers. Nature Genetics. 1994;6:152–6.
41. Easton DF, Ford D, Peto J. Inherited susceptibility to breast cancer. Cancer Surv. 1993;18:95–113.
42. Lane D, Crawford L. T-antigen is bound to a host protein in SV40 transformed cells. Nature. 1979;278:261–3.
43. Isobe M, Emanuel B, Givol D, Oren M, Croce C. Localisation of the gene for human p53 tumour antigen to band 17p13. Nature. 1986;320:84–5.
44. Eliyahu D, Michalovitz D, Oren M. (1985). Overproduction of p53 antigen makes established cells highly tumorigenic. Nature (London). 1985;316:158–60.
45. Hinds P, Finlay C, Levine A. Mutation is required to activate the p53 gene for co-operation with the ras oncogene and transformation. J Virol. 1989;63(2):739–46.
46. Lavigueur A, Maltby V, Mock D, Rossant J, Pawson T, Bernstein A. High incidence of lung, bone, and lymphoid tumours in mice overexpressing mutant alleles of the p53 oncogene. Mol Cell Biol. 1989;9(9):3982–91.
47. Malkin D, Li F, Strong L, *et al.* Germ line p53 mutations in a familial syndrome of breast cancer, sarcomas and other neoplasms. Science. 1990;250:1233–8.
48. Srivistava S, Zou Z, Pirollo K, Blattner W, Chang E. Germ-line transmission of a mutated p53 gene in a cancer prone family with Li-Fraumeni syndrome. Nature (London). 1990;348:747–9.
49. Li FP, Fraumeni JF. Soft tissue sarcomas, breast cancer and other neoplasms. A familial syndrome? Ann Intern Med. 1969;71:747–52.
50. Birch JM, Hartley AL, Tricker KJ *et al.* Prevelance and diversity of constitutional mutations in the p53 gene among 21 Li-Fraumeni families. Cancer Res. 1994;54(5):1298–304.
51. Warren W, Eeles R, Ponder BA *et al.* No evidence for germline mutations in the p53 gene in 25 breast cancer families. Oncogene. 1992;7(5):1043–6.
52. Prosser J, Elder P, Condie A, MacFadyen I, Steel CM, Evans HJ. Mutations in p53 do not account for heritable breast cancer: a study in five affected families. Br J Cancer. 1991;63:181–4.
53. Borresen A-L, Andersen TI, Garber J *et al.* Screening for germ-line TP53 mutations in breast cancer patients. Cancer Res. 1992;52:3234–6.
54. Sidransky D, Tokino T, Helzlsouer K *et al.* Inherited p53 gene mutations in breast cancer. Cancer Res. 1992;5(10):2984–6.
55. Lidereau R, Soussi T. Absence of p53 germline mutations in bilateral breast cancer patients. Hum Genet. 1992;89:250–2.
56. Toguchida J, Yamaguchi T, Dayton S *et al.* Prevalence and spectrum of germline mutations of the p53 gene among patients with sarcomas. N Engl J Med. 1992;326:1301–8.
57. Malkin D, Jolly K, Barbier N *et al.* Germline mutations of the p53 tumour-suppressor in children and young adults with second malignant neoplasms. N Engl J Med. 1992;326:1309–15.
58. Lane DP. p53, guardian of the genome. Nature (London). 1992;358:15–16.
59. Birch JM, Easton D, Ponder B, Spurr N, Lane D, Craft A, Hopwood P, on behalf of the UK Cancer Families Study Group. Guidelines for testing for germline p53 mutations and the management of families with such mutations. [Prepared December 1993] Available from Dr JM Birch, The Christie Hospital, Manchester, UK.
60. Boder E. Ataxia–telangiectasia: an overview. In: Giatii RA, Swift M, eds. Ataxia–telangiectasia: genetics, neuropathology, and immunology of a degenerative disease of childhood. New York: Alan Liss; 1985:1–63.

61. Spector BD, Filipovich AH, Perry GS III, Kersey JH. Epidemiology of cancer in ataxia–telangiectasia. In: Bridges BA, Harnden G, eds. Ataxia–telangiectasia: a cellular and molecular link between cancer, neuropathology and immune deficiency. Chichester, England: John Wiley; 1982:103–38.
62. Morrell D, Cramatie E, Swift M. Mortality and cancer incidence in 263 patients with ataxia–telangiectasia. J Natl Cancer Inst. 1986;77:89–92.
63. Pippard EC, Hall AJ, Barker DJP, Bridges BA. Cancer in homozygotes and heterozygotes of ataxia–telangiectasia and xeroderma pigmentosum in Britain. Cancer Res. 1988;48:2929–32.
64. Swift M, Morrell D, Cromatie E, Chamberlain AR, Skolnick MH, Bishop DT. The incidence and gene frequency of ataxia–telangiectasia in the United States. Am J Hum Genet. 1986;39:573–83.
65. Swift M, Morrell D, Massey RB, Chase C. Incidence of cancer in 161 families affected by ataxia–telangiectasia. N Engl J Med. 1991;325:1831–6.
66. Swift M, Sholman L, Perry M, Chase C. Malignant neoplasms in families of patients with ataxia–telangiectasia. Cancer Res. 1976;36:209–15.
67. Swift M, Reitnauer PJ, Morrell D, Chase CL. Breast and other cancers in families with ataxia–telangiectasia. N Engl J Med. 1987;316:1289–94.
68. Borresen A-L, Andersen Ti, Treti S, Heiberg A, Moller P. Breast cancer and other cancers in Norwegian families with ataxia–talangiectasia. Genes Chromosomes Cancer. 1990;2:339–40.
69. Easton DE. Some problems of the genetic epidemiology of cancer [PhD thesis]. University of London; 1992.
70. Gatti RA, Berkel I, Boder E *et al.* Localisation of an ataxia–telangiectasia gene to chromosome 11q22-23. Nature (London). 1988;336:577–80.
71. Foroud T, Wei S, Zvi Y *et al.* Localisation of an ataxia–telangiectasia locus to a 3cM interval on chromosome 11q22-q23: linkage analysis of 11 families by an international consortium. Am J Hum Genet. 1991;49:1263–79.
72. Wooster R, Ford D, Mangion J *et al.* Absence of linkage to ataxia–telangiectasia locus in familial breast cancer. Hum Genet. 1993;92:91–4.
73. Jehgers H, McKusick V, Katz KH. Generalised intestinal polyposis and melanin spots of the oral mucosa, lips and digits. N Engl J Med. 1979;241:993–1005.
74. Konishi F, Wyse NE, Muto T *et al.* Peutz-Jehgers polyposis associated with carcinoma of the digestive organs. Dis Colon Rectum. 1987;30:790–9.
75. Spiegelman AD, Murday V, Phillips RKS. (1989). Cancer and the Peutz-Jehgers syndrome. Gut. 1989;30:1588–90.
76. Utsunomiya J, Gocho T, Miyanaga E *et al.* Peutz-Jehgers syndrome; its natural course and management. Johns Hopkins Med J. 1974;136:71–82.
77. Giardello FM, Welsh SB, Hamilton SR *et al.* Increased risk of cancer in the Peutz-Jehgers syndrome. N Engl J Med. 1987;316:1511–14.
78. Bagan JV, Penarrocha M, Vera-Sempere F. Cowden syndrome: clinical and pathological considerations in two new cases. Oral Maxillofacial Surg. 1989;47:289–94.
79. Carlson GJ, Nivatvongs S, Snover DC. Colorectal polyps in Cowden's disease (multiple hamartomatous syndrome). Am J Pathol. 1984;8:763–9.
80. Guerin V, Bene MC, Judlin P, Beurey J, Landes P, Faure G. Cowden disease in a young girl; gynaecologic and immunologic overview in a case and in the literature. Obstet Gynecol. 1989;73:890–2.
81. Lloyd KM, Dennis M. Cowden's disease; a possible new symptom complex with multiple system involvement. Ann Intern Med. 1963;58:136–42.
82. Mallory SB. Genodermatoses with malignant potential. In: Alper JC, ed. Genetic disorders of the skin. St Louis: Mosby Year Books; 1990:224–66.
83. Russell Jones R, O'Brien M, Wells RS. Cowden's syndrome. Br J Dermatol. 1981;105 (suppl 19):57–8.
84. Brownstein MH, Mehregan AH, Bikowski JB *et al.* The dermatopathology of Cowden's disease. Br J Dermatol. 1979;100:667–73.
85. Starink TM, Vander Veen JPW, Arwert F *et al.* The Cowden syndrome; a clinical and genetic study in 21 patients. Clin Genet. 1986;29:223–33.
86. Gardner DJ. Case of the season. Semin Roentgenol. 1990;25:223–4.
87. Chilovi F, Zancaella L, Perino F *et al.* Cowden's disease with gastrointestinal polyposis. Gastrointest Endosc. 1990;36:323–4.

88. Starink TM, James WD, Rodman OC *et al.* (1986). Multiple hamartoma syndrome (Cowden's disease) associated with non-Hodgkins lymphoma. Arch Dermatol. 1986;122:572–5.
89. Willard W, Borgen P, Bol R, Tiwari R, Osbourne M. Cowden's disease; a case report with analysis at the molecular level. Cancer. 1992;69:2969–74.
90. Eeles RA, Warren W, Knee G *et al.* Constitutional mutation in exon 8 of the p53 gene in a patient with multiple primary tumours; molecular and immunohistochemical findings. Oncogene. 1993;8:1269–76.
91. Eng C, Murday V, Mohammed S *et al.* Cowden syndrome and Lhermitte-Duclos disease in a family; a single genetic syndrome with pleiotropy? J Med Genet. 1994;31:458–61.
92. Rosenblatt KA, Thomas DB, McTieman A *et al.* Breast cancer in men: aspects of familial aggregation. J Natl Cancer Inst. 1991;83:849–53.
93. Stratton MR, Ford D, Neuhasen S *et al.* Familial male breast cancer is not linked to the BRCAI locus on chromosome 17q. Nature Genet. 1994;7:103–7.
94. Wooster R, Mangion J, Eeles R *et al.* A germline mutation in the androgen receptor gene in two brothers with breast cancer and Reifstein syndrome. Nature Genet. 1992;2:132–4.
95. Lobaccaro J-M, Lumbroso S, Belon C *et al.* Male breast cancer and the androgen receptor gene. Nature Genet. 1993;5:109–10.
96. Adami H-O, Adams G, Boyle P *et al.* Report of a working party for the Nordic Cancer Union. Breast cancer etiology. Int J Cancer. 1990;Suppl 5:22–39.
97. Sellers TA, Kushi LH, Potter JD *et al.* Effect of family history, body fat distribution, and reproductive factors on the risk of post-menopausal breast cancer. N Engl J Med. 1992;326:1323–9.
98. Feinleib M. Breast cancer and artificial menopause: a cohort study. JNCI. 1968;41:315–29.
99. Biggs PJ, Warren W, Venitt S, Stratton M. (1993). Does a genotoxic carcinogen contribute to human breast cancer? The value of mutational spectra in unravelling the aetiology of cancer. Mutagenesis. 1993;8:275–83.
100. UK National Case-Control Study Group. Oral contraceptive use and breast cancer risk in young women: subgroup analysis. Lancet. 1990;335:1507–9.
101. Steinberg K, Thacker SB, Smith L *et al.* A meta-analysis of the effect of oestrogen replacement therapy on the risk of breast cancer. JAMA. 1991;265:1985–90.
102. Kaufman DW, Palmer JR, de Mouzon J, *et al.* Estrogen replacement therapy and the risk of breast cancer: results from the case control surveillance study. Am J Epidemiol. 1991;134:1375–85.
103. Higginson J, Muir CS, Munoz N. Human cancer: epidemiology and environmental causes. Cambridge monographs on cancer research. Cambridge: Cambridge University Press; 1992:39–44.
104. Lincoln DW. Contraception for the year 2020 [review]. Br Med Bull. 1993;49:222–36.
105. Lange K, Weeks D, Boelinke M. Programs for pedigree analysis: MENDEL, FISHER and dGene. Genetic Epidemiol. 1988;5:471–2.
106. Bishop DT. Familial predisposition to cancer. Cancer Topics. 1992:66–68.
107. Wooster R, Neuhausen SL, Mangion J, *et al.* Localization of a breast cancer susceptibility gene, BRCA2, to chromosome 13q12–13. Science. 1994;265:2088–90.

2
The genetics of lung cancer

N.E. Caporaso

INTRODUCTION

Lung cancer occupies a place of central importance among malignant neoplasia because of worldwide rising incidence, high mortality rates and the potential for prevention through curtailment of smoking[1]. It is the leading cause of cancer deaths in the United States[2] and perhaps worldwide. While early-stage lung cancer is amenable to surgical cure, 70% of patients have regional or distant spread at the time of diagnosis, and overall five-year survival rates are only 5–10%[3]. The American Cancer Society estimated that 157 000 new lung cancer cases arose in the United States in 1990 with 142 000 deaths. Four pathological types account for more than 90% of cases: epidermoid cancer (35%), adenocarcinoma (30%), and large cell carcinoma (15%), these three being collectively referred to as non-small cell lung cancer (NSCLC). The fourth category, small cell carcinoma (20%), is characterized by specific pathological and molecular findings, as well as distinct clinical features, such as early metastasis and an initial responsiveness to chemotherapy[4].

While lung cancer is the malignancy most clearly associated with external exposures (i.e. tobacco) and therefore is a model for chemical carcinogenesis, evidence will be reviewed which supports a hereditary component of risk. In addition, (molecular) genetic events that accompany the malignant process have been convincingly described. With both a distinct environmental component and hereditary aspects to consider, it is not surprising that gene–environment interaction has been proposed to account for differences in susceptibility. Pharmacogenetic risk factors (hereditary traits that code the enzymes that metabolize carcinogens, repair DNA damage, or control other relevant pathways) will be reviewed. To set the stage for a consideration of these issues, the central role of tobacco in lung carcinogenesis must first be considered.

TOBACCO SMOKE AND LUNG CARCINOGENESIS

Lung cancer is thought to arise from long-term exposure to carcinogens in a susceptible host. Tobacco smoke contains an array of biologically active components. Major toxins or carcinogens in tobacco include carbon monoxide, benzene, nicotine, polycyclic aromatic hydrocarbons, aromatic amines, *N*-nitrosamines, heavy metals and radioelements, such as polonium 210[5]. Mainstream smoke (generated by puff-drawing through the cigarette) and side-stream smoke (emitted by the smouldering tobacco into the ambient air) differ in the relative content of these compounds. Environmental tobacco smoke consists of side-stream smoke and exhaled mainstream smoke.

Both the type of tobacco and the method of tobacco curing influences the chemical content: air-cured tobacco (no artificial heat in drying) differs from flue-cured tobacco (dried by artificial heat) in that a darker tobacco (Cuba, France) is produced, with a higher content of aromatic amines and certain other carcinogens. Most of the tobacco smoked in the United States is flue-cured. A description of selected biologically active components of tobacco smoke with relevance to lung cancer is given in Table 2.1. A comprehensive review of tobacco constituents may be found in the IARC Monograph on tobacco smoke[6].

Numerous studies have confirmed the strong and consistent association between cigarette smoking and lung cancer[7]. In the 1930s, mass-manufactured cigarettes gained popularity and, by the early 1950s, case-control studies in the United States[8] and Great Britain[9] demonstrated the association of smoking with lung cancer. Cohort studies[10,11] clearly established a greater than ten-fold risk for male cigarette smokers. In 1964, the first Surgeon General's report declared smoking to be the major cause of lung cancer among American men. Approximately 85% of lung cancer can be attributed to cigarette smoking[12] and

Table 2.1 Biologically active constituents of tobacco smoke possibly associated with lung cancer

Compound	*Role*
Nitrogen oxides	Formed from nitrates and nitrogenous compounds in tobacco[112], these compounds are probably precursors to carcinogenic *N*-nitrosamines
Hydrogen cyanide (HCN)	Nitrate is a precursor for HCN, which is metabolized in the liver to thiocyanate, an indicator for uptake of tobacco smoke[113]. Thiocyanate catalyses *N*-nitrosamine formation[114].
Benzene (also toluene, hydrazine, vinyl chloride and others)	These carcinogens are present to a greater extent in sidestream than in mainstream smoke[115].
Polycyclic aromatic hydrocarbons (PAH)	A number of compounds, including benzo [a] pyrene, a prototype carcinogen which forms DNA adducts in pulmonary tissue. These compounds are prominent in sidestream smoke.
Nicotine	Accounts for almost 90% of the alkaloids in smoke; the addictive agent in tobacco.
N-Nitrosamine	Highest concentrations of *N*-nitrosamines are found in French 'black' tobacco. Includes volatile, non-volatile and tobacco-specific nitrosamines (TSNA). TSNA are the most abundant carcinogens in tobacco smoke.
Metals	Metal constituents of tobacco smoke which are either human or animal carcinogens include: arsenic, chromium, nickel, cadmium, lead and cobalt.
Radioelements	^{210}Po is an α-emitter present in tobacco smoke[116].

public health strategies to control lung cancer have focused on efforts to reduce smoking (banning sales to minors, taxation, limiting tobacco use in public areas, smoking cessation efforts, and professional and public education). Chemoprevention targeted at inhibiting tobacco carcinogenesis has been studied[13].

Age-adjusted lung cancer death rates in men in the United States rose steadily from 11 per 100 000 population in 1940 to 74 per 100 000 in 1987, parallelling the rise in cigarette smoking. In women, a similar trend was observed with rates of 6 per 100 000 in the early 1960s to 28 per 100 000 in 1987. In the late 1960s, the percentage of US males who smoked began to decline (with a slower decline beginning in women a decade later) and this has resulted in a decline in lung cancer incidence and mortality in younger age groups, consistent with a decrease in smoking in this age group[14].

All the histological types follow a normal dose–response relationship with increased smoking, but adenocarcinoma is least associated with smoking[15]. A curious and unexplained observation is a worldwide increase in the proportion of adenocarcinoma over the past 25 years. In Japan, the proportion of adenocarcinoma increased from 26% to 45% in males and from 45% to 69% in females from 1970 to 1989[16].

OTHER TOBACCO USE

A great variety of tobacco products are used worldwide. Cigars, for instance, generally consist of air-cured and fermented tobaccos. Generally, epidemiological studies have found an intermediate level of risk (between cigarette smokers and non-smokers) for smokers of cigars and pipes. The relative risks for three large cohort studies in the United States are shown in Table 2.2.

ENVIRONMENTAL AND OCCUPATIONAL AGENTS

A multiplicative (synergistic) relationship between exposure to tobacco and certain respiratory carcinogens has been observed for asbestos[17], uranium[18] and polycyclic hydrocarbons[19]. Exposure to radon has been identified as a cause for lung cancer in miners working underground and a consistent dose–response has

Table 2.2 Relative risk from smoking tobacco in US cohort studies

Study	*Cigarettes only*	*Cigars only*	*Pipes only*
American Cancer Society Nine-State Study[117, 118]	9.9	1.0	3.0
American Cancer Society 25-State Study[119]	9.2	1.9	2.2
US Veterans Study[120]	12.1	1.7	2.1

been observed[20–23], while the role of residential radon exposure remains controversial[24,25].

Japanese workers in a factory manufacturing mustard gas between 1929 and 1940 had a greater than 30-fold excess of lung cancer mortality[26]. Asbestos fibres are well-established causative agents in asbestosis, mesothelioma and lung cancer. Coke-oven workers have an excess mortality from lung cancer compared with other steel workers[27], based on polycyclic aromatic hydrocarbon exposure. An excess of lung and nasal cancers in nickel refinery workers was observed in workers employed before 1925[28] while workers who process chromium (but not chromite-ore miners or those engaged in the chrome pigment industry) have exhibited an excess mortality from lung cancer[29]. An excess of lung cancer has been observed in workers exposed to arsenic, including manufacturers of sheep dip containing arsenic compounds, vineyard workers exposed to arsenical insecticides, and Japanese copper smelters exposed to arsenic[30].

Exposure to environmental tobacco smoke is increasingly appreciated as a lung cancer risk factor. The results of a multicentre case-control study found a 30% increased risk of lung cancer in non-smoking females with a smoking spouse. While tobacco is a risk factor for all histological types, it is worth noting that occupational exposures may favour certain histologies[31].

A wide variety of recognized occupational lung carcinogens is evident from Table 2.3.

GENETIC FACTORS AND MOLECULAR INVESTIGATIONS

A general argument for a role for heritable factors in lung cancer is based on classical approaches including the study of familial aggregations, twin studies and segregation analyses. Increasingly, the evidence is supplemented by molecular investigations, including specific chromosome abnormalities associated with histological subtypes, tumour suppressor and oncogene studies, and pharmacogenetic association studies.

CLASSICAL GENETIC APPROACHES

Familial aggregations

Familial clustering may reflect shared risk factors that are genetic or environmental. Systematic population-based studies of cancer risk in first-degree relatives consistently demonstrate increased risk in those relatives. For instance, Goldgar *et. al.'s* study, based on the Utah Population Database, reported a 2.6 (2.1–3.1) relative risk of lung cancer in first-degree relatives of probands[32]. Such studies are particularly challenging to interpret with regard to lung cancer as smokers are more common among relatives of lung cancer patients. While certain studies have included adjustment for smoking, or analysed smokers and non-smokers separately, other shared risks in lung cancer relatives, such as passive smoking exposure, occupational exposure, or a common high-risk diet, might provide alternative explanations to a genetic factor as a means of explaining the consist-

Table 2.3 Occupational lung carcinogens[121]

Carcinogen	*Level of evidence for association*	*Occupations*
Acrylonitrile	Probable	Textile-fibre, rubber
Arsenic	Definite	Arsenic-related, sheep-dip, wool-fibre, mining, smelting, vineyard workers
Asbestos	Definite	Asbestos mining, insulating, shipyard workers[122], plumbing, cement, pipe-fitters
BCME, CMME	Definite	Chemical industry
Beryllium	Probable	Beryllium-related
Cadmium	Definite	Alkaline battery, cadmium-related
Chromium (hexavalent)	Definite	Chromate related
Coal tar	Probable	Roofers, slaters, aluminium, coal gasification, coke production
Diesel engine exhaust	Probable	Railroad workers, drivers, dock workers, mechanics
Nickel	Definite	Nickel-related, welding
Silica	Probable	Ore mining, granite and stone industries
Soots	Definite	Chimney sweeps
Talc (with asbestos fibres)	Definite	Talc mining[123], milling, pottery workers
Vinyl chloride	Probable	Vinyl chloride workers

ent finding of increased risk in relatives of affected individuals. Early investigators observed excess risk of lung cancer in relatives of probands compared with control relatives after adjustment for risk factors[33–36]. More recent studies have extended these findings using a retrospective case-control design[37–39].

Twin studies

Joishy *et al.*[40] reported on a set of identical twins with alveolar cell carcinoma and similar clinical features. Formal twin studies in registries, notably the Swedish and Finnish, have generally not revealed large excess concordance for lung cancer in monozygotic twins compared with dizygotic twins.

We have recently reported[41] a study of lung cancer in the NAS Veterans Twin Registry that included 15 924 twin pairs: virtually all the twins who served in the US Military in World War II. Interestingly, overall, there was an excess of concordant pairs with lung cancer for all zygosity groups. The observed to expected frequency of concordant pairs was 3.99 in DZ twins and 2.98 in MZ twins. The ratio of observed to expected concordance among monozygotic twins (MZ) did not exceed that among dizygotic twins (DZ) (overall rate ratio 0.75

(95% confidence interval 0.35–1.61)), in spite of the likelihood that MZ pairs are more likely to be concordant for smoking than DZ pairs. This finding is consistent with a familial, but not necessarily genetic, component to lung cancer. A cohort analysis of lung cancer mortality that accounted for age, sex, race and smoking intensity in 300 person-years of follow-up among 47 MZ twins whose smoking twins had died of lung cancer found no lung cancer deaths (expected 0–4.09). Overall, these data do not provide support for a genetic component of lung cancer, at least within males aged 50 or older[41].

Segregation analysis

Segregation analysis tests whether the pattern of phenotypes (i.e. lung cancer) in families is consistent with Mendelian inheritance. In a study by Sellers *et al.*[42], in an area of Louisiana with a high rate of lung cancer, there was some consistency with the twin study cited above in that the putative genetic effect was prominent in younger affected individuals, i.e. 70% of those under age 50 were predicted to have some genetic component, while 70% of cases older than 70 were due solely to smoking. This study was consistent with the existence of a major gene that influences the age of onset of lung cancer[42].

MOLECULAR INVESTIGATIONS

Cytogenetic studies

While classical cytogenetic studies were crucial in the identification of specific chromosome defects that characterize most of the haematological malignancies, findings in solid tumours have been much less specific. In the case of lung cancer, deletion of the short arm of chromosome 3 is observed in virtually all small cell carcinomas and many non-small cell cancers[43], and a tumour suppressor gene on this chromosome arm is postulated. Loss of heterozygosity has been noted on 8p[44], 11p[45], 5q[46] and 9p[47,48] as well as other loci[49] (see below). Clonal abnormalities have been observed on virtually every chromosome[50].

Tumour suppressor genes

Tumour suppressor genes encode proteins that regulate cell growth, and many tumours exhibit loss of these genes at various stages in the carcinogenic process.

p53

The product of the p53 gene is a protein that negatively regulates growth and therefore cell proliferation.

Loss of heterozygosity on the short arm of chromosome 17 in the region of the p53 gene has been detected in tumour samples taken from many malignancies, including those of the lung[51,52]. In subjects with loss of heterozygosity in the region of p53, most exhibit mutations in p53 when the mutational hot spots (exons 4–8) are sequenced[53], with the highest percentage observed in small cell histology (70%) and the lowest in adenocarcinoma (33%). The most common mutation observed is a transversion (i.e. purine to pyrimidine or *vice versa)* while the frequency of transitions (purine to purine or pyrimidine to pyrimidine) is lower than in almost any other cancer. This may reflect the predominance of exogenous mechanisms (i.e. tobacco smoke carcinogen exposure) in the origin of p53 mutations in this tumour type[54]. It is thought that these mutations act by eliminating the normal growth suppressive activity of the p53 gene product.

rb

Abnormalities in another tumour suppressor gene, retinoblastoma (rb), mapped to the long arm of chromosome 13, have been detected in small cell primary tumours[55] and cell lines[56].

Dominant oncogenes

Oncogenes are derived from normal cellular genes (proto-oncogenes). When these genes are altered by mutation, malignancy can result. An example is the bcl/abl translocation (Philadelphia chromosome) in chronic myelogenous leukaemia.

ras

A GTP-binding protein that is involved in signal transduction is encoded by *ras*. Well-characterized point mutations in codons 12, 13 or 61 confer transforming activity. *ras* mutations are observed at an early stage in animal systems but their role in early bronchial lesions is unclear. New highly sensitive molecular techniques, such as the polymerase chain reaction (pcr) and single strand conformational polymorphism (sscp), can be employed to detect such mutational changes in early lesions. Thus, these types of markers offer the theoretical potential for screening high-risk groups and for early detection via sputum sampling.

K-*ras* mutations have been observed in 30% of smokers with adenocarcinoma and are associated with a poor prognosis. The mutations are less frequent in non-smokers and in other histologies[57].

bcl-2

bcl-2 is a proto-oncogene that produces a protein that may protect cells from apoptosis (programmed cell death). The 14:18 chromosome translocation observed in most follicular lymphomas means that this gene is associated with the immunoglobulin heavy-chain promoter[58]. An immunochemical analysis using a monoclonal antibody specific for bcl-2 protein was tested on a surgical series and 25% (20/80) of squamous cell and 12% (5/42) adenocarcinomas expressed the abnormal antigen. There was a survival benefit in subjects with the protein[59].

Others

Altered expression, amplification or overexpression of erb1 and -2[60], HER2/*neu*[61,62], *jun*, *myc* family[63], c-*myb*[54] and c-*raf*-1[65] have all been observed.

In contrast to the specific gene mutations observed in most haematological malignancies, in general, the mutations seen are neither observed in all cases nor specific to lung cancer.

Other gene defects

Retinoic acid receptor

Retinoids are vitamin A analogues that influence the growth of epithelial tissue and have been proposed as possible chemopreventive agents because of studies indicating suppression of carcinogenesis in animals. *trans*-retinoic acid has been used successfully as a treatment for promyelocytic leukemia[66]. During the development of lung cancer, mucociliary differentiation is impaired, similar to the effects of vitamin A deprivation. A deletion on chromosome 3p maps close to the retinoic acid receptor ß, and is frequently observed in human lung cancer. It has been reported recently that this receptor loses retinoic acid responsiveness in lung cancer cell lines, a feature that may contribute to neoplastic progression[67].

Association studies/candidate genes

Lung cancer is an ideal condition for the study of gene-environment interactions as a strong case can be made for the participation of both environmental exposures (tobacco) and genetic factors (based on the above discussion). Thus, case-control studies have been used to test hypotheses regarding genes that are involved in pathways thought to be mechanistically plausible. These studies have recently been reviewed[68].

Toxic chemicals do not exert carcinogenic effects by themselves but require activation to electrophilic forms before detrimental effects will result[69,70]. Phase 1 enzymes, mostly belonging to the P450 group, perform the initial biotransformation, while Phase 2 enzymes participate in further steps that typically precede elimination. It is convenient to consider candidate genes in each of these categories.

Phase 1

CYP2D6 (Debrisoquine phenotype)

An important area of investigation in lung cancer involves polymorphic genes that catalyse carcinogen activation. The prototype enzyme is debrisoquine hydroxylase, coded by the P450 gene, CYP2D6. Debrisoquine is an antihypertensive drug used in Great Britain, and individuals deficient in its metabolism on a genetic basis (approximately 10% in Western populations) were observed to have an exaggerated response to the drug, i.e. hypotension. Debrisoquine phenotyping studies (based on the ratio of drug to metabolite excreted in an aliquot of urine following a subtherapeutic test dose of the drug) have generally indicated excess risk in 'extensive metabolizers', meaning homozygous dominant or heterozygous individuals compared with homozygous recessive 'poor metabolizers'. The enzyme participates in the metabolism of at least 30 common medications, but the question of whether it actually activates a major carcinogen in tobacco smoke remains unclear. A mechanism for the association remains speculative, but, if nicotine is a substrate for CYP2D6[71], poor metabolizers might require less substrate to satisfy tobacco addiction. A review of risk in extensive metabolizers from all published studies indicates significant heterogeneity. Given this, a summary odds ratio cannot be calculated (Table 2.4). A number of well-designed studies currently in the field as well as a metanalysis that we are conducting should help resolve these issues. Critical methodological difficulties in these studies are reviewed at the end of this section.

CYP1A1 (Aryl Hydrocarbon Hydroxylase Inducibility)

Polycyclic aromatic hydrocarbons are metabolized to mutagenic DNA-binding compounds by members of the P4501A family of enzymes. The respiratory carcinogen, benzo[a]pyrene is the best known carcinogen substrate. Variability in metabolic activity with respect to these compounds concordant with cancer susceptibility has been well described in the mouse. The ability to induce the carcinogen metabolizing enzyme varies widely in humans, and a three-model phenotype consistent with autosomal dominant inheritance has been demonstrated[72,73]. Aryl hydrocarbon hydroxylase inducibility (coded by the gene CYP1A1) has been linked with lung cancer susceptibility in a study by Kellerman *et al.*[74] and confirmed in subjects with other smoking-related cancers, such as laryngeal[75] and oral cavity[76], as well as lung[77,78], although not all studies were supportive[79]. Methodological difficulties have been blamed for heterogeneity in some studies, e.g. seasonal variation in the assay, poor reproducibility, effect–cause bias, and poor cell survival in lung cancer patients. In the light of this, there has been great interest in developing a genotype marker that accurately reflects the human variation in this trait.

A restriction fragment length polymorphism (RFLP) based an a MspI site 3′ to the CYP1A1 gene has been studied in lung cancer patients and controls. To

Table 2.4 Studies of debrisoquine phenotype and lung cancer by histology

Author and year	*Lung cancer*	*Control*	*Odds ratio (95% CI)*
Ayesh *et al.* 1984[124],1989[125]	EM 241 PM 4	EM 215 PM 19	5.3 (1.9–1.5)
Roots *et al.* 1988[126]	EM 251 PM 19	EM 240 PM 30	1.7 (0.9–3.0)
Caporaso *et al.* 1990[127]	EM 88 PM 1	EM 80 PM 12	13.2 (2.1–8.0)
Benitez *et al.* 1991[128]	EM 80 PM 4	EM 123 PM 10	1.6 (0.5–5.1)
Wolf *et al.* 1992[129]	EM 348 PM 13	EM 689 PM 31	1.2 (0.6–2.3)
Horsmans *et al.* 1991[130]	EM 86 PM 5	EM 155 PM 12	1.3 (0.5–3.7)
Puchetti *et al.* 1994[131]	EM 115 PM 1	EM 809 PM 45	6.3 (1.1–37)
Duche *et al.* 1991[132]	EM 143 PM 10	EM 234 PM 20	1.2 (0.6–2.6)
Tefre *et al.* 1994[133]	EM 184 PM 20	EM 111 PM 6	0.5 (0.2–1.2)
Law *et al.* 1989[134]	EM 102 PM 2	EM 95 PM 9	4.8 (1.1–20)
Shaw *et al.* 1994[135]	EM 306 PM 29	EM 346 PM 27	0.8 (0.5–1.4)
Hirvonen *et al.* 1993[136]	EM 105 PM 1	EM 115 PM 7	6.4 (1.0–40)
Summary (% PM)	EM 1199 PM 47 (3.7)	EM 1617 PM 121 (7.0)	No summary odds ratio Heterogeneity χ^2 $= 33.8, p = 0.0004$

date, four studies in Western populations have revealed no association, while studies from Japan have found evidence for an association. As a general caution in the interpretation of this work, both the Oriental reports derive from one hospital (Saitama Cancer Center Hospital, Japan) (Table 2.5).

The association of an MspI polymorphism with lung cancer in Japan is especially interesting as the association with the genetic marker is strongest in those

Table 2.5 Studies of P4501A1polymorphism in an Oriental population

Study	*Cases n (%)*	*Controls n (%)*	*Odds ratio (95% CI)*
Nakachi *et al.* 1991[144]	32 (21)	40 (11)	2.1 (1.3–3.4)
Hayashi *et al.* 1992[145]	26 (12)	17 (5) 13 (4)	3.0 (1.6–5.6)

with low to moderate tobacco exposure. This suggests that the genetic co-factor acts predominantly within a certain exposure range. Below that range, exposure is insufficient to cause cancer in sufficient numbers to detect. Above that range, the genetic factor is less important because the enzyme is 'saturated' and little additional carcinogenic effect results.

CYP2E1

The CYP2E1 (nitrosamine) trait is associated with an enzyme which catalyses oxidation and DNA adduct formation by nitrosamines, and is therefore a plausible candidate for a susceptibility factor in lung cancer. A variety of polymorphisms of this gene, located in the transcription regulation area (PstI, RsaI) or adjoining intron (DraI), have been examined in relation to lung cancer in man[80–83]. Although weak excess risk has been observed in a few of the studies, the lack of a convincing relationship between the RFLP and gene expression and activity has lessened enthusiasm. CYP2E1 is inducible by ethanol and therefore is a plausible candidate for tumours jointly associated with tobacco and alcohol, such as those of the oesophagus.

CYP1A2 (*N*-oxidation phenotype)

Arylamines and heterocyclic amines are substrates for this enzyme. Phenotyping is accomplished by administration of caffeine and quantitation of metabolites (either in expired air[84] or urine[85]). This marker has not been extensively studied in relation to cancer because of methodological problems. First, it is not clear how much of the variability in enzyme levels is due to induction and how much reflects the postulated genetic component[86]; second, the enzyme is induced by smoking, resulting in confounding[87]; third, the enzyme is restricted to the liver, making its role in the lung less plausible than is the case for CYP1A1, with which it shares 80% homology.

CYP3A4

CYP3A4 metabolizes certain medications, including cyclophosphamide, ifosfamide, vinblastine, nifedipine[88], erythromycin and cyclosporine, as well as the compounds, aflatoxin B_1 and benzo[a]pyrene (3-hydroxylation)[89]. To date, there have been no human cancer studies.

CYP2A6

This enzyme activates certain carcinogens, the most important of which is the tobacco-derived respiratory carcinogen, 4-(methylnitrosoamino)-1-(3-pyridyl)-1-butanone (NKK)[90]. Phenotyping and genotyping methods are under investigation but, as yet, a method suitable for field investigation is not available.

Phase 2

Phase 2 enzymes detoxify compounds through conjugation with moieties that increase their solubility and therefore promote excretion, although, in some cases, they may activate carcinogens.

GSTM1

Genetic deficiency of the glutathione-*S*-transferase μ gene, present in 50% of Western populations, might increase lung cancer risk through reduced ability to conjugate and detoxify (or enhance elimination) of carcinogenic electrophiles, such as the metabolites of tobacco-derived polycyclic aromatic hydrocarbons, e.g. diol-epoxides. A role in tumour promotion is also possible through increased vulnerability to lipid peroxidation. There is evidence that GSTM1 null individuals have more sister chromatid exchanges in their lymphocytes[91].

Table 2.6 Glutathione S-transferase μ locus and lung cancer by histology

Authors and year	*Lung cancer (% null)*	*Control (% null)*	*Odds ratio (95% CI)*
Zhong *et al.* 1991[137]	130+ 98– (43%)	131+ 94– (42%)	1.1 (0.7–1.5)
Brockmoller *et al.* 1993[138]	55+ 62– (53%)	73+ 82– (53%)	1.0 (0.6–1.6)
Hayashi *et al.* 1992[139]	94+ 118– (56%)	191+ 167– (47%)	1.4 (1.0–2.0)
Nazar–Stewart *et al.* 1993[140]	9+ 16– (64%)	15+ 14– (48%)	1.9 (0.6–5.6)
Heckbert *et al.* 1992[141]	35+ 64– (65%)	42+ 58– (58%)	1.3 (0.7–2.3)
Kihara *et al.* 1994[142]	70+ 108– (61%)	110+ 91– (45%)	1.9 (1.2–2.8)
Seidegard *et al.* 1986[143]	23+ 43– (65%)	46+ 32– (41%)	2.7 (1.4–5.3)
Alexandrie *et al.* 1994[106]	131+ 161– (55%)	195+ 213– (52%)	1.1 (0.8–1.5)
Summary	547+ 610– (53%)	803+ 751– (48%)	1.3 (1.1–1.5) Note: heterogeneity χ^2 is not significant

For GSTM1, there are currently eight published studies which evaluate a GSTM1 null/lung cancer association (Table 2.6). Three studies found significantly increased risk, while the others reported some increased lung cancer risk in null subjects that did not reach statistical significance. Overall, for null individuals, with all histological types of lung cancer, a summary odds ratio of 1.3 (1.1–1.5, 95% CI) is observed. The heterogeneity χ^2 is not significant, indicating reasonable agreement among the studies, in spite of differences in design, control selection, etc. However, if adenocarcinoma is considered independently (only in studies where histology and GST were enumerated), no increased risk whatsoever is found; the odds ratio is 1.0 (0.7–1.4). In contrast, the remaining non-adenocarcinoma subjects exhibit elevated risk with an odds ratio equal to 1.5 (1.2–1.9). GST immunohistochemical staining has been observed in the lung, varies among individuals, and is most intense in the central bronchial epithelium (the site of the more certainly smoking-related histologies, as opposed to adenocarcinoma that occurs more frequently in the periphery), consistent with increased risk associated with the null genotype in these histologies[92]. Finally, another smoking-related tumour, bladder cancer, has been studied in five case-control studies (data not shown) and exhibits an almost identically increased risk. These findings indicate that it is quite likely that a GSTM1 null genotype constitutes at least a weak risk factor for lung cancer. While the relative risk is small, the population-attributable risk is likely to be considerable.

NAT2

N-acetyl-transferase (the acetylation phenotype) has been extensively studied in relation to bladder cancer, based on the functional role of this enzyme in the metabolism of arylamines. No association has been observed with lung cancer[109].

Others

UDP-glucuronyltransferase, cysteine conjugate ß-lysase, and epoxide hydrolase are other Phase 2 enzymes that have been studied in human populations.

Other polymorphisms

A miscellaneous group of candidate genes involved in modulation of oncogene or tumour suppressor activity, metabolism of nutrients, non-specific or unknown mechanisms of initiation of promotion, DNA or macromolecule repair, or immune function has been described.

Hras vtr rare alleles

This gene is the best studied of the miscellaneous group. A variable tandem repeat (VTR) DNA-RFLP is located 3′ to the HRAS-1 structural genes. A weak association of 'rare alleles' with lung cancer has been observed in a few studies[93–95].

p53, L-myc polymorphisms

Germ-line polymorphisms that might theoretically influence the expression or activity of these genes have not led to convincing associations in Caucasians[96–98].

GSTT1, glutathione S-transferase-θ

The soluble glutathione transferases comprise four families. In addition to the μ (GSTM1) polymorphism discussed above, another genetic polymorphism is responsible for a phenotype that catalyses glutathione-dependent conjugation of halomethanes, and determines 60% of the population as conjugators and 40% as non-conjugators. Products of dihalomethanes are mutagenic (resulting in increased SCE in non-conjugators[99]), may cause lung tumours in mice, and may be human carcinogens. This polymorphism awaits epidemiological testing in humans[100].

Poly(ADP-ribose) polymerase polymorphism

This DNA-binding protein on chromosome 13 is divided in DNA processing and a two-allele polymorphism has exhibited an increase in the minor allele in lung cancer in at least one study[101,102].

METHODOLOGICAL ISSUES IN INTERDISCIPLINARY STUDIES

Experience has taught that association studies that incorporate genetic susceptibility markers are fraught with pitfalls. Basic tenets of sound epidemiological study design are not reviewed here but cannot be overemphasized. A few succinct points of special relevance are summarized as the 'ten commandments' of metabolic studies:

1. Exposure assessment
   It is not likely that any gene causes lung cancer in the absence of smoking or some other exogenous exposure. Unless careful assessment of exposure to suspected or known carcinogens is included, human population studies will be uninterpretable. There must be a distinction between exposures that contribute to cancer (remote) and exposures that influence the biomarker measured (recent). Interaction with exposure is implicit in the postulated mechanism for the influence of these genes (see Nos. 9 and 10) and will require the pertinent data.
2. Genotype/phenotype[103]
   Reliable genotyping approaches that can assign the genotype based on detection of germ-line mutations using the polymerase chain reaction

(PCR) are increasingly substituting for traditional phenotyping approaches. These approaches are hampered by allelic herogeneity, as evidenced with CYP2D6. Complexities that can render genotype interpretation difficult include:

a. Inability of PCR to detect all the relevant mutations, e.g. in the case of CYP2D6, no PCR approach is yet available to detect complete deletion of the gene ('D' mutation) a mutation accounting for 15% or so of mutant alleles in Western populations. A Southern blot is required for reliable detection[104].

b. Variability of mutation type and frequency in different ethnic groups (see No. 3) is expected. Interpretation of a genotype may not be straightforward since certain 'mutations' may have variable effects or increase enzyme activity[105].

An advantage of more efficient genotyping is that larger studies and examination of multiple markers simultaneously will improve efficiency[106].

3. Misclassification[107]
Misassignment of the genotype/phenotype can result in degradation of study power and bias (usually towards the null), especially at extremes of prevalence of the 'at-risk' polymorphism.

4. Ethnic variation[108]
All genetic traits exhibit ethnic variation. Serious bias results if cases and controls are drawn from different ethnic groups. Another common problem is low power due to low marker prevalence (see No. 5).

5. Power
A common error occurs when a small study finds a risk magnitude similar to other positive studies, however, lacking statistical significance, the study is reported as 'negative' (Type II error). While sample size is often constrained in studies that incoporate biomarkers, power calculations should be an integral part of these study design.

6. Cause–effect bias
Certain biomarkers are related to the presence of disease in the host, i.e. tumour markers. A distinction must be made between a tumour marker and a (genetic) host susceptibility factor that specifies a phenotype. In fact, any phenotype may theoretically be affected by a variety of factors that can be influenced by the presence of tumour or its treatment. Studies employing a probe drug and subsequent measurement of metabolism must be alert to this source of bias (see Nos. 3 and 6).

7. Incident versus prevalent cases
Study of prevalent cases can introduce bias if a marker is related to survival, or if a marker only predisposes to 'aggressive' tumours.

8. Biospecimens
Traditionally, blood samples have served as a source of genetic material for germ-line DNA. Increasingly, less invasive methodologies are

becoming feasible, e.g. buccal scraping or tests on archival tissue, etc. More problematic are phenotype determinations, subject to distortion due to improper storage, processing or assay. Phenotyping requires measurement of a ratio of metabolites from a tracer dose of a specific metabolic probe (e.g. caffeine, dextromethorphan).

9. Qualitative interaction
   The enzyme–substrate specificity implicit in these associations suggests that risk will be altered in the host bearing a specific gene only when the host is exposed to the relevant environmental agent.

10. Quantitative interaction
    There is likely to be a range of exposure over which a given gene will alter risk. Recent studies have been more attentive to the collection of high-quality exposure data, and this has allowed exploration of a number of gene–cancer[110] or gene–exposure[111] effects.

    Studies which incorporate careful exposure assessment with investigation of these molecular lesions in appropriate populations (i.e. smokers, asbestos-exposed, miners, etc.) are crucial in order to elucidate lesions on the causal pathway. If heritable genetic susceptibility genes are identified, individuals at risk may be targeted for special intervention (e.g. to stop smoking). Important ethical problems will arise as our appreciation of genetic determinants of the aetiology of lung cancer are clarified.

CONCLUSIONS

Since lung cancer is rare in non-smokers (especially when other occupational exposures are excluded), it is important to preface any discussion of the 'genetic' component of susceptibility to lung cancer by observing that any plausible genetic factor must act in concert with tobacco to alter the probability of developing the disease. It is worth recalling the data of Adler[146] (see Wynder and Hoffman for review[147]) that, in 1912, prior to the era of common cigarette smoking, primary lung cancer constituted less than 0.5% of all cancer. Given the high mortality and high incidence of this disease, the clear relationship to smoking, the fact that smoking causes many other serious diseases (heart disease, chronic obstructive lung disease, stroke, etc.), and the evidence that stopping results in health benefits at any age, efforts to oppose smoking by clinicians, educators policy makers and scientists are mandatory. Especially important, in view of the addictive nature of tobacco smoking, are concerted efforts to oppose advertising directed at younger age groups. Nevertheless, even if a major decline in tobacco consumption occurs, mortality rates are unlikely to decline much during the next two decades because there is a large cohort of smokers already exposed. Thus, efforts to develop effective chemoprevention are worthwhile.

A molecular genetic component to the risk of lung cancer does seem to exist and some hereditary component appears likely. Efforts to understand the mechanism better should have practical applications, although the merits of screening or early diagnosis remain undemonstrated. Occupational risk factors, though less important in terms of attributable risk, have relevance because of the existence of high exposures in certain subpopulations, the involuntary nature of the exposure, synergistic effects in smokers, and the potential for prevention. In the genetic context, it should be appreciated that certain agents may act through pathways mediated by specific enzymes and thus may be distinctively associated with putative genetic risk factors.

Improved understanding of aetiology through biochemical and molecular epidemiological approaches has the potential to revolutionize our strategy towards this malignancy. New insights which emerge should provide alternative approaches to the prevention, control and therapy of lung cancer.

References

1. A Report of the Surgeon General. The Health Consequence of Smoking: Cancer, DHHS (PHS) 82-50179. Rockville, MD: Office on Smoking and Health, US Department of Health and Human Services; 1982.
2. Boring CC, Squires TS, Tong T. Cancer statistics 1991. CA. 1991;41:19–36.
3. Minna JD, Higgins GA, Glatstein EJ. Cancer of the lung. In: DeVita VT, Hellman S, Rosenberg S, eds. Principles and practice of oncology. Philadelphia: JB Lippincott Co; 1982:396–474.
4. Lubin JH, Blot WJ. Assessment of lung cancer risk factors by histologic category. JNCI. 1984;73:383–9.
5. Hoffmann D, Hecht SS. Advances in tobacco carcinogenesis. In: Cooper CS, Grover PL, eds. Handbook of experimental pharmacology. Vol 94. Heidelberg: Springer-Verlag; 63.
6. IARC monographs on the evaluation of the carcinogenic risk of chemicals to human, tobacco smoking. Vol 38. Lyon, France: IARC; 1986.
7. Doll R, Peto R. Cigarette smoking and bronchial carcinoma: dose and time relationships among regular smokers and lifelong non-smokers. J Epid Commun Health. 1978;32(4):303–13.
8. Levin ML, Goldstein H, Gerhardt PR. Cancer and tobacco smoking: A preliminary report. JAMA. 1950;143:336–8.
9. Doll R, Hill AB. A study of the aetiology of carcinoma of the lung. Br Med J. 1952;2:1271–86.
10. Hammond EC. Smoking in relation to the death rates of one million men and women. Natl Cancer Inst Monogr. 1966;19:127–204.
11. Doll R, Peto R. Mortality in relation to smoking: 20 years' observations on male British doctors. Br Med J. 1976;2:1525–36.
12. US Surgeon General. The health consequences of smoking: cancer. NIH Publication 82-50179. Washington, DC: US DHHS; 1982.
13. Castonguay A. Methods and strategies in lung cancer control. Cancer Res. 1992;52 (Suppl):2641–51.
14. Department of Health and Human Services. Reducing the Health Consequences of Smoking: 25 Years of Progress: A Report of the Surgeon General, DHHS Publication No (CDC) 89-8411. Washington, D.C.: US Department of Health and Human Services, Center for Chronic Disease Prevention and Health Promotion, Office on Smoking and Health; 1989.
15. Wynder EL, Covey LS. Epidemiologic patterns in lung cancer by histologic types. Eur J Clin Oncol. 1987;23:1491–6.
16. Ikeda T, Kurita Y, Inutsuka S, Tanaka K, Nakanishi Y, Shigematsu N, Nobutomo K. The changing pattern of lung cancer by histologic type – a review of 1151 cases from a University hospital in Japan, 1970–1989. Lung Cancer. 1991;7:157–64.
17. Hammond EC, Selikoff IJ. Asbestos exposure, cigarette smoking, and death rates. Ann NY Acad Sci. 1979;330:473.
18. Archer VE. Enhancement of lung cancer by cigarette smoking in uranium and other miners. Carcinog Compr Surv. 1985;8:23.
19. Mossman BT, Craighead JE. Mechanisms of asbestos carcinogenesis. Environ Res. 1981;25:269–80.

20. National Council on Radiation Protection and Measurements. Evaluation of occupation and environmental exposures to radon and radon daughters in the United States. NCRP Report 78. Bethesda MD: National Council on Radiation Protection and Measurements; 1984.
21. National Research Council, Committee on the Biological Effects of Radiation. Health risks of ionizing radiation. Health risks of radon and other internally-deposited alpha emitters: BEIR IV. Washington, DC: National Academy Press; 1988.
22. Samet JM, Kutvirt DM, Waxweiler RJ, Key CR. Uranium mining and lung cancer in Navajo men. NEJM. 1984;310:1481–4.
23. Lubin HJ, Boice JD Jr, Edling C, *et al.* Radon and lung cancer risk: a joint analysis of 11 underground miners studies. NIH Publication no. 94-3644. Rockville, MD: National Institute of Health; 1994.
24. Schoenberg JB, Klotz JB, Wilcox HB, *et al.* Case-control study of residential radon and lung cancer among New Jersey women. Cancer Res. 1990;50:6520–4.
25. Letourneau EG, Krewski D, Choi NW, *et al.* Case-control study of residential radon and lung cancer in Winnipeg, Manitoba, Canada. Am J Epidemiol. 1994;140(4):310–22.
26. Wada S, Nishimoto Y, Miyanishi M, *et al.* Mustard gas as a cause of respiratory neoplasia in man. Lancet 1968;1:1161–3.
27. Lloyd J. Long-term mortality of steelworkers. V. Respiratory cancer of coke plant workers. J Occup Med. 1971;13:53–68.
28. Doll R, Morgan L, Speizer F. Cancer of the lung and nasal sinuses in nickel workers. Br J Cancer. 1970;24:623–32.
29. Machle W, Gregorius F. Cancer of the respiratory system in the United States chromate-producing industry. US Public Health Reports. 1948;63:1114–27.
30. Fraumeni JF Jr. Chemicals in the induction of respiratory tract tumors. In: Proceedings of the XI International Cancer Congress, Florence, 1974. Excerpta Medica International Congress Series No. 351, Vol. 3. Cancer Epidemiology, Environmental Factors. Amsterdam: Exerpta Medica; 1974.
31. Vena JE, Byers TE, Cookfair D, Swanson M. Occupation and lung cancer risk. Cancer 1985;56:910–17.
32. Goldgar DE, Easton DF, Cannon-Albright LA, Skolnick MH. Systematic population-based assessment of cancer risk in first-degree relatives of cancer probands. JNCI. 1994;86(21):1600–7.
33. Tokuhata GK, Lillienfeld AM. Familial aggregation of lung cancer risk in humans. JNCI. 1963;30:289.
34. Ooi WL, Elston RC, Chen VW, Bailey-Wilson JE, Rothschild H. Increased familial risk for lung cancer. JNCI. 1986;76:217.
35. Tokuhata GK, Lilienfeld AM. Familial aggregation of lung cancer in humans. JNCI. 1963;30:289–312.
36. Ooi WL, Elston RC, Chen VW, Bailey-Wilson JE, Rothschild H. Increased familial risk for lung cancer. JNCI. 1986;76:217–22.
37. Sellers TA, Elston RC, Stewart C, Rothschild H. Familial risk of cancer among randomly selected cancer probands. Genet Epidemiol. 1988;4:381–92.
38. Ooi WL, Elston RC, Chen VW, Bailey-Wilson JE, Rothschild H. Increased familial risk of lung cancer. JNCI. 1986;76:217–22.
39. Shaw GL, Falk RT, Pickle LW, Mason TJ, Buffler PA. Lung cancer risk associated with cancer in relatives. J Clin Epidemiol. 1991;44:429–37.
40. Joishy SK, Cooper RA, Rowley PT. Alveolar cell carcinoma in identical twins: similarity in time of onset, histochemistry, and site of metastasis. Ann Intern Med. 1977;87:447.
41. Braun M, Caporaso N, Page W, Hoover R. Genetic component of lung cancer: cohort study of twins. Lancet. 1994;344:440–1.
42. Sellers TA, Bailey-Wilson JE, Elston RC, Wilson AE, Elston RC, Rothschild H. Evidence for Mendelian inheritance in the pathogenesis of lung cancer. JNCI. 1990;82:1272–9.
43. Brauch H, Johnson B, Hovis J, Yano T, Gazdar A, Minna JD. Molecular analysis of the short arm of chromosome 3 in small-cell and non-small cell carcinoma of the lung. NEJM. 1987;317:1109–13.
44. Ohata H, Emi M, Fujiwara Y, *et al.* Deletion mapping of the short arm of chromosome 8 in non-small cell lung carcinoma. Genes Chromosome Cancer. 1993;7:85–8.
45. Ludwig CU, Raefle G, Dalquen P, Stulz P, Stahel R, Obrecht JP. Allelic loss on the short arm of chromosome 1 in non-small cell lung carcinoma. Int J Cancer. 1991;49:661–5.

46. Hosoe S, Ueno K, Shigedo Y, *et al.* A frequent deletion of chromosome 5q21 in advanced small cell and non-small cell carcinoma of the lung. Cancer Res. 1994;54:1787–90.
47. Center R, Lukeis R, Dietzsch E, Gillespie M, Garson OM. Molecular deletion of 9q sequances in non-small cell cancer and malignant mesothelioma. Genes Chromosome Cancer. 1993;7:47–53.
48. Mead LJ, Gillespie MT, Irving LB, Campbell LJ. Homozygous and hemizygous deletions of 9p centromeric to the inteferon genes in lung cancer. Cancer Res. 1994;54:2307–9.
49. Shiseki M, Kohno T, Nishikawa R, Sameshima Y, Mizoguchi H, Yokoda J. Frequent allelic losses on chromosome 2q, 18q, 22q in advanced non-small cell lung cancer. Cancer Res. 1994;54:5643–8.
50. Lukeis R, Irving L, Garson M, Hasthorpe S. Cytogenetics of non-small cell lung cancer: analysis of consistent non-random abnormalities. Genes Chromosome Cancer. 1990;2:116–24.
51. Yokota J, Wada M, Shimosato Y, Terada M, Sugimura T. Loss of heterozygosity on chromosomes 3, 13, and 17 in small-cell lung cancer and chromosome 3 in adenocarcinoma of the lung. PNAS USA. 1987;84:9252–6.
52. Weston A, Willey JC, Modali R, *et al.* Differential DNA sequence deletions from chromosomes 3, 11, 13 and 17 in squamous cell carcinoma, large-cell carcinoma, and adenocarcinoma of the human lung. PNAS USA. 1989;86:5099–103.
53. Miller CW, Simon K, Aslo A, *et al.* p53 Mutations and lung tumors. Cancer Res. 1992;52:1695–8.
54. Greenblatt MS, Bennett WP, Hollstein M, Harris CC. Mutations in the p53 tumor suppressor gene: Clues to cancer etiology and molecular pathogenesis. Cancer Res. 1994;54: 4855–78.
55. Horowitz JM, Yandell DW, Park S-H, *et al.* Point mutational inactivation of the retinoblastoma antioncogene. Science. 1989;243:937–40.
56. Horowitz JM, Park S-H, Bogenmann E, *et al.* Frequent inactivation of the retinoblastoma antioncogene is restricted to a subset of human tumor cells. PNAS USA. 1990;87:2775–9.
57. Rodenhuis S, Slebos RJC. Clinical significance of ras oncogene activation in human lung cancer. Cancer Res. 1992; 52(Suppl):2665–9.
58. Tsujimoto Y, Croce CM. Analysis of the structure, transcripts and protein products of bcl 2, the gene involved in human follicular lymphoma. Proc Natl Acad Sci USA. 1986;83:5214–18.
59. Pezzella F, Turley H, Kuzu I, *et al.* bcl-2 Protein in non-small-cell lung carcinoma. NEJM. 1993;329:690–4.
60. Paakko P, Nuorva K, Kamel D, Soinin Y. Evidence by in situ hybridization that c-erbB-2 proto-oncogene expression is a marker of malignancy and is expressed in lung adenocarcinoma. Am J Resp Cell Mol Biol. 1992;7:325–34.
61. Yokota T, Toyoshima K, Sugimura T, *et al.* Amplification of c-erb-B2 oncogene in human adenocarcinomas in vivo. Lancet. 1986;1:765–7.
62. Sozzi G, Miozzo M, Tagliabue E, *et al.* Cytogenetic abnormalities and overexpression of receptors for growth factors in normal bronchial epithelium and tumor samples of lung cancer patients. Cancer Res. 1991;51:400–4.
63. Little CD, Nau MM, Carney DN, Gazdar AF, Minna JD. Amplification and expression of the c-myc oncogene in human lung cancer cell lines. Nature (London). 1983;306:194–6.
64. Grifin C, Baylin S. Expression of the c-myb oncogene in human small cell lung carcinoma. Cancer Res. 1985;45:272–5.
65. Pfeifer AMA, Jones RT, Bowden PE, *et al.* Human bronchial epithelial cells transformed by the c-raf-1 and c-myc protooncogenes induce multidifferentiated carcinomas in nude mice: A model for lung carcinogenesis. Cancer Res. 1991;51:3793–801.
66. Huang M, Ye YC, Chen SR, *et al.* Use of *all-trans* retinoic acid in the treatment of acute promyelocytic leukemia. Blood 1988;72:567–72.
67. Zhang X, Liu Y, Lee M-O, Pfahl M. A specific defect in retinoic acid response associated with human lung cancer cell lines. Cancer Res. 1994;54:5663–9.
68. Caporaso N, Landi MT, Vineis P. Relevance of metabolic polymorphisms to human malignancy. Pharmacogenet. 1991;1:4–19.
69. Guengerich FP, Shimada T. Oxidation of toxic and carcinogenic chemicals by human cytochrome P-450 enzymes. Chem Res Toxicol. 1991;4(4):391–407.
70. Miller EC, Miller JA. Mechanisms of chemical carcinogenesis. Cancer. 1981;47(5):1055–64.
71. Cholerton S, Arpanahi A, McCraken N, *et al.* Poor metabolizers of nicotine and CYP2D6 polymorphism. Lancet. 1994;343:62–3.

72. Trell L, Korsgaard R, Janzon L, Trell E. Distribution and reproducibility of aryl hydrocarbon hydroxylase inducibility in a prospective population study of middle-aged male smokers and non-smokers. Cancer. 1985;56:1988–94.
73. Kellerman G, Luyte-Kellerman M, Shaw CR. Genetic variation of aryl hydrocarbon hydroxylase in human lymphocytes. Am J Hum Genet. 1973;25:327–31.
74. Kellermann G, Shaw CR, Luyten-Kellermann M. Aryl hydrocarbon hydroxylase inducibility and bronchogenic carcinoma. NEJM. 1973;289:934–7.
75. Trell E, Korsgaard R, Hood B, Kitzing P, Norden G, Simonsson BG. Aryl hydrocarbon hydroxylase inducibility and laryngeal carcinomas. Lancet. 1976;2:140.
76. Trell E, Bjorlin G, Andreasson L, Korsgaard R, Mattiasson I. Carcinoma of the oral cavity in relation to aryl hydrocarbon hydroxylase inducibility, smoking, and dental status. Int J Oral Surg. 1981;10:93.
77. Kouri RE, McKinney CE, Slomiany DJ, Snodgrass DR, Wray NP, McLemore TL. Positive correlation between high aryl hydrocarbon hydroxylase activity and primary lung cancer as analyzed in cryopreserved lymphocytes. Cancer Res. 1982;42:5030–7.
78. Gurgis HA, Lynch HT, Mate T, *et al.* Aryl hydrocarbon hydroxylase activity in lymphocytes from lung cancer cases and normal controls. Oncology. 1976;33:105.
79. Paigen B, Gurtoo HL, Minowada J, *et al.* Questionable relation of aryl hydrocarbon hydroxylase to lung-cancer risk. NEJM. 1977;297:346–50.
80. Uematsu F, Kikuchi H, Motomiya M, *et al.* Association between restriction fragment length polymorphism of the human cytochrome P450IIE1 gene and susceptibility to lung cancer. Jpn J Can Res. 1991;82:254–6.
81. Hirvonen A, Husgafvel-Pursiainen K, Anttila S, Karjalainen A, Vainio H. The human CYP2E1 gene and lung cancer: DraI and RsaI restriction fragment length polymorphisms in a Finnish study population. Carcinogenesis. 1993;14(1):85–8.
82. Persson I, Johansson I, Bergling H, *et al.* Genetic polymorphism of cytochrome P4502E1 in a Swedish population. FEBS Lett. 1993;319:207–11.
83. Kato S, Shields PG, Caporaso NE *et al.* Cytochrome P450IIE1 genetic polymorphisms, racial variation, and lung cancer risk. Cancer Res. 1992;52:6712–15.
84. Kotake AN, Schoeller DA, Lambert GH, Baker AL, Schaffer DD, Josephs H. The caffeine CO_2 breath test: Dose response and route of *N*-demethylation in smokers and nonsmokers. Pharmacol Ther. 1982;32(2):261–9.
85. Butler MA, Lang NP, Young JF, *et al.* Determination of CYP1A2 and NAT2 phenotypes in human populations by analysis of caffeine urinary metabolites. Pharmacogenetics. 1992;2(3):116–27.
86. Vincent-Viry M, Pontes ZB, Gueguen R, Galteau M-M, Siest G. Segregation analyses of four urinary caffeine ratios implicated in the determination of human acetylation phenotype. Genet Epidemiol. 1994;11:115–29.
87. Bock KW, Schrenck D, Forester A, Griese E-U, Morike K, Brockmeier D, Eichelbaum M. The influence of environmental and genetic factors of CYP2D6, CYP1A2, and UDP-glucuronosyltransferases in man using sparteine, caffeine, and paracetamol probes. Pharmacogenetics. 1994;4:209–18.
88. Shimada T, Guengerich FP. Evidence for cytochrome P-45ONF, the nifedipine oxidase, being the principal enzyme involved in the bioactivation of aflatoxins in human liver. Proc Natl Acad Sci USA. 1989;86:462–5.
89. Yun C-H, Shimada T, Guengerich FP. Roles of human liver cytochrome P4502C and 3A enzymes in the 3-hydroxylation of benzo (a) pyrene. Cancer Res. 1992;52:1868–74.
90. Crespi CL, Penman BW, Leakey JAE, *et al.* A tobacco-smoke derived nitrosamine, NNK, is activated by multiple human cytochrome P450s including the polymorphic CYP2D6. Carcinogenesis. 1991;12:1197–201.
91. Poppel G, Verhagen H, Veer P, van Bladeren PJ. Markers for cytogenetic damage in smokers: Association with plasma antioxidants and glutathione *S*-transferase μ. Cancer Epidemiol Biomarkers Prev. 1993;2:441–7.
92. Anttila S, Hirvonen A, Vainio H, Husgafvel-Pursiainen K, Hayes JD, Ketterer B. Immunohistochemical localization of glutathione *S*-transferase in human lung. Cancer Res. 1993;53:5643–8.
93. Sugimura H, Caporaso N, Hoover RN, *et al.* Association of rare alleles of the Harvey *ras* proto oncogene locus with lung cancer. Cancer Res. 1990;50:1857–62.

94. Krontiris TG, Devlin B, Karp DD, Robert NJ, Risch N. An association between the risk of cancer and mutations in the Hras1 minisatellite locus. NEJM. 1993;329(8):517–23.
95. Heighway J, Thatcher N, Cerny T, Hasleton PS. Genetic predisposition to human lung cancer. Br J Cancer. 1986;53:453–7.
96. Weston A, Ling-Cawley HM, Caporaso NE, *et al.* Determination of the allelic frequencies of an L-myc and a p53 polymorphism in human lung cancer. Carcinogenesis. 1994;15(4):583–7.
97. Weston A, Perrin LS, Forrester K. *et al.* Allelic frequency of a p53 polymorphism in human lung cancer. Cancer Epidemiol Prev. 1992;1(6):481–4.
98. Tamai S, Sugimura H, Caporaso N, *et al.* Restriction fragment length polymorphism analysis of the L-myc gene locus in a case-control study of lung cancer. Int J Cancer. 1990;46:411–15.
99. Hallier E, Langhof T, Dannappel D, Polymorphism of glutathione conjugation of methyl bromide, ethylene oxide and dichloromethane in human blood: influence on the induction of sister chromatid exchanges (SCE) in lymphocytes. Arch Toxicol. 1993;67:173–8.
100. Pemble S, Schroeder KR, Spencer SR, *et al.* Human glutathione *S*-transferase theta (GSTT1): cDNA cloning and the characterization of a genetic polymorphism. Biochem J. 1994;300:271–6.
101. Lyn D, Cherney BW, Lalande M, *et al.* A duplicated region is responsible for the poly(ADP-ribose) polymerase polymorphism on chromosome 13, associated with a predisposition to cancer. Am J Hum Genet. 1993;52:124–34.
102. Bhatia KG, Cherney BW, Huppi K, *et al.* A deletion linked to a poly(ADP-ribose) polymerase gene on chromosome 13q33-qter occurs frequently in the normal black population as well as in multiple tumor DNA. Cancer Res. 1990;50:5406–13.
103. Caporaso NE, Shields PG, Landi MT, *et al.* The debrisoquine metabolic phenotype and DNA-based assays: implications of misclassification of lung cancer and the debrisoquine metabolic phenotype. Environ Health Perspect. 1992;98:101–5.
104. Saxena R, Shaw GL, Relling MV, *et al.* Identification of a new variant CYP2D6 allele with a single base deletion in exon 3 and its association with the poor metabolizer phenotype. Hum Mol Genet. 1994;3(6):923–6.
105. Johansson I, Lundquist E, Bertilsson L, Dahl M-L, Sjoquist F, Ingelman-Sunberg M. Inherited amplification of an active gene in the cytochrome P450 CYP2D6 locus as a cause of ultrarapid metabolism of debrisoquine. PNAS USA. 1993;90:11825–9.
106. Alexandrie A-K, Sundberg MI, Seidegard J, Tornling G, Rannug A. Genetic susceptibility to lung cancer with special emphasis on CYP1A1 and GSTM1: a study on host factors in relation to age at onset, gender and histological cancer types. Carcinogensis. 1994;15(9):1785–90.
107. Rothman N, Stewart WF, Caporaso NE, Hayes RB. Misclassification of genetic susceptibility biomarkers: Implications for case-control studies and cross-population studies. Cancer Epidemiol Biomarkers Prev. 1993;2:299–303.
108. Lin HJ, Han C-Y, Lin BK, Hardy S. Ethnic distribution of slow acetylator mutations in the polymorphic *N*-acetyltransferase (NATs) gene. Pharmacogenetics. 1994;4:125–34.
109. Philip PA, Fitzgerald DL, Cartwright RA, Peake MD, Rogers HJ. Polymorphic N-acetylation in lung cancer. Carcinogenesis. 1988;9:491–3.
110. Kihara M, Kihara M, Noda K. Lung cancer risk of GSTM1 null genotype is dependent on the extent of tobacco smoke exposure. Carcinogenesis. 1994;15(2):415–18.
111. Vineis P, Bartsch H, Caporaso N, *et al.* Genetically based *N*-acetyltransferase metabolic polymorphism and low-level environmental exposure to carcinogens. Nature (London). 1994;369:154–6.
112. Johnson WR, Hale RW, Clough SC, Chen PH. Chemistry of conversion of nitrate nitrogen to smoke products. Nature (London). 1973;243:223–5.
113. Benowitz NL. The use of biological fluid analysis in assessing tobacco smoke consumption (National Institute on Drug Abuse, Research Monograph No. 48; DHHS Publ. No (ADM) 83–1285). Rockville, MD: DHHS.
114. Boyland E, Nice E, Williams K. The catalysis of nitrosation by thiocyanate from saliva. Food Cosmet Toxicol. 1971;9:639–43.
115. Wynder EL, Hoffmann D. Tobacco and tobacco smoke. Studies in experimental carcinogenesis. New York, NY: Academic Press; 1967.
116. Bodgen JD, Kemp FW, Buse M, *et al.* Composition of tobaccos from countries with high and low incidences of lung cancer. I. Selenium, polonium-210. JNCI. 1981;66:27–31.

117. Hammond EC, Horn D. Smoking and death rates – report on forty-four months of follow-up of 187,783 men. I. Total mortality. JAMA. 1958;166:1159–72.
118. Hammond EC, Horn D. Smoking and death rates – report on forty-four months of follow-up of 187,783. II. Death rates by cause. JAMA 1958;166:1294–308.
119. Hammond EC. Smoking in relation to death rates of one million men and women. NCI Monogr. 1966;19:127–204.
120. Rogut E, Murray JL. Smoking and causes of death among US veterans : 16 years of observation. Publ Health Rep. 1980;95:213–22.
121. Siemiatycki J. Introduction to occupational cancer. In: Siemiatycki J. ed. Risk factors for cancer in the workplace. CRC Press; 1991.
122. Blot WJ, Morris LE, Stroube R, *et al.* Lung and laryngeal cancer in relation to shipyard employment in coastal Virginia. JNCI. 1980;65:571–5.
123. Thomas TL, Stewart PA. Mortality from lung cancer and respiratory disease among pottery workers exposed to silica and talc. Am J Epidemiol. 1987;125:35–43.
124. Ayesh R, Idle JR, Ritchie JC, Crothers MJ, Hetzel MR. Metabolic oxidation phenotypes as markers for susceptibility to lung cancer. Nature (London). 1984;312:169.
125. Caporaso N, Pickle LW, Bale S, Ayesh R, Hetzel M, Idle J. The distribution of debrisoquine metabolic phenotypes and implications for the suggested association with lung cancer risk. Genet Epidemiol. 1989;6:517–24.
126. Roots I, Drakoulis N, Ploch M, *et al.* Debrisoquine hydroxylation phenotype, acetylation phenotype, and ABO blood groups as genetic host factors of lung cancer risk. Klin Wochenschr. 1988;66:87–97.
127. Caporaso NE, Tucker MA, Hoover RN, *et al.* Lung cancer and the debrisoquine metabolic phenotype. JNCI. 1990;82:1264–72.
128. Benitez J, Ladero JM, Jara C, *et al.* Polymorphic oxidation of debrisoquine in lung cancer patients. Eur J Cancer. 1991;27:2,158–61.
129. Wolf RC, Smith CAD, Gough AC, *et al.* Relationship between debrisoquine hydroxylase polymorphism and cancer susceptibility. Carcinogenesis. 1992;13:1035–8.
130. Horsmans Y, Desager JP, Harvengt C. Is there a link between debrisoquine oxidation phenotype and lung cancer susceptibility? Biomed Pharmacother. 1991;45:359–62.
131. Puchetti V, Faccini GB, Micciolo R, Ghimenton F, Bertrand C, Zatti N. Dextromethorphan test for evaluation of congenital predisposition to lung cancer. Chest. 1994;105:449–53.
132. Duche JC, Joanne C, Barre J, *at al.* Lack of relationship between the polymorphism of debrisoquine oxidation and lung cancer. Br J Clin Pharmac. 1991;31:533–6.
133. Tefre T, Daly A, Armstrong M, *et al.* Genotyping of the CYP2D6 gene in Norwegian lung cancer patients and controls. Pharmacogenetics. 1994;4 (2):47–57.
134. Law MR, Hetzel MR, Idle JR. Debrisoquine metabolism and genetic predisposition to lung cancer. Br J Can. 1989;59:686–7.
135. Shaw GL, Falk RT, Tucker MA, *et al.* Debrisoquine metabolism and lung cancer risk. Proc AACR. 1994;35:1753.
136. Hirvonen A, Husgafvel-Pursiainen K, Anttila S, Karjalainen A, Pelkonen O, Vainio H. PCR-based CYP2D6 genotyping for Finnish lung cancer patients. Pharmacogenetics. 1993;3:19–27.
137. Zhong S, Howie AF, Ketterer B, *et al.* Glutathione *S*–transferase mu locus: use of genotyping and phenotyping assays to assess association with lung cancer susceptibility. Carcinogenesis. 1991;12:1533–7.
138. Brockmoller J, Kerb R, Drakoulis N, Nitz M, Roots I. Genotype and phenotype of glutathione *S*-transferase class mu isozyme and x in lung cancer patients and controls. Cancer Res. 1993;53:1004–11.
139. Hayashi S, Watanabe J, Kawajiri K. High susceptibility to lung cancer analyzed in terms of combined genotypes of PA50IA1 and mu-class glutathione *S*-transferase genes. Jpn J Cancer Res. 1992;83:866–70.
140. Nazar-Stewart V, Motulsky AG, Eaton DL, *et al.* The glutathione *S*-transferase μ polymorphism as a marker for susceptibility to lung cancer. Cancer Res. 1993;53:2313–18.
141. Heckbert SR, Wiess NS, Hornung SK, Eaton DL, Motulsky AG. Glutathione *S*-transferase and epoxide hydrolase activity in human leukocytes in relation to risk of lung cancer and other smoking related cancers. JNCI. 1992;84:414–22.
142. Kihara M, Kihara M, Noda K. Lung cancer risk of GSTM1 null genotype is dependent on the extent of tobacco smoke exposure. Carcinogenesis. 1994;15 (2):415–18.

143. Seidegard J, DePierre J, Pero RW. Hereditary interindividual differences in glutathione transferase activity towards trans-stilbene oxide in resting human mononuclear leukocytes are due to a particular isoenzyme(s). Carcinogenesis. 1985;6:1211–16.
144. Nakachi K, Imai K, Hayashi S, Watanabe J, Kawajiri K. Genetic susceptibility to squamous cell carcinoma of the lung in relation to cigarette smoking dose. Cancer Res. 1991;51:5177–80.
145. Hayashi S, Watanabe J, Kawajiri K. High susceptibility to lung cancer in terms of combined genotypes of P450IA1 and mu–class glutathione *S*-transferase gene. Jpn J Cancer Res. 1992;83:866–70.
146. Adler I. Primary malignant growths of the lung and bronchi. A pathological and clinical study. New York: Longmans, Green and Co.; 1912.
147. Wynder EL, Hoffman D. Smoking and lung cancer: Scientific challenges and opportunities. Cancer Res. 1994;24:5284–95.

3
Colorectal cancer

J.D. Potter, T.A. Sellers and S.S. Rich

DESCRIPTIVE EPIDEMIOLOGY

Colorectal cancer is the third most common cancer worldwide (after breast and cervix in women and lung and stomach in men); it accounts for approximately 9% of all cancers[1]. Incidence varies approximately 20-fold around the world[2,3]. Highest rates are seen largely in the developed world – western Europe, North America, Australasia – with age-adjusted (world standard) incidence rates of 25 to 35 per 100 000 in the late 1980s. It is notable that rates in northern Italy (>30 per 100 000 for males) are now higher than in England and Wales (<20 per 100 000). The formerly low rates in Japan have now risen to a level comparable to those in England and Wales. The lowest rates are seen in India (1–3 per 100 000)[3].

Up to the 1970s, colon cancer was the only cancer that occurred with approximately equal frequency in women and men[4]. In North America and Australia (high rates) and Japan and Italy (rapidly rising rates) in particular, the age-adjusted rates for men now exceed those for women, in some cases by more than 20%. The sex differences are less marked in England and Wales. The male and female rates in New Zealand *pakeha* (non-Maoris; around 30 per 100 000) are equal. There is a tendency for the rates to be similar between the sexes or to show a female excess before the age of 50 years and, consistently, to show a male excess after 50[2–4]. The risk of cancer varies by subsite within the colon[2,3,5]; Correa and Haenszel[5] noted that this variation itself differed between high- (greater predominance of left-sided lesions) and low-risk countries. The subsite risk varies between the sexes and, further, by age; women have higher rates of right-sided neoplasms than men and tend to develop their cancers at an earlier age[4,6].

Rates of colon cancer vary by race and ethnic status[2,3]. High rates are seen in Caucasians of northern European origin – both in their native countries and in the areas to which they have migrated; lower rates are seen in those of southern European background but these tend to rise with migration. Rates in Asia and Africa are lower but rise consistently with migration to higher risk areas and with westernization. Overall, migrant data suggest that the 20-fold international variation in incidence may be largely explained by dietary and environmental differences. The one interesting exception appears to be the Maoris (Polynesians) who show an unexpectedly low incidence rate in New Zealand (11.4 per 100 000 in males and 13.7 per 100 000 in females) despite the apparent similarity of their dietary behaviour with their *pakeha* (of white European origin) compatriots[3,7]. The Hawaiian Hawaiians (also Polynesians) were previously also reported to be at lower risk, similar to that seen in New Zealand. By the late 1980s, these low rates were seen only in women (13.7 per 100 000) with the male Hawaiians showing a rate more than twice that (28.0 per 100 000)[3]. This is the largest sex difference ever reported for colon cancer in any group. While there are male–female differences in gut function and metabolism (see below), if this is an accurate description of the situation (i.e. not an artifact of reporting), the rapidity with which the increase has occurred suggests that there has been a major change in male compared with female behaviour in this population; this may prove extremely important in understanding gene–environment interactions in the genesis of colon cancer.

More than 90% of cancers of the colon are adenocarcinomas[8]. Very little is known about the aetiology of colonic lymphomas and carcinoids which comprise almost all of the remaining histological types[8]. Similarly, little is known about the relationship of specific histological subtypes of adenocarcinoma to the risk factors, physiological processes, or molecular changes discussed below.

Migrant studies, as suggested above, as well as the above-mentioned rapid changes in Italy, Japan and male Polynesians in Hawaii, have shown that the disease is particularly sensitive to changes in environment. Incidence rates reach those of the host country within one or two generations, even within the migrating generation[9–12]. Additionally, colon cancer has long been known to occur more frequently in families of those with the disease than in those without[13] and there are several rare genetic syndromes that carry an excess risk of colon cancer[14–16]. While the data argue strongly for an environmental explanation for the international variation, in any one population, there appear to be clear differences in susceptibility to the relevant environmental exposures.

PROBABLE CAUSAL ENVIRONMENTAL FACTORS

Ecological findings suggest that diets high in fat, protein and meat, and low in plant foods increase the risk of developing colon cancer[17]. Epidemiological studies in which individual patterns of behaviour are measured, both cohort and case-control, have provided support for these observations; dietary factors have been shown to be important risk factors for colon cancer but the strength of associations varies by sex and age[17].

The finding that vegetable consumption is inversely associated with risk is the most consistent observation. This association with lower risk may be a manifestation of a general phenomenon whereby risks of cancer at almost all epithelial sites are diminished in the presence of a diet high in plant foods and the bioactive phytochemicals that they contain[18,19]. Of the 28 individual-level studies in the literature that have discussed findings for vegetables, 23 found an inverse association[17]. If attention is confined to studies with the best methods, there are 15 that have reported on vegetables[20–33], of which only one[31] failed to find a reduced risk in association with elevated levels of one or more measures of vegetable intake. For colorectal cancer in particular, however, the related conclusion, that foods high in fibre (often a measure of vegetable as well as grain intake) are protective, has been shown in a formal meta-analysis of 13 case-control studies[34] with odds ratios of 1.0, 0.8, 0.7, 0.6, 0.5 from lowest to highest quintile of consumption. Nevertheless, in those populations where cereal consumption is high – southern Europe and Asia, particularly – it is puzzling that the risk is higher in individuals with a higher consumption of rice (Japanese)[35] or of pasta and rice (southern Europe)[23,36].

Meat, protein and fat are consistently, almost universally, positively related to risk[17]. Of the 16 studies that have reported on the association with fat and protein, 13 have shown an increased risk. Sixteen of 27 studies have reported an increase in risk associated with higher meat consumption[17]. When attention is confined to the better-conducted studies, eight[21,22,25,29,31,37–9] out of eleven[21,22,25,28,29,31,32,37–40] studies show a positive association with meat intake. High consumption of fat or meat, i.e. being in the top 20–30% of consumers, vs. the lowest 20–30% is frequently associated with a greater than 2-fold increase in risk of colon cancer[17]. A preference for heavily cooked meat has been shown to be associated with an elevated risk: approaching a 3-fold risk for colon cancer and 6–fold for rectal cancer[41].

Finally, in relation to food and dietary practices, the epidemiological literature can be considered weakly supportive of the hypothesis that relatively high intakes of calcium and vitamin D protect against colon cancer[17,42] perhaps via the mechanism originally proposed by Newmark and colleagues[43].

Physical inactivity, originally shown to be a risk factor by Garabrant and colleagues[44], has emerged as one of the most consistent indicators of an elevated risk for colon cancer; all but one of 17 individual-level studies in the literature have shown a higher risk for the less active[17]. Most studies have focused on job-related activity. Nevertheless, studies examining total activity, leisure time activity, and participation in college athletics also show that risk of colon cancer is reduced among more active individuals of both sexes[17].

Several recent studies have suggested that use of aspirin and a variety of other non-steroidal anti-inflammatory drugs (NSAIDS) reduces risk of colon cancer[45,46].

Stocks[47] first reported in 1957 an elevated, though not statistically significant, risk of colorectal cancer among daily beer drinkers compared with abstainers. Although cross-cultural, ecological comparisons appear to suggest a positive association between alcohol consumption (mostly beer) and colorectal cancers, cautious interpretation of these results is clearly warranted. In studies of alcoholics or brewery workers, the risk of colon cancer was elevated (non-significantly) in three of nine studies. The risk of rectal cancer was elevated in four of seven studies[17]. Of the 14 cohort and case-control studies that have examined alcohol and colon cancer, 7 have reported a positive association; 12 of the 21 alcohol–rectal cancer studies show a positive association. Beer appears to be positively related to colon cancer but perhaps less consistently than to rectal cancer[17].

FAMILIAL PREDISPOSITION

Individuals with a family history of colorectal cancer are at approximately 2-fold increased risk of the disease; in women, a family history of breast, ovarian and endometrial cancer may also be related to an increased risk of colon cancer[48–50]. There appears to be an approximately 2-fold increase in the risk of ovarian cancer if a first-degree relative has had colorectal cancer[51,52] and a more weakly elevated risk of colon cancer if a first-degree relative has had breast cancer[53]. A problem in interpreting clearly the effects of family history on colorectal cancer risk is the difficulty in separating out genetic from environmental effects, since even dietary behaviour remains more uniform among family members than can be explained solely by living in the same culture[54].

There are also several genetic syndromes that carry an excess risk of colon cancer, including familial adenomatous polyposis (FAP) and Gardner syndrome. FAP is characterized by the development, as early as childhood, of multiple colo rectal adenomas, numbering from a few to several thousand and a lifetime risk of adenocarcinoma that approaches 100%[15]. It is inherited in a Mendelian dominant fashion but accounts for less than 1% of all colon cancer. Gardner syndrome is similar but includes both polyposis and soft-tissue manifestations[14].

Another form of colorectal neoplasia that shows familial aggregation is hereditary non-polyposis colorectal cancer (HNPCC)[55]. This disorder is not readily distinguished from 'sporadic' neoplasia on physical examination (there is no tendency to extensive polyposis) but accounts for a larger proportion of all colon cancer cases than FAP. The most clear distinguishing features of the family history are the tendency to early onset and the pattern of other cancers in the family – particularly those of the endometrium, urinary tract, stomach and biliary system[56].

Colorectal cancer is thus a disease for which there exist both genetic predisposition and causal environmental exposures. How these are related is not understood in any detail but, as the following data suggest, there are some promising leads.

SPECIFIC SYNDROMES AND THEIR GENETIC ORIGINS

FAP

As noted above, FAP and Gardner syndrome are inherited as Mendelian dominant disorders[14,15]. The localization of the FAP gene, *APC*, was independently determined by Leppert *et al.*[57] and Bodmer *et al.*[58] in 1987 and mapped to chromosome 5q. Subsequently, it was demonstrated that the same genetic locus is also involved in Gardner syndrome[59]. The relevant gene has now been sequenced and a variety of germ-line mutations in individuals with FAP and Gardner syndrome have been described[60–63].

Mutations/polymorphisms have also been described in the germ-line of individuals with 'sporadic' adenoma and carcinoma although the significance of these remains to be determined[64]. Somatic deletions in the 5q21 region are also well established as early events in sporadic colon cancer[64] (also see below). The

APC gene was the second in this region of 5q to be identified as mutated in colon cancer, and abnormalities of the *APC* gene are now believed to be a crucial and early step in most colonic neoplasia – either as a result of an inherited mutation or as a somatic mutation in colonic epithelial cells. Somatic mutations in this gene have also been described in a number of other cancers[65–66].

In December 1993, two reports appeared[68,69], identifying, for the first time, the possible functions of the APC protein. In both somatic and germ-line abnormalities, the mutation results in a stop codon and thus a truncated or absent protein. Until recently, nothing was known about the function of the protein and gene homology had not been established. Although much remains to be clarified, these papers show that the protein product of *APC* associates in the cell with proteins called catenins. It has been demonstrated that the APC protein contains a series of three imperfect 15-amino-acid repeats between amino acids 1014 and 1210, and that any one of these repeats is sufficient to bind catenins[68]. The catenins are known to interact in a different manner with E-cadherin, one of a family of cell-adhesion molecules, although no 3-way complexes have been identified. This, nonetheless, provides evidence that *APC* is involved in some manner with cell adhesion – of importance perhaps both early in carcinogenesis (via disruption of cell communication or impairment of sloughing of cells at the luminal surface) and late (via changes in metastatic potential). Intriguingly, β-catenin (with which the APC protein interacts) has been shown to have 70% homology with a gene – *armadillo* – known to be involved in the development of the fruit fly[70–72]. The relationship between catenins/*armadillo* and *APC* adds to the growing evidence for the interconnection between important developmental genes and the biology of carcinogenesis.

HNPCC

Hereditary non-polyposis colon cancer was first noted to be a familial disorder by Warthin in 1913 and was subsequently studied in great detail by Lynch *et al.*[55,56] who suggested that there were two forms of the disease – one involving colorectal cancer only, and the other, as noted above, including a wider group of tumours, such as those of the endometrium, urinary tract and stomach. More recent thinking has inclined to the view that these are not distinct syndromes, and the molecular genetics appears to confirm that they have common origins in inherited mutations of a class of genes.

A linkage analysis involving two large HNPCC kindreds was recently reported by a group led jointly by de la Chappelle and Vogelstein[73,74]. They found strong linkage to anonymous microsatellite markers (D2S123, D2S119) on chromosome 2p16-15[73] and postulated a mechanism different from that associated with the inherited abnormality of tumour suppressor genes – perhaps involving a predisposition to genetic instability and manifest as widespread alterations in short repeated DNA sequences[74,75]. In an additional 14 smaller kindreds, linkage could be excluded in three, and the remaining 11 displayed both positive and negative Lod scores, suggesting genetic heterogeneity.

Three papers[76–78] were subsequently published on the identity and function of the gene on 2p. At that stage, this gene had been tentatively identified as the cause of the genomic instability seen in some but not all[73] of the cancers in these patients. Other workers[75,79] had traced the genomic instability to other genes associated with colon cancer. The 2p gene has now been cloned and sequenced[76,77]. It *(hMSH2)* is a homologue of the *mutS* gene found in yeast and is a member of the family of genes that code for mismatch repair enzymes. *mutS* has been shown to cause genomic instability in yeast[80]. Four other members of this family of genes have been identified in the human genome, largely on the basis of their homology to known mismatch repair enzymes in yeast. One of these *(hMLH1)* has been localized to 3p23-21 and linked to other families with HNPCC[81,82]. Again, none of the colon tumours showed loss of heterozygosity (LOH) for any markers on 3p; however, increases in band sizes were detected, suggesting a mechanism similar to that associated with the gene on 2p. This effect was traced to an inherited heterozygous deletion and the finding has recently been replicated[83]. *hMSH3* is located on chromosome 5 (de la Chappelle, personal communication). The other two genes (*PMS1* and *PMS2*) appear to be strong candidates as susceptibility genes for colon cancer but have not, to date, been linked to HNPCC families[82]. At least one abnormality of *hMSH2* – the 6-bp splice-site polymorphism – does not appear to occur more commonly in those with sporadic colon cancer than those without cancer (Bishop, personal communication; Potter *et al.*, unpublished observations).

Another rare probably Mendelian dominant syndrome with a pattern of internal malignancy (frequently colorectal cancer) and at least one sebaceous tumour is Muir–Torre syndrome. This has now been shown to be associated with a similar pattern of microsatellite instability[84] and to be linked to the same region of 2p as some of the HNPCC families[85].

OTHER PREDISPOSING FACTORS

Acetylator Status

Sugimura and Sato[86] originally proposed that specific heterocyclic amines, which are potent mutagens and present in cooked protein, were important in the aetiology of colon cancer. Several classes of these compounds have been identified[87] and have been shown to be carcinogenic in animals[88]. Relevant human evidence has accumulated from a number of sources. Firstly, the observations on the role of meat, fat and protein, noted above, are consistent with there being a more specific causal exposure that is strongly associated with these dietary factors. Secondly, there is a 3–6-fold elevated risk associated with a preference for heavily cooked meat[41]. Thirdly, the capacity to metabolize arylamines (and therefore the extent to which colonic DNA may be exposed) is under the control of a polymorphic enzyme – NAT2. As described by Turesky and colleagues[89], the mechanism appears to be as follows: heterocyclic arylamines readily undergo hepatic *N*-oxidation (itself a function of the activity of $P450_{1A2}$ – which is phenotypically polymorphic) and subsequently *N*-glucuronidation. The resulting conjugated *N*-hydroxy metabolites are transported to the colonic lumen, deconjugated (by bacterial β-glucuronidases) and reabsorbed. In the mucosa, the *N*-hydroxy derivatives are good substrates for *O*-acetylation (via

NAT2), producing *N*-acetoxy arylamines which are potent DNA-adduct formers. Kadlubar and colleagues[90] have recently shown that both acetylator status (NAT2) *and* *N*-oxidation status ($P450_{1A2}$) predict risk and that fast acetylators who are also fast *N*-oxidizers are at nearly three times the risk of those who are slow acetylators/slow *N*-oxidizers.

SOMATIC GENETICS

Vogelstein and colleagues[91–95] have provided extensive evidence that there are accumulating (but not linear) somatic genetic changes that accompany (and perhaps cause) the transition from normal colonic mucosa to carcinoma. A crucial early observation that Vogelstein's group made was that there were a very large number of changes in the genetic complement of colon cancer cells[92]. Beginning with this finding, these workers chose a number of the most common changes – those involving one known oncogene, K*ras* – and loss of heterozygosity on 5q (already known by then to be the site of the APC gene) and on chromosomes 18q and 17q (the latter was recognized early as plausibly the p53 tumour suppressor gene)[91]. One of the problems that this entirely sensible approach has produced is that those genes that were chosen for further study from the whole allelotype[92] (a neologism coined by Vogelstein to capture the partially consistent multiplicity of genetic changes observed) have largely become accepted as the whole story of somatic genetic change in colon cancer rather than a crucial part. It is not yet clear what the earliest changes are, but aberrant crypt foci (see below) show mutations of *ras* at a rate not much different from that found in adenomatous polyps and cancer[96]. Nonetheless, approximately 50% of tumours show no abnormality of *ras* at all, arguing strongly that there are at least two separate pathways to colon neoplasia or, at least, that there is an alternative step to the mutation of K*ras*.

If the carcinogenic sequence is regarded as beginning with small polyps, the earliest described change, at present, is an abnormality of the APC gene on chromosome 5q21[64]. As with individuals who have inherited abnormalities of the gene (see above), almost all somatic mutations in this gene appear to produce stop codons and therefore to result in an absent or truncated protein product. As already noted, this protein appears to be involved in cell–cell communication and cell adhesion via interactions with catenins and, indirectly, cadherins[68,69]. The way in which the mutations and loss of protein contribute to carcinogenesis remains unclear, but as many as 80% (perhaps even 100%) of early lesions show abnormalities of this gene, underlining its crucial role early in the process[64].

One of the first DNA changes to be described in colonic neoplastic lesions was the extensive loss of methyl groups[97]. This observation is important for a number of reasons. Firstly, it suggests a pathway via which exogenous agents may influence the carcinogenic process without being directly genotoxic (see below for more on this). Secondly, the control of expression of many genes is via the integrity of methylation patterns[98]; loss of methylation provides a mechanism for the expression of inappropriate genes in the colon cell and for suppression of appropriate ones (if what becomes expressed is a negative regulator). This plausibly leads to changes in replication via alteration of growth regulatory pathways or other important aspects of cell function or regulation. A hypothesis has also been advanced suggesting that loss of methyl groups makes DNA more sticky, thereby increasing the likelihood of breaks, sister chromatid exchanges, etc. Finally, DNA methylation is itself under complex genetic control, raising some questions regarding the role of mutation and expression of these genes in colon neoplasia[99].

ras genes were first identified as the transforming genes of known sarcoma viruses[100]. The early observations of widespread mutations of several of the *ras* proto-oncogenes in tumours at a large number of sites confirmed the important role of these genes in growth control and tumorigenesis[101–103]. The finding that the lesions in colon neoplasia were not random but involved a very limited number of quite specific changes (see below) suggested very strongly that such changes are an intimate and crucial part of the process of carcinogenesis and not simply epiphenomena or by-products of the process[104,105]. (This specificity is true of *ras* mutations in other cancers but the patterns of mutations and the *ras* proto-oncogenes involved differ from tumour to tumour[106–109].) Ras is a 21-kDa protein and a member of a widespread family of proteins involved in growth regulation in normal and neoplastic tissue[110,111]. The members of this family are GTPases and are central to the monitoring and control of a large segment of the information flow in eukaryotic cells, involving not only growth and differentiation but also control of the cytoskeleton and traffic between membrane-bound cellular compartments. They function as binary switches bound alternately to GDP (the inactive state) and GTP (the active state). This process is, in turn, controlled by three classes of protein that catalyse the on-switch (the GDP to GTP step), the off-switch, or protect Ras from switching[111]. The major result of the mutations seen in colon tumours is a change in the tertiary structure of the protein so that it becomes permanently locked into the active configuration. Accordingly, there is no regulation of all the downstream events, one major consequence of which is a loss of control of growth and differentiation[110,111]. The *ras* mutations seen in colon neoplasia almost always involve condons 12, 13 and 61 of K*ras* located on chromosome 12[104,105]. The mutations frequently involve transversions and transitions (about 60%)[112] and, as noted above, are found in about half of all colonic neoplastic lesions from the smallest polyps to metastatic tumours. It is unclear what differentiates those polypoid tumours that do and do not show *ras* mutations; there is one identified group of tumours, however, that do not appear to show *ras* mutations at all – the flat adenomas[113]. Much more on the cause and role of *ras* mutations in cancers arising in adenomatous polyps, and of the process of tumorigenesis in lesions without *ras* mutations, remains to be clarified. The ability to detect mutated *ras* in faeces raises the possibility of detecting colonic neoplasia in its early stages but the 50% of tumours that have a normal *ras* would remain undetected – an unacceptably high false negative rate. However, combining this test with other (yet-to-be-developed) molecular screening techniques may ultimately yield a screening battery with useful sensitivity and specificity.

One of the genes involved later (apparently) in the progression of neoplasia is DCC (deleted in colon cancer)[94]. This is the gene on 18q. The initial LOH seen in neoplastic lesions identified it as a tumour suppressor gene. This plausibly codes for a cell-adhesion molecule – a member of the IgG superfamily[94]. As with a number of the other genes singled out for further study by Vogelstein and colleagues, DCC has been shown to be involved in a number of other gastrointestinal carcinomas[114,115]. Why cell-adhesion molecules function as tumour suppressors remains to be established. Nonetheless, it is clear that this is a crucial issue in colon neoplasia as at least two of the molecular changes, one early (APC) and one later (DCC), involve cell adhesion.

The last of the initial Vogelstein genes is p53, found on chromosome 17p. Originally thought to be an oncogene (because of the dominant negative role of mutated forms), p53 became established as the second (after Rb) clear example of a tumour suppressor gene[116]. This gene is known to be important, when lost via somatic mutation, in the progression of almost all human cancers[117]. p53 is a DNA-binding protein with transcriptional activational activity[118] and plays an important role in the cellular response to DNA damage[119]. It is thought that one of its most important functions is as a negative regulator of the cell cycle[120]. Further, it is now known also to be the gene involved, as a germ-line mutation, in a significant proportion (though not all) of the families with inherited predisposition to the Li-Fraumeni syndrome[121]. It is interesting to note, and remains unexplained, that colon cancer is not part of this syndrome.

ASSOCIATIONS WITH HISTOPATHOLOGY

The earliest pathological model of colorectal carcinogenesis proposed that the disease progressed from small adenomatous polyps through larger ones to cancer and thence to metastasis[122]. An important observation of Fearon and Vogelstein[95] was the correlation between the somatic molecular changes and the degree of dysplasia/neoplasia seen at histological examination. Figure 3.1 is

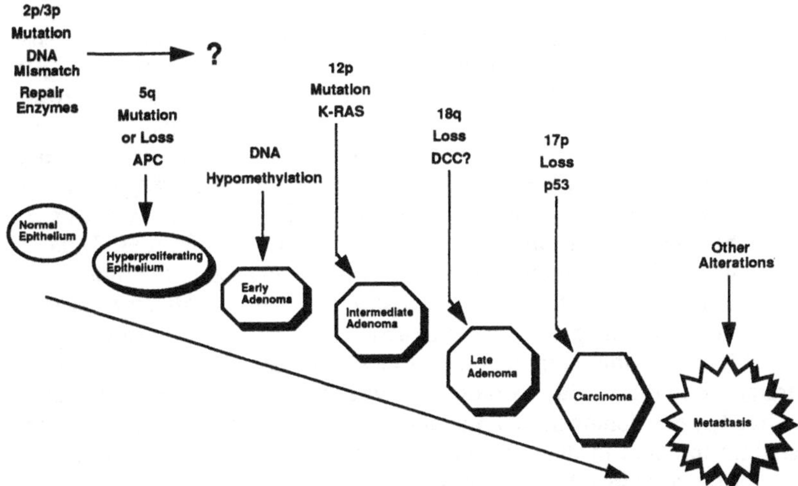

Figure 3.1 Germ-line and somatic genetic changes in the development of colorectal cancer. (After Fearon and Vogelstein. Cell. 1990;61:763[95])

modified and updated from that originally presented by those workers. It is worth emphasizing again that the associations between the DNA/gene changes and the histopathology are probabilistic and correlational, not deterministic; further, these changes are cumulative not linear. Indeed, an alternative hypothesis to the creeping (and unintended) dogma of a one-to-one correspondence between specific allelic losses and mutations on the one hand and histopathology on the other might be more tenable – namely that, as somatic changes accumulate, the genome becomes more disordered within the cell, and this results in increasingly greater degrees of disorder in cell behaviour and tissue architecture.

Interesting findings that tie the molecular events to perhaps even earlier stages of the observable cellular/tissue progression are those involving the aberrant crypt focus (ACF)[123–126]. ACFs possibly represent an earlier microscopic change seen in both mouse and man, and are 200 times more common in the mucosa of individuals with familial polyposis than in normal mucosa[127]. These lesions are inducible in mice by known colon carcinogens, are promotable by cooked protein and sugar, and give rise to polyps[124,128–131]. ACFs show some molecular changes, particularly mutations in *ras*, that are compatible with these tissue abnormalities being a very early stage of the process of carcinogenesis[96].

As with most known patterns of progression, it appears probable that additional mutational events arise within an existing focus of abnormal cells. Consistent with this is the observation that ACFs are more common than small polyps, and that these, in turn, are more common than large polyps.

ANIMAL MODEL – THE MIN MOUSE

Most models of colon carcinogenesis have relied on systemic or local delivery of one of a few carcinogens to rodents. These models have been used largely to examine the role of diet and bile acids in carcinogenesis. Recently, as a result of transplacental carcinogenesis experiments with ethylnitrosourea, a mouse with a previously unknown phenotype was observed; this dominantly transmitted phenotype includes shortened lifespan and severe intestinal bleeding as a result of multiple intestinal neoplasia (MIN)[132]. Although the histology is not an exact replica of human familial polyposis, there are marked similarities. It has now been established that this mouse has a stop codon mutation in the mouse homologue of the *APC* gene[132]. It is expected that further study on dietary, other environmental, and possible gene–gene interactions in the MIN mouse will provide considerable insight into both the process of carcinogenesis and possible preventive strategies, in those with sporadic as well as familial, even FAP, tumours[133]. It has already been demonstrated that genetic background influences the number of intestinal tumours in the MIN heterozygote. When a postulated modifying gene, *MOMI*, was mapped[134], it was shown that this modifier appeared to control nearly 50% of the genetic variation in tumour numbers in some strains. *MOMI* is found in a region of synteny with human 11p36-35, a site of frequent LOH in colon tumours.

PROBABLE LINKS BETWEEN ENVIRONMENTAL FACTORS, GENETIC PREDISPOSITION AND THE PROGRESSION OF THE DISEASE

A number of explanations for the way in which dietary and other factors influence the development of colorectal cancer have been proposed. While these hypotheses often account for some of the major influences on the risk of large bowel carcinogenesis, there is, as yet, no complete and coherent explanation for all of the known epidemiology, pathophysiology and molecular biology.

The earliest proposed pathophysiological mechanism to account for the increased risk associated with fat and meat – the bile acid hypothesis[135] – has been modified more recently by an increased understanding of colonic fermentation, volatile fatty acid production, and a variety of resultant anticarcinogenic effects[136,137]. This can reasonably be called the bile acid/volatile fatty acid hypothesis. In its simplest form, what is proposed is that a high dietary fat intake provokes greater hepatic production of bile acids; these, on reaching the large bowel, are converted to their secondary forms by intestinal bacteria; secondary bile acids are tumour promoters. Volatile fatty acids, on the contrary, are produced by the colonic fermentation of plant fibres, and tend (particularly butyrate) to be antipromotional. They may be a preferential fuel for healthy colonic mucosa. A further physiological hypothesis invokes the effect of cooking and heating on food, resulting in both potential carcinogens, such as heterocyclic arylamines[86,87], and promoters such as hydroxymethylfuraldehyde[128].

What is important about these physiological hypotheses is that they are neither mutually exclusive nor incompatible with (though they provide different interpretations of) the epidemiological data described above. Specifically, fat increases bile acid production, ultimately increasing the exposure of the bowel mucosa to the toxic, trophic and promoting effects of (particularly secondary) bile acids. Fibre binds bile acids, reduces transit time, increases stool bulk, and ferments to volatile fatty acids which may be directly anticarcinogenic and which, by lowering pH, may reduce the conversion of primary to secondary bile acids. A role for calcium as a saponifying agent, that therefore reduces the exposure of the colonic mucosa to bile acids, has also been proposed[43]. Alcohol may have an effect like that of fat on the hepatic production of bile acids. The original eating-frequency hypothesis[138] (greater number of meals is associated with increased risk) was proposed on the basis that a higher frequency of eating is associated with a greater degree of bile-acid recirculation and therefore a higher proportion of secondary bile acids. Thus the fat/fibre etc. hypothesis and the bile acid/volatile fatty acid hypothesis appear to represent a simple mapping of epidemiological on physiological models.

There is a further effect of plant foods at the physiological and biochemical level that is not, apparently, immediately involved in the fat-and-fibre story. Vegetables contain a large number of substances – both micronutrients, such as ascorbate and carotenoids, and 'non-nutrients' such as flavonoids, isothiocyanates, phenols and indoles – with potent anticarcinogenic properties[19,139,140]. The biochemical/molecular steps from cell exposure to a procarcinogen to cell replication in an abnormal manner can be considered as follows: procarcinogen is activated to ultimate carcinogen (either form may be solubilized and excreted); carcinogen passes through cell and nuclear membranes; carcinogen interacts with DNA; DNA synthesis and replication (or DNA repair) occur; cell replication with abnormal DNA and abnormal protein synthesis (or cell differentiation) result. One or more known phytochemicals, at almost every one of these steps, can alter the likelihood of carcinogenesis, usually in a favorable direction but sometimes in a way that increases the risk of cancer. For example, there are a number of substances – glucosinolates and indoles, isothiocyanates and thiocyanates, phenols, and coumarins – that induce a variety of solubilizing and (usually) inactivating enzymes; ascorbate and phenolic compounds block the formation of carcinogens, such as nitrosamines; carotenoids and flavonoids act as antioxidants; lipid-soluble compounds, such as sterols and carotenoids, could alter membrane structures; some of the sulphur-containing compounds can suppress DNA and protein synthesis; and carotenoids suppress DNA synthesis and enhance differentiation[19,139,140]. Is there a plant anticarcinogen that enhances DNA repair?

One of the concomitants (possibly casual precursors) of carcinogenesis is a higher rate of cell replication. Calcium has ameliorated the proliferative changes in rodents[141–143] and in some[144,145], but not all[146], controlled trials in humans. Possible mechanisms include not only, as note above, the binding of bile acids and fatty acids to form inert soaps[43] but also direct effects on the cell cycle, reducing proliferation and inducing terminal differentiation of epithelial cells[147–149]. To date, clear evidence for these mechanisms from human studies is scarce.

Several mechanisms by which physical activity could reduce risk have been proposed. The most widely held hypothesis is that physical activity stimulates colonic peristalsis, thereby decreasing the time that the mucosa is exposed to the colonic contents; however, transit time is not a well-established risk factor for colon neoplasia. Activity also modifies immune responses; acute exercise has favourable effects upon T and B cells and produces an increase in the number and activity of NK cells[150–152] and interleukin-1 levels[153,154]: it may thus produce less favourable conditions for tumour growth. Exercise has been shown to have endocrine effects, both acute and chronic: oestradiol, progesterone, prolactin, LH and FSH are reported to increase during and after exercise[155–157].

Indeed, aspects of endocrine function may be more generally important in colonic carcinogenesis. As noted above, subsite and age differences in colon cancer risk vary between the sexes: there is a female excess of right-sided colon cancers at all ages, and a male excess of left-sided cancers[6,158]. Further, there are physiological correlates for these observations: males and females show differences, under controlled experimental conditions, in transit time, stool bulk, volatile fatty acid production, and bile acid metabolism, that are largely consistent with epidemiological observations[158–160]. These data provide support for metabolic differences between men and women that may be mediated ultimately by hormones but also are consistent with differences in colonic bacterial populations, fermentation rates and general colonic milieu. Gut neuropeptides are important in bile acid secretion and motility and there is a small amount of evidence, in animals, that sex hormones can influence these ubiquitous mediators. Production of galanin mRNA fluctuates with the oestrus cycle in rats[161], and diet can affect the expression of some of the peptide hormone genes[162].

There is *prima facie* evidence, then, that our current models of colon carcinogenesis are relatively consistent at epidemiological and physiological levels. However, the influences of dietary factors, of cooking food, of reproduction and hormones, of alcohol, and of exercise each seem to work through multiple and different but, in some cases, overlapping pathways to carcinogenesis. One way to encapsulate this is to suggest that the variety of exposures, the host responses, and physiological states primarily determine what the colon epithelial cell sees. That is, these factors determine, modify and condition the 'growth media'[163], both luminal and plasma, in which the colonic cells are bathed. Thus, each of the risk factors operates through a variety of pathways that can be thought of as physiological cascades[163–165]. For example, vegetables increase the capacity of the large bowel contents to bind bile acids to increase bacterial mass and volatile fatty acid production. These conditions, in turn, produce effects on cell turnover and maturation and inhibit production of secondary bile acids by reducing intraluminal pH. Meanwhile, the water-holding capacity of fibre and the higher bacterial mass increase stool bulk, increase the work-load of gut musculature, and reduce transit time. Plant-derived anticarcinogens and carcinogens (respectively decreasing and increasing the likelihood of carcinogenesis) add further complexity to the growth medium.

Ingested meat and fat, on the other hand, are respectively a source of carcinogens and a stimulus to hepatic bile acid production. Other factors, including bacterial species and pattern of bacterial enzyme production, as well as transit time, will alter the production rate and concentration of secondary bile acids, thereby modifying the degree of cell damage and repair and influencing gut surface area. The increase in cellular damage may increase cell proliferation rates.

The tissue side of the colonic cells is exposed to plasma-borne carcinogens and anticarcinogens; further, there is the likelihood that specific relationships – both accelerating and controlling growth – exist between fibroblasts and epithelial cells, particularly those mediated by endogenous growth factors[166,167]. The recently described inverse association with NSAIDs plausibly operates via this mechanism. Whether growth factor paracrine/autocrine loops are also related to some other risk factors (e.g. alcohol and exercise) seems to be a reasonable and testable question[168].

Risk of colon cancer, in this model, might be regarded as the summation, over long periods of time, of the moment-to-moment consequences of such physiological cascades and molecular loops.

For the purpose of understanding the relationship between the epidemiological and molecular data, it is important to note that there are several exciting lines of inquiry that, currently, do more than hint at relationships with the molecular findings; nonetheless, they do give insights into the sorts of questions it is increasingly possible to answer.

DNA hypomethylation is an early step in colon carcinogenesis[97]. Of particular interest is the question of whether DNA methylation is influenced by environmental or dietary factors. Chronic deficiency of both methionine and choline results in alterations of DNA methylation and produces tumours in rodents[98]. More importantly for the human situation, deficiency of folate (major dietary sources include green vegetables) may have similar effects[69]. Animal studies have shown that isothiocyanates, found in large amounts in cruciferous vegetables, inhibit both carcinogenesis and DNA methylation[19,139,140]. Willett's group has recently shown that low folate, low methionine and high alcohol (itself often associated with low folate) are all correlated with increased risk of colonic adenomatous polyps, suggesting strongly that the abnormalities of methylation seen in early colon neoplasia are plausibly directly related to dietary factors[170]. The animal data from studies of isothiocyanates and the human observations may appear potentially contradictory but both hypo- and hypermethylation of DNA are hallmarks of the early stages of the carcinogenesis. These data may point to mechanisms by which substances without the capacity to mutate DNA are nonetheless involved in the expression or development of the malignant phenotype.

Further, there is evidence of dietary influences on other processes at the molecular level: one of the most interesting is the hypothesis that fat is important in colon carcinogenesis because it is a source of diacylglycerol, normally an intracellular messenger leading to protein kinase C activation, protein phosphorylation and cell turnover. Weinstein and colleagues[171,172] have proposed that the interaction of fat, bile acids and bacteria produces excess *intraluminal* diacylglycerol which will mimic and amplify such cell-replication signals.

It is also possible that dietary constituents could influence both early and later stages of the carcinogenic process via effects on gene expression. For instance, the level of dietary fat has been shown, in experimental animals, to alter both the production of eicosanoids[173,174] (which, in turn, can influence DNA synthesis and tumour promotion) and the induction of genes coding for Phase I and II metabolizing enzymes[175,176]. In one experiment, however, dietary fat did not influence the expression of *myc* or H*ras* in normal or neoplastic colonic tissue[177]. Further, fasting and refeeding are followed by structural changes in chromatin at the site of genes involved in metabolic regulation and the degree and kinds of changes are dependent on the amount of fat and protein in the diet[178]; this, via endocrine and paracrine mechanisms, could have a major effect on cell replication rates.

Dietary variables with the capacity for direct DNA-damaging effects include arylamines described above. It is worth noting that the transversion and transition mutations seen with high frequency in K*ras* are plausibly related to the interaction between arylamines and DNA[179]. To take one additional step (but one for which there are, as yet, no data), it seems plausible that the lesions resulting from interaction of arylamines and other carcinogens with genomic DNA are more poorly repaired, or less frequently repaired, in individuals with abnormalities of DNA repair. This could provide a link between carcinogenic dietary exposures and the germ-line abnormalities in DNA mismatch repair enzymes seen in HNPCC.

The suggestion that there is some coherence among the epidemiology, the physiology and the molecular biology is exciting. Perhaps more importantly, this kind of integration across aetiological models suggests ideas that may be generalized to the aetiology of other diseases. Finally, on a philosophical note, it is worth bearing in mind that seeking coherence across aetiological hypotheses is not a reductionist pursuit; rather, it is powered by a belief that there are different levels of explanation of carcinogenesis that cast light each upon the others, and that overall understanding will be incomplete without such integration.

References

1. Parkin DM, Läärä E, Muir CS. Estimates of the worldwide frequency of sixteen major cancers in 1980. Int J Cancer. 1988;41:184–97.
2. Muir C, Waterhouse J, Mack T *et al.* Cancer incidence in five continents. Vol 5, IARC Sci Publ 88. Lyon: International Agency for Research on Cancer; 1987.
3. Parkin DM, Muir CS, Whelan SL *et al.* Cancer incidence in five continents. Vol 6, IARC Sci Publ 120. Lyon: International Agency for Research on Cancer; 1992.
4. McMichael AJ, Potter JD. Reproduction, endogenous and exogenous sex hormones, and colon cancer: A review and hypothesis. J Natl Cancer Inst. 1980;65:1201–7.
5. Correa P, Haenszel W. The epidemiology of large bowel cancer. Adv Canc Res. 1978;26:2–141.
6. McMichael AJ, Potter JD. Host factors in carcinogenesis. Certain bile-acid profiles that selectively increase the risk of proximal colon cancer. J Natl Cancer Inst. 1985;75:185–91.
7. Smith AH, Pearce NE, Joseph JG. Major colorectal cancer aetiological hypotheses do not explain mortality trends among Maori and non-Maori New Zealanders. Int J Epidemiol. 1985;14:79–85.
8. Schottenfeld D, Winawer SJ. Large intestine. In: Schottenfeld D, Fraumeni JF, eds. Cancer epidemiology and prevention. Philadelphia: WB Saunders Co; 1982:703–27.
9. Haenszel W. Cancer mortality among the foreign born in the United States. J Natl Cancer Inst. 1961;26:37–132.
10. Wynder EL, Shigematsu T. Environmental factors of cancer of the colon and rectum. Cancer. 1967;20:1520–61.
11. McMichael AJ, McCall MG, Hartshorne JM, Woodings TL. Patterns of gastrointestinal cancer in European migrants to Australia: the role of dietary change. Int J Cancer. 1980;25:431–7.
12. McMichael AJ, Giles GG. Cancer in migrants to Australia: extending the descriptive epidemiological data. Cancer Res. 1988;48:751–6.
13. Macklin MT. Inheritance of cancer of the stomach and large intestine in man. J Natl Cancer Inst. 1969;24:551–71.
14. Gardner EJ. A genetic and clinical study of intestinal polyposis, a predisposing factor for carcinoma of the colon and rectum. Am J Human Genet. 1951;3:167–76.
15. Veale AMO. Intestinal polyposis. Cambridge: Cambridge University Press; 1965.
16. Utsunomiya J, Lynch HT. Hereditary colorectal cancer. New York: Springer-Verlag; 1990.
17. Potter JD, Slattery ML, Bostick RM, Gapstur SM. Colon cancer: a review of the epidemiology. Epidemiol Rev. 1993;15:499–545.
18. Steinmetz K, Potter J. Vegetables, fruit, and cancer. I. Epidemiology. Cancer Cause Cont. 1991;2:325–57.
19. Steinmetz K, Potter J. Vegetables, fruit, and cancer. II. Mechanisms. Cancer Cause Cont. 1991;2:427–42.
20. Haenszel W, Locke FB, Segi M. A case-control study of large bowel cancer in Japan. J Natl Cancer Inst. 1980;64:17–22.
21. Miller AB, Howe GR, Jain M, *et al.*. Food items and food groups as risk factors in a case-control study of diet and colorectal cancer. Int J Cancer. 1983;32:155–61.
22. Manousos O, Day NE, Trichopoulos D, *et al.* Diet and colorectal cancer: A case-control study in Greece. Int J Cancer. 1983;32:1–5.
23. Macquart-Moulin G, Riboli E, Cornée J, *et al.* Case-control study on colorectal cancer and diet in Marseilles. Int J Cancer. 1986;38:183–91.
24. Steinmetz KA, Potter JD. Food group consumption and colon cancer in the Adelaide Case-control Study. I. Vegetables and fruit. Int J Cancer. 1993;53:711–19.
25. Kune S, Kune GM, Watson F. Case-control study of dietary etiologic factors: The Melbourne Colorectal Cancer Study. Nutr Cancer. 1987;9:21–42.
26. Tuyns AJ, Kaaks R, Haelterman M. Colorectal cancer and the consumption of foods: a case-control study in Belgium. Nutr Cancer. 1988;11:189–204.
27. Graham S, Marshall J, Haughey B *et al.* Dietary epidemiology of cancer of the colon in western New York. Am J Epidemiol. 1988;128:490–503.
28. West DW, Slattery ML, Robison LM *et al.* Dietary intake and colon cancer: Sex and anatomic site-specific associations. Am J Epidemiol. 1989;130:883–94.

29. Lee HP, Gourley L, Duffy SW *et al.* Colorectal cancer and diet in an Asian population – a case control study among Singapore Chinese. Int J Cancer. 1989;43:1007–16.
30. Benito E, Stiggelbout A, Bosch FX *et al.* Nutritional factors in colorectal cancer risk: A case-control study in Majorca. Int J Cancer. 1991;49:161–7.
31. Peters RK, Pike MC, Garabrant D, Mack TM. Diet and colon cancer in Los Angeles County, California. Cancer Cause Cont. 1992;3:457–73.
32. Zaridze D, Filipchenko V, Kustov V *et al.* Diet and colorectal cancer: results of two case-control studies in Russia. Eur J Cancer. 1993;29A:112–15.
33. Steinmetz KA, Kushi LH, Bostick RM, Folsom AR, Potter JD. Vegetables, fruit and colon cancer in the Iowa Women's Health Study. Am J Epidemiol. 1994;139:1–15.
34. Howe GR, Benito E, Castellato, R *et al.* Dietary intake of fiber and decreased risk of cancers of the colon and rectum: evidence from the combined analysis of 13 case-control studies. J Natl Cancer Inst. 1992;84:1887–96.
35. Tajima K, Tominga S. Dietary habits and gastro-intestinal cancers: A comparative case-control study of stomach and large intestinal cancers in Nagoya, Japan. Jpn J Cancer Res. 1985;76:705–16.
36. LaVecchia C, Negri E, Decarli A *et al.* A case-control study of diet and colorectal cancer in northern Italy. Int J Cancer. 1988;41:492–8.
37. Steinmetz KA, Potter JD. Food group consumption and colon cancer in the Adelaide Case-control Study. II. Meat, poultry, seafood, dairy foods, and eggs. Int J Cancer. 1993;53:720–7.
38. Benito E, Obrador A, Stiggelbout A *et al.* A population-based case-control study of colorectal cancer in Majorca. I. Dietary factors. Int J Cancer. 1990;45:69–76.
39. Willett WC, Stampfer MJ, Colditz GA *et al.* Relation of meat fat and fiber intake to the risk of colon cancer in a prospective study among women. N Engl J Med. 1990;323:1664–72.
40. Bostick RM, Potter JD, Kushi LH *et al.* Sugar, meat, and fat intake, and non-dietary risk factors for colon cancer incidence in Iowa women (United States). Cancer Cause Cont. 1994;5:38–52.
41. Gerhardsson de Verdier M, Hagman U, Peters RK *et al.* Meat cooking methods and colorectal cancer: a case-referent study in Stockholm. Int J Cancer. 1991;49:520–5.
42. Bostick RM, Potter JD, Sellers TA *et al.* Relation of calcium, vitamin D, and dairy food intake to incidence of colon cancer among older women. Am J Epidemiol. 1993;137:1302–17.
43. Newmark HL, Wargovich MJ, Bruce WR. Colon cancer and dietary fat, phosphate, and calcium: a hypothesis. J Natl Cancer Inst. 1984;72:1323–5.
44. Garabrant DH, Peters JM, Mack TM, Bernstein L. Job activity and colon cancer risk. Am J Epidemiol. 1984;119:1005–14.
45. Thun MJ, Namboodiri MM, Heath CW. Aspirin use and reduced risk of fatal colon cancer. N Engl J Med. 1991;325:1593–6.
46. Rosenberg L, Palmer JR, Zauber AG *et al.* A hypothesis: nonsterodial anti-inflammatory drugs reduce the incidence of large-bowel cancer. J Natl Cancer Inst. 1991;83:355–8.
47. Stocks P. Cancer incidence in North Wales and Liverpool region in relation to habits and environment. 35th Annual Report, Suppl to Part 2. London: British Empire Cancer Campaign; 1957: 1–127.
48. Lovett E. Family studies in cancer of the colon and rectum. Br J Surg. 1976;63:13–18.
49. Bale SJ, Chakravarti A, Strong LC. Aggregation of colon cancer in family data. Genet Epidemiol. 1984;1:53–61.
50. Burt RW, Bishop DT, Cannon LA *et al.* Dominant inheritance of adenomatous colonic polyps and colorectal cancer. N Engl J Med. 1985;312:1540–4.
51. Schildkraut JM, Thompson WD. Relationship of epithelial ovarian cancer to other malignancies within families. Genet Epidemiol. 1988;5:355–67.
52. Cramer DW, Hutchinson GB, Welch WR *et al.* Determinants of ovarian cancer risk. I. Reproductive experiences and family history. J Natl Cancer Inst. 1983;71:711–16.
53. Andrieu N, Calvel F, Auquier A, *et al.* Association between breast cancer and family malignancies. Eur J Cancer. 1991;27:224–8.
54. Sellers TA, Kushi L, Potter JD. Can dietary intake patterns account for the familial aggregation of disease? Evidence from adult siblings living apart. Genet Epidemiol. 1991;8:105–12.
55. Lynch PM, Lynch HT. Colon cancer genetics. New York: Van Nostrand Rheinhold; 1985.
56. Lynch HT, Lynch JF, Cristofaro G. Genetic epidemiology of colon cancer. In: Lynch HT, Hirayama T, eds. Genetic epidemiology of cancer. Boca Raton, FL: CRC Press; 1989:251–77.

57. Leppert M, Dobbs M, Scambler P *et al.* The gene for familial polyposis coli maps to the long arm of chromosome 5. Science. 1987;238:1411–13.
58. Bodmer WF, Bailey CJ, Bodmer J *et al.* Localization of the gene for familial adenomatous polyposis on chromosome 5. Nature (London). 1987;328:614–16.
59. Leppert M, Burt R, Hughes J *et al.* Genetic analysis of an inherited predisposition to colonic cancer in a family with a variable number of adenamatous polyps. N Engl J Med. 1990;32:904–8.
60. Nishisho I, Nakamura Y, Miyoshi Y *et al.* Mutations of chromosome 5q21 genes in FAP and colorectal cancer patients. Science. 1991;253:665–9.
61. Groden J, Thliveris A, Samowitz W *et al.* Identification and characterization of the familial adenomatous polyposis coli gene. Cell. 1991;66:589–600.
62. Kinzler K, Nilbert M, Su L-K *et al.* Identification of FAP locus genes from chromosome 5q21. Science. 1991;253:661–5.
63. Joslyn G, Carlson M, Thliveris A *et al.* Identification of deletion mutations and three new genes at the familial polyposis locus. Cell. 1991;66:601–13.
64. Powell, SM, Nathan Z, Beazer-Barclay Y *et al.* APC mutations occur early during colorectal tumorigenesis. Nature (London). 1992;359:253–7.
65. Tamura G, Maesawa C, Suzuki Y *et al.* Mutations of the *APC* gene occur during early stages of gastric adenoma development. Cancer Res. 1994;54:1149–51.
66. Hosoe S, Ueno K, Shigedo Y *et al.* A frequent deletion of chromosome 5q21 in advanced small cell and non-small cell carcinoma of the lung. Cancer Res. 1994;54:1787–90.
67. Horii A, Nakatsuru S, Miyoshi Y *et al.* Frequent somatic mutations of the *APC* gene in human pancreatic cancer. Cancer Res. 1992;52:6696–8.
68. Su LK, Vogelstein B, Kinzler KW. Association of the APC tumor suppressor protein with catenins. Science. 1993;262:1734–7.
69. Rubinfeld B, Souza B, Albert I *et al.* Association of the apc gene product with β-catenin. Science. 1993;262:1731–4.
70. Peifer M. Cancer, catenins, and cuticle pattern: a complex connection. Science. 1993;262:1667–8.
71. Siegfried E, Wilder E, Perrimon N. Components of *wingless* signalling in *Drosophila.* Nature (London). 1994;367:76–80.
72. Nordemeer J, Klingensmith J, Perrimon N, Nusse R. *dishevelled* and *armidillo* act in the wingless signalling pathway in Drosophila. Nature (London). 1994;367:80–3.
73. Peltomaki P, Aaltonen LA, Sistonen P *et al.* Genetic mapping of a locus predisposing to human colorectal cancer. Science. 1993;260:810–12.
74. Aaltonen LA, Peltomaki P, Leach FS *et al.* Clues to the pathogenesis of familial colorectal cancer. Science. 1993;260:812–16.
75. Thibodeau SN, Bren G, Schaid D. Microsatellite instability in cancer of the proximal colon. Science. 1993;260:816–19.
76. Fishel R, Lescoe MK, Rao MRS *et al.* The human mutator gene homolog *MSH2* and its association with hereditary nonpolyposis colon cancer. Cell. 1993;75:1027–38.
77. Leach FS, Nicolaides NC, Papadopoulos N *et al.* Mutations of a *mutS* homolog in hereditary nonpolyposis colorectal cancer. Cell. 1993;75:1215–26.
78. Parsons, R, Li G-M, Longley MJ *et al.* Hypermutability and mismatch repair deficiency in RER+ tumor cells. Cell. 1993;75:1227–36.
79. Ionov Y, Peinado MA, Malkbosyan S *et al.* Ubiquitous somatic mutations in simple repeated sequences reveal a new mechanism for colonic carcinogenesis. Nature (London). 1993;363:558–61.
80. Strand M, Prolla TA, Liskay PM, Potes T. Destabilization of tracts of simple repetitive DNA in yeast by mutations affecting DNA mismatch repair. Nature (London). 1993;365:274–6.
81. Lindblom A, Tannergard P, Werelius B, Nordenskjold M. Genetic mapping of a second locus predisposing to hereditary non-polyposis colon cancer. Nature Genet. 1993;5:279–82.
82. Papadopoulos N, Nicolaides NC, Wei Y-F *et al.* Mutation of a *mutL* homolog in hereditary colon cancer. Science. 1994;263:1625–9.
83. Bronner CE, Baker SM, Morrison PT *et al.* Mutation in the DNA mismatch repair gene homologue hMLH1 is associated with hereditary non-polyposis colon cancer. Nature (London). 1994;368:258–61.
84. Honchel R, Halling KC, Schaid DJ *et al.* Microsatellite instability in Muir-Torre syndrome. Cancer Res. 1994;54:1159–63.

85. Hall NR, Murday VA, Chapman P *et al.* Genetic linkage in Muir-Torre syndrome to the same chromosomal region as cancer family syndrome. Eur J Cancer. 1994;30A:180–2.
86. Sugimura T, Sato S. Mutagens–carcinogens in foods. Cancer Res. 1983;43:2415s–21s.
87. Jägerstad M, Reuterswärd AL, Grivas S *et al.* Effects of meat composition and cooking conditions on the formation of mutagenic imidazoquinoxalines (MeIQx and its methyl derivatives). In: Hayashi Y, Nagao M, Sugimura T *et al.*, eds. Diet, nutrition and cancer. Tokyo, Japan, 1985. Tokyo, Japan: Japan Scientific Societies Press; 1986:87–96.
88. Ohgaki H, Hasegawa H, Kato T *et al.* Carcinogenicities in mice and rats of IQ, MeIQ, and MeIQx. In: Hayashi Y, Nagao M, Sugimura T *et al.*, eds. Diet, nutrition and cancer. Tokyo, Japan, 1985. Tokyo, Japan: Japan Scientific Societies Press; 1986:97–105.
89. Turesky, RJ, Lang, N, Butler, MA *et al.* Metabolic activation of carcinogenic heterocyclic aromatic amines by human liver and colon. Carcinogenesis. 1991;12:1417–22.
90. Kadlubar FF, Butler MA, Kaderlik KR *et al.* Polymorphisms for aromatic amine metabolism in humans: relevance for human carcinogenesis. Environ Health Persp. 1992;98:69–74.
91. Baker S, Fearon E, Nigro J *et al.* Chromosome 17 deletions and p53 gene mutations in colorectal carcinomas. Science. 1989;244:217–22.
92. Vogelstein B, Fearon E, Kern S *et al.* Allelotype of colorectal carcinomas. Science. 1989;244:207–12.
93. Kinzler K, Nilbert M, Vogelstein B *et al.* Identification of a gene located at chromosome 5q21 that is mutated in colorectal cancers. Science. 1991;251:1366–70.
94. Fearon E, Cho K, Nigro J *et al.* Identification of a chromosome 18q gene that is altered in colorectal cancers. Science. 1990;247:49–56.
95. Fearon ER, Vogelstein B. A genetic model for colorectal tumorigenesis. Cell. 1990;61:759–67.
96. Pretlow TB, Basitus TA, Fulton NC *et al.* K-ras mutations in putative preneoplastic lesions in human colon. J Natl Cancer Inst. 1993;85:2004–7.
97. Feinberg A, Vogelstein B. Hypomethylation of *ras* oncogenes in primary human cancers. Biochem Biophys Res Commun. 1983;111:47–54.
98. Hoffman RM. Altered methionine metabolism, DNA methylation and oncogene expression in carcinogenesis. Biochim Biophys Acta. 1984;738:49–87.
99. El-Deiry WS, Nelkin BD, Celano P *et al.* High expression of the DNA methyltransferase gene characterizes human neoplastic cells and progression stages of colon cancer. Proc Natl Acad Sci. 1991;88:3470–4.
100. Ellis R, DeFeo D, Shih T *et al.* The p21 *src* genes of Harvey and Kirsten sarcoma viruses originate from divergent members of a family of normal vertebrate genes. Nature (London). 1981;292:506–11.
101. Reddy E, Reynolds R, Santos E, Barbacid M. A point mutation is responsible for the acquisition of transforming properties by the T24 human bladder carcinoma oncogene. Nature (London). 1982;300:149–53.
102. Tabin C, Bardley S, Bargmann C *et al.* Mechanism of activation of a human oncogene. Nature (London). 1982;300:143–9.
103. Taparowsky E, Suard Y, Fasano O *et al.* Activation of the T24 bladder carcinoma transforming gene is linked to a single amino acid change. Nature (London). 1982;300:762–5.
104. Bos JL, Fearon ER, Hamilton SR *et al.* Prevalence of *ras* gene mutations in human colorectal cancers. Nature (London). 1987;327:293–7.
105. Bos JL. *ras* oncogenes in human cancer: a review. Cancer Res. 1989;49:4682–9.
106. Almoquera C, Shibata D, Forrester K *et al.* Most human carcinomas of the exocrine pancreas contain mutant c-K-*ras* genes. Cell. 1988;53:549–54.
107. Smit VTHBM, Boot AJM, Smits AMM *et al.* K-*ras* codon 12 mutations occur very frequently in pancreatic adenocarcinomas. Nucleic Acids Res. 1988;16:7773–87.
108. Rodenhuis S, Van De Wetering ML, Mooi WJ *et al.* Mutational activation of the K-*ras* oncogene, a possible pathogenetic factor in adenocarcinoma of the lung. N Engl J Med. 1987;317:929–35.
109. Shi Y, Zou M, Schmidt H *et al.* High rates of *ras* codon 61 mutation in thyroid tumors in an iodide-deficient area. Cancer Res. 1991;51:2690–3.
110. Haubruck H, McCormick F. Ras p21: effects and regulation. Biochim Biophys Acta. 1991;1072:215–29.
111. Boguski MS, McCormick F. Proteins regulating Ras and its relatives. Nature (London). 1993;366:643–54.

112. Burmer GC, Rabinovitch PS, Loeb LA. Frequency and spectrum of c-Ki-ras mutations in human sporadic colon carcinoma, carcinomas arising in ulcerative colitis, and pancreatic adenocarcinoma. Environ Health Perspect. 1991;93:27–31.
113. Fujimori T, Satonaka K, Yamamura-Idei Y *et al.* Non-involvement of *ras* mutations in flat colorectal adenomas and carcinomas. Int J Cancer. 1994;57:51–5.
114. Höhne MW, Halatsch M-E, Kahl GF, Weinel RJ. Frequent loss of expression of the potential tumor suppressor gene DCC in ductal pancreatic adenocarcinoma. Cancer Res. 1992;52:2616–19.
115. Uchino S, Tsuda H, Noguchi M *et al.* Frequent loss of heterozygosity of the *DCC* locus in gastric cancer. Cancer Res. 1992;52:3099–102.
116. Vogelstein B. A deadly inheritance. Nature (London). 1990;348:681–2.
117. Hollstein M, Sidransky D, Vogelstein B, Harris CC. p53 mutations in human cancers. Science. 1991;253:49–53.
118. Farmer G, Bargonetti J, Zhu H *et al.* Wild-type p53 activates transcription *in vitro*. Nature (London). 1992;358:83–6.
119. Kastan MB, Onyekwere O, Sidransky D *et. al.* Participation of p53 protein in the cellular response to DNA damage. Cancer Res. 1991;51:6304–11.
120. Levine AJ, Momand J, Finlay CA. The p53 tumour suppressor gene. Nature (London). 1991;351:453–6.
121. Malkin D, Li FP, Strong LC *et al.* Germ line p53 mutations in a familial syndrome of breast cancer, sarcomas, and other neoplasms. Science. 1990;250:1233–8.
122. Hill MJ, Morson BC, Bussey HJR. Aetiology of adenoma–carcinoma sequence in large bowel. Lancet. 1978;1:245–7.
123. Bird RP. Observation and quantification of aberrant crypts in the murine colon treated with a colon carcinogen; preliminary findings. Cancer Lett. 1987;37:147–51.
124. Tudek B, Bird RP, Bruce WR. Foci of aberrant crypts in the colons of mice and rats exposed to carcinogens associated with foods. Cancer Res. 1989;49:1236–40.
125. Roncucci L, Medline A, Bruce WR. Classification of aberrant crypt foci and microadenomas in human colon. Cancer Epidemiol Biol Prev. 1991;1:57–60.
126. Pretlow TP, Barrow BJ, Ashton WS *et al.* Aberrant crypts: putative preneoplastic foci in human colonic mucosa. Cancer Res. 1991;51:1564–7.
127. Roncucci L, Stamp D, Medline A *et al.* Identification and quantification of aberrant crypt foci and microadenomas in the human colon. Hum Pathol. 1991;22:287–94.
128. Corpet DE, Stamp D, Medline A *et al.* Promotion of colonic microadenoma growth in mice and rats fed cooked sugar or cooked casein and fat. Cancer Res. 1990;50:6955–8.
129. Zhang X-M, Stamp D, Minkin S *et al.* Promotion of aberrant crypt foci and cancer in rat colon by thermolyzed protein. J Natl Cancer Inst. 1992;84:1026–30.
130. Pretlow TP, O'Riordan MA, Somich GA *et al.* Aberrant crypts correlate with tumor incidence in F344 rats treated with azoxymethane and phytate. Carcinogenesis. 1992;13:1509–12.
131. Moser AR, Pitot HC, Dove WF. A dominant mutation that predisposes to multiple intestinal neoplasia in the mouse. Science. 1990;247:322–4.
132. Su LK, Kinzler KW, Vogelstein B *et al.* Multiple intestinal neoplasia caused by a mutation in the murine homolog of the APC gene. Science. 1992;256:668–70.
133. Moser AR, Dove WF, Roth KA, Gordon JI. The *Min* (multiple intestinal neoplasia) mutation: its effect on gut epithelial cell differentiation and interaction with a modifier system. J Cell Biol. 1992;116:1517–26.
134. Dietrich WF, Lander ES, Smith JS *et al.* Genetic identification of MOM-1, a major modifier locus affecting Min-induced intestinal neoplasia in the mouse. Cell. 1993;75:631–9.
135. Hill MJ, Aries VC. Faecal steroid composition and its relationship to cancer of the large bowel. J Path. 1971;104:129–39.
136. Stephen A, Cummings J. Mechanism of action of dietary fibre in the human colon. Nature (London). 1980;284:283–4.
137. Cummings J. Fermentation in the human large intestine: evidence and implications for health. Lancet. 1983;1:1206–9.
138. Potter JD, McMichael AJ. Diet and cancer of the colon and rectum: A case-control study. J Natl Cancer Inst. 1986;76:557–69.
139. Wattenberg, LW. Inhibition of chemical carcinogenesis. J Natl Cancer Inst. 1987;60:11–18.

140. Wattenberg LW. Inhibition of carcinogenic effects of polycyclic hydrocarbons by benzyl isothiocyanate and related compounds. J Natl Cancer Inst. 1977;58:195–8.
141. Wargovich MJ, Eng VWS, Newmark H. Calcium inhibits the damaging and compensatory proliferative effects of fatty acids on mouse colon epithelium. Cancer Lett. 1984;23:253–8.
142. Bird RP, Schneider R, Stamp D *et al.* Effect of dietary calcium and cholic acid on the proliferative indices of murine colonic epithelium. Carcinogenesis. 1986;7:657–61.
143. Wargovich MJ, Eng WWS, Newmark HL *et al.* Calcium ameliorates the toxic effect of deoxycholic acid on colonic epithelium. Carcinogenesis. 1983;4:1205–7.
144. Wargovich MJ, Isbell G, Shabot M *et al.* Calcium supplementation decreases rectal epithelial cell proliferation in subjects with sporadic adenoma. Gastroenterology 1992;103:92–7.
145. Bostick RM, Fosdick L, Wood JR *et al.* Calcium normalizes distribution of proliferating cells but does not affect proliferation rate in colorectal mucosa of sporadic adenoma patients: A randomized, double-blind, placebo-controlled clinical trial. JNCI. 1995 (in press).
146. Bostick RM, Potter JD, Fosdick L *et al.* Calcium and colorectal epithelial cell proliferation: Findings from a preliminary randomized double-blind placebo-controlled clinical trial. J Natl Cancer Inst. 1993;85:132–41.
147. Hennings J, Michael D, Chang C *et al.* Calcium regulation of growth and differentiation of mouse epidermal cells in culture. Cell. 1980;19:245–54.
148. Yuspa SH, Koehler B, Kulesz-Martin M *et al.* Clonal growth of mouse epidermal cells in medium with reduced calcium concentration. J Invest Dermatol. 1981;76:144–6.
149. Lechner JF, Haugen A, McClendon IA *et al.* Clonal growth of normal adult human bronchial epithelial cells in a serum-free medium. In Vitro. 1982;18:633–42.
150. Yu DTY, Clements J, Pearson CM. Effect of sport stress on lymphocyte transformation and antibody formation. Clin Exp Immunol. 1977;28:326–31.
151. Mackinnon LT. Exercise and natural killer cells. What is the relationship? Sports Med. 1989;7:141–9.
152. Shephard RJ. Physical activity and cancer. Int J Sports Med. 1990;11:413–20.
153. Simon HB. The immunology of exercise: a brief review. JAMA. 1984;252:2735–8.
154. Ravikumar T, Rodrick M, Steele G *et al.* Interleukin generation in experimental colon cancer of rats: effects of tumor growth and tumor therapy. J Natl Cancer Inst. 1985;74:893–8.
155. Cumming DC, Vickovic MM, Wall SR *et al.* The effect of acute exercise on pulsatile release of luteinizing hormone in women runners. Am J Obstet Gynecol. 1985;153:482–5.
156. Bonen A, Ling WH, MacIntyre KP *et al.* Effects of exercise on the serum concentrations of FSH, LH, progesterone and estradiol. Eur J Appl Physiol. 1979;42:15–23.
157. Jurkowski JE, Joanes NL, Walker WC *et al.* Ovarian hormonal responses to exercise. Med Sci Sports Exerc. 1981;13:109–14.
158. McMichael AJ, Potter JD. Do intrinsic sex differences in lower alimentary tract physiology influence the sex-specific risks for bowel cancer and other biliary and intestinal diseases? Am J Epidemiol. 1983;118:620–7.
159. Stephen AM, Wiggins HS, Englyst HN *et al.* The effect of age, sex and level of intake of dietary fibre from wheat on large-bowel function in thirty healthy subjects. Br J Nutr. 1986;56:349–61.
160. Lampe JW, Slavin JL, Potter JD. Sex differences in colonic function: a randomized trial. Gut. 1993;34:531–6.
161. Kaplan L, Spindel E, Isselbacher K, Chin W. Tissue-specific expression of the rat galanin gene. Proc Natl Acad Sci. 1988;85:1065–9.
162. Lund PK. Nutritional control of gastrointestinal hormone gene expression. In: Berdainer CD, Hargrove JL, eds. Nutrition and gene expression. Boca Raton, FL: CRC Press; 1993:91–116.
163. McMichael AJ, Potter JD. Dietary influences upon colon carcinogenesis. In: Hayashi Y, Nagao M, Sugimura T *et al.*, eds. Diet, nutrition and cancer. Tokyo, Japan, 1985. Tokyo, Japan: Japan Scientific Societies Press; 1986:275–90.
164. Potter JD. Large bowel cancer: epidemiology and biology. Ergeb Gastroenterol. 1989; 24:137–40.
165. Potter JD. Colon cancer: reconciling the epidemiology, physiology, and molecular biology. JAMA. 1992;268:1573–7.
166. Anzano MA, Riemann D, Pritchett W, *et al.* Growth factor production by human colon carcinoma cell lines. Cancer Res. 1989;49:2898–904.
167. Mukaida H, Hirabayashi N *et al.* Significance of freshly cultured fibroblasts from different tissue in promoting cancer cell growth. Int J Cancer. 1991;48:423–7.

168. Ross JA, Potter JD, Severson RK. Platelet-derived growth factor and the epidemiology of colorectal cancer: a hypothesis. Eur J Canc Prev. 1993;2:197–210.
169. Yunis JJ, Soreng AL. Constitutive fragile sites and cancer. Science. 1984;226:1199–204.
170. Giovanucci E, Stampfer MJ, Colditz GA *et al.* Folate, methionine, and alcohol intake and risk of colorectal adenoma. J Natl Cancer Inst. 1993;85:875–84.
171. Morotomi M, Guillem J, LoGerfo P, Weinstein IB. Production of diacylglycerol, an activator of protein kinase C, by human intestinal microflora. Cancer Res. 1990;50:3595–9.
172. Guillem JG, Weinstein IB. The role of protein kinase C in colon neoplasia. In: Herrera L, ed. Familial adenomatous polyposis. New York: Alan R. Liss; 1990:325–32.
173. Rosenthal MD. Fatty acid metabolism of isolated mammalian cells. Prog Lipid Res. 1987;26:87.
174. Nicosia S, Patrono C. Eicosanoid biosynthesis and action: novel opportunities for pharmacological intervention. FASEB J. 1989;3:1941.
175. Rutten AAJJL, Flake HE. Influence of high dietary levels of fat on rat hepatic phase I and II biotransformation enzyme activities. Nutr Rep Int. 1987;36:109.
176. Kim HJ, Choi ES, Wade AE. Effect of dietary fat on the induction of hepatic microsomal cytochrome P450 isozymes by phenobarbital. Biochem Pharmacol. 1990;39:1423.
177. Guillem JG, Hsieh LL, O'Toole KM *et al.* Changes in expression of oncogenes and endogenous retroviral-like sequences during colon carcinogenesis. Cancer Res. 1988;48:3964.
178. Castro EC. Nutrient effects on DNA and chromatin structure. Annu Rev Nutr. 1987;7:407.
179. Beland FA, Kadlubar FF. Formation and persistence of arylamine DNA adducts *in vivo*. Environ Health Perspect. 1985;62:19–30.

4
The genetics of prostate cancer

R.A. Eeles

INTRODUCTION

Prostate cancer is a significant public health problem. There are 10 000 cases per year in England and Wales, and 8000 deaths[1]. In the USA, it is the most common malignancy and the second most common cause of cancer deaths[2], with 132 000 cases per year and 34 000 deaths[3]. Furthermore, the incidence is increasing by 10–20% every 5 years[4]. Conversely, histological evidence of asymptomatic prostate cancer is found frequently at autopsy[5]. Therefore, it seems that a large proportion of men harbour disease which will remain asymptomatic, whilst, in others, it progresses to cause substantial morbidity and mortality. One of the main goals of research into the genetics of prostate cancer is to identify those lesions which will progress to clinically significant disease.

Prostate cancer has special features which need to be examined at the molecular level, namely the tendency for prostate cancer to occur in the outer part of the gland[6] and the relationship of prostatic intra-epithelial neoplasia to invasive cancer[7].

The disease is usually asymptomatic until it is advanced. In the UK, where there is no active screening programme, the disease has often metastasized at presentation. Only 13% of cases with disease localized to the pelvis, treated at The Royal Marsden Hospital, UK from 1970–89, presented with stage T1 disease confined to the prostate (Eeles *et al.*, in preparation). Even in the USA, where, in the last few years, there has been a greater emphasis on earlier detection, at least 40% of cases currently have metastases at presentation. This proportion may decrease as screening becomes more widespread. The five-year survival rate for all stages is 55–78% depending on the series reported, but for T1 overall is 74–95%[8], the higher grade tumours having the lower survival rate. The improved survival rate for those with disease at an earlier stage provides a rationale for early detection. However, the argument against screening the general population is that large numbers of people would have to be screened to detect a few cancers. For example, prostate-specific antigen screening in the general population detects histological cancer in about 2–4% of those screened[9,10]. If a predisposing gene or genes could be characterized, men at increased risk of prostate cancer could be identified and offered targeted screening and prevention. If genetic studies could detect which tumours will progress, early treatment which is potentially curative could then be offered selectively to patients who have a risk of progression within their lifetime.

THE AETIOLOGY OF PROSTATE CANCER

Epidemiological studies of the aetiology of prostate cancer suggest many causal factors, of which genetic predisposition is one (see later). The disease is rare in young men; only 1% of cases occur before 55 years old[11]. It is more common in certain racial groups, particularly negroes[12] where the prognosis is also worse. This is still apparent, even when corrected for socioeconomic status[13]. Just as in breast cancer, it is a relatively uncommon disease in Japan, but there is a higher mortality in Japanese immigrants to the USA[14], suggesting an environmental component. Some studies suggest that this is dietary fat[15] and that the effect occurs via hormonal changes[16].

Hormonal factors have been studied with conflicting results. Levels of testosterone and its derivatives are not consistently different between cases and controls. However, it has been shown by twin studies that the production of testosterone and dihydrotestosterone is under genetic influences[17]. Prostate cancer risk is also associated with higher fertility rate[18] and influenced by marital status[19]. The effects of sexual factors, such as age at puberty and first sexual intercourse, are not consistent between studies. The effect of vasectomy is controversial, some studies suggesting an associated increased risk of prostate cancer, and others refuting this[20].

It has been suggested that an infectious agent may be involved since higher prostate cancer rates are correlated with crude measures of increased sexual activity, for example, ever-married men versus single men[21], lower age at first sexual intercourse and first marriage[22], and venereal disease[19]. Virus-like particles have been found in prostatic cancer tissue[23] and antiviral antibody titres are higher in cases than controls[24].

The disease is more common in urban than rural areas[21] but socioeconomic factors are unrelated[25] and there is no significant relationship to previous diseases, height, circumcision, smoking or alcohol consumption[26]. Some occupations carry an increased risk, namely those in the cadmium[27] and rubber industries[28].

It may be possible to study the interactions of these factors with genetic predisposition once predisposing genes have been identified.

EVIDENCE FOR GENETIC PREDISPOSITION TO PROSTATE CANCER

The first piece of evidence is that prostate cancer may be familial in some instances. The best examples of familial clustering are the large Utah kindreds, some containing over 20 cases (Reference 29 and Cannon-Albright, personal communication) for example Figure 4.1. Woolf[30] first described an increased incidence of prostate cancer in the relatives of cases. He studied the incidence of

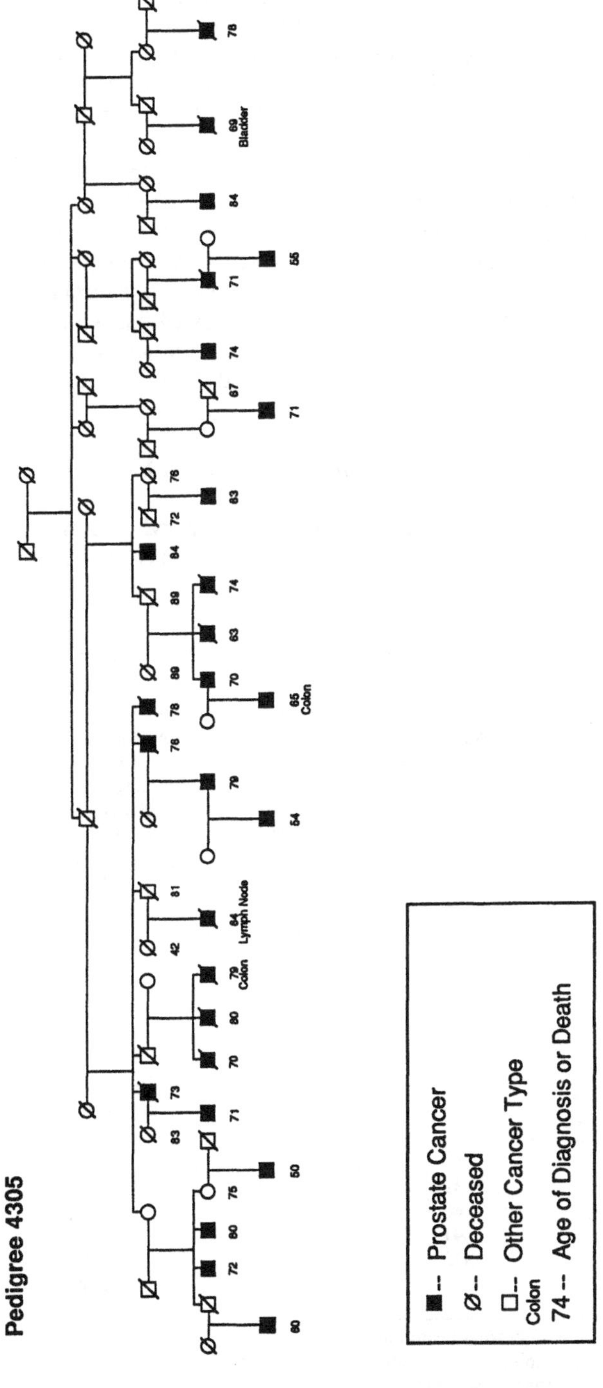

Figure 4.1 Example of one of the large Utah pedigrees (courtesy of Dr Cannon-Albright)

prostate cancer in the first-degree relatives (fathers and brothers) of 228 individuals with prostate cancer in the Utah Mormon population and age-matched controls. Using death certificate data, he found that first-degree relatives of prostate cancer cases had a relative risk of 3 of developing prostate cancer. This is similar to the relative risks that have been in the other common cancers where there is a genetic component.

There have been two types of studies to demonstrate whether there is an increased risk of prostate cancer in relatives of cases. Both have a case-control study format; one type compared the number of prostate cancer cases in relatives of cases versus controls, and the other compared the percentage of cases versus controls with a positive family history. These studies are summarized in Table 4.1. The relative risk values in first-degree relatives of cases range from 3–11 with the first study type, and from 0.64–7.5 with the second type. Only one study[19] had a reduced relative risk in relatives, and it only included 39 cases.

Studies of familial prostate cancer in the Utah population, USA

Utah has a 1.2-times increased rate of prostate cancer when compared with the rest of the USA[38]. Studies of familial cancer in Utah have been revolutionized

Table 4.1 Summary of studies investigating whether there is an increased risk of prostate cancer in relatives of cases

References (authors)	*No. of cases*	*No. of cases in first-degree relatives of cases*	*No. of cases in first-degree relatives of controls*	*Relative risk*
31 (Morganti *et al.*)[a]	183	11	1	11
30 (Woolf)[b]	228	15	5	3
32 (Krain)[a]	221	12	2	6
33 (Fincham *et al.*)[a]	382	58	31	3.2
29 (Cannon)[b]	2824	*	*	2.4
34 (Meikle *et al.*)[b]	150	11 (brothers only)	1	4 (at age 80) 16.6 (at age < 49)
		Cases with +ve family history	*Controls with +ve family history*	
19 (Steele *et al.*)[a]	39	12.8%	20.0%	0.64
22 (Schuman *et al.*)[a]	40	16.7%	7.3%	2.3
35 (Steinberg *et al.*)[a]	691	15.0%	8.0%	1.9
36 (Spitz *et al.*)[a]	378	13.0%	5.7%	2.3
37 (Ghadirian *et al.*)[a]	140	15.0%	2.0%	7.5

[a] Information from patient/control questionnaire only.
[b] Diagnosis verified by hospital records, cancer registration or death certificate.
* Measured genealogical index – see text

by three data sources: the computerized genealogy records of the church of Jesus Christ of Latter Day Saints (LDS or Mormons), the Utah SEER Cancer Registry, and the Utah Death Certificates. Together, these data comprise the Utah Population Data Base or UPDB[39].

Genealogical work is central to membership in the LDS church. The extended family unit is very important, both for a sense of identity and because it is believed that ancestors can be solemnized posthumously into membership of the LDS church. Pioneers from much of Northern Europe emigrated to the USA in the nineteenth century and persecution drove them west in the USA until they came to the Salt Lake valley in Utah and built Salt Lake City. This is now the centre for the LDS church and houses the Family History Library containing computer records of the Mormon genealogy which was started in 1894. Each family compiles family group sheets and the library contains 8 million of these. All those family group sheets which contain at least one birth or death date in Utah or along the pioneer Western trail have been obtained from the society and form the basis of the Utah Genealogical Database[40]. The data, which relate to 185 000 families (1.5 million individuals), have been computerized and all individuals linked into a genealogy representing the Utah descendants of the Mormon pioneers[39]. The relatives of a given individual can therefore be traced.

The Utah Cancer Registry was made statewide in 1966, and, in 1973, became one of eleven population-based registries of the Surveillance, Epidemiology and End Results (SEER) Program of the National Cancer Institute in America. The registry maintains abstracts of clinical records and follow-up data on all cancer cases. The Utah death certificates have been computerized for all individuals who have died since 1955. The computerized genealogy, death records and Cancer Registry have been linked to create the Utah Population Database (UPDB).

The advantage of this population for genetic studies is that early polygamy (occurring in 10–20% of the male pioneers until 1890), high fertility, low non-paternity and a high degree of cooperation result in very large well-documented extended families with low levels of inbreeding in which the gene pool is large because the original Mormon poineers were unrelated and numerous. Many Mormons have remained in Utah, and those that have migrated are still often traceable through family reunions, a Mormon custom.

The genetic make-up is very similar to that of Northern Europeans, as has been shown from gene frequency studies[41] and, due to a continued influx of immigrants, there are normal levels of inbreeding[42].

Genealogical index

The genealogical index (GI) uses the UPDB to assess the relationship between a pair of individuals. All cases of a particular cancer are considered and the degree of relatedness between the affected individuals is measured. The degree of relatedness is quantified by the Malecot coefficient of kinship[43]. This expresses the probability that randomly selected homologous genes from two individuals are identical by descent from a common ancestor. In the absence of inbreeding, it is

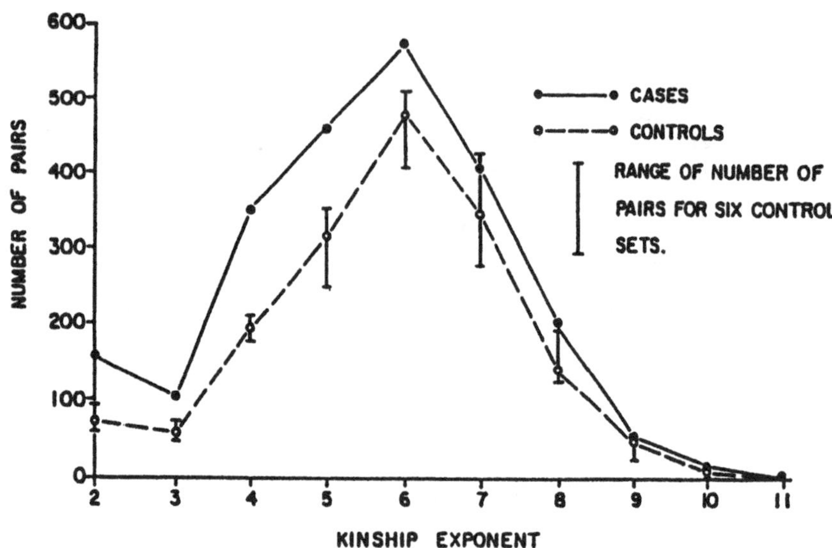

Figure 4.2 Kinship distribution of prostate cancer showing statistically significant excess familiality in cases extending to seventh-degree relatives

calculated in integral powers of 1/2 (the power of 1/2 is the kinship component). For example, for siblings, since there are two genetic steps between them, the coefficient is $1/2)^2$; for uncle–nephew, it is $(1/2)^3$, with kinship exponents 2 and 3, respectively. Tens of thousands of pairs of cases have been analysed to assess the kinship components, and these were then averaged to obtain a figure for the disease site. This figure is called the genealogical index (GI) and is expressed as a figure ($\times 10^{-5}$). In 1982, Cannon *et al.*[29] measured the GI in extended prostate-cancer kindreds traceable, within each of the kindreds, back to a common ancestor in the UPDB. The GI was 2.57 for prostate cancer cases and 1.45 for controls. This excess familiality extended out to seventh-degree relatives, many of whom will not even know each other, indicating that it is likely that a common gene has given a predisposition to these cancers to distantly related relatives (Figure 4.2). A potential bias, that cases within the UPDB have more complete information than controls, was excluded by studying accidental death records.

This analysis has recently been updated using 41 940 Cancer Registry records linked to the UPDB genealogy[44]. The GI is now known as the GIF which stands for genealogical index of familiality. Of the common cancers, prostate cancer is one of the most familial (GIF of 3.70 in cases vs. 2.76 in controls). It is surpassed by melanoma (4.06 vs. 2.64) and is followed by colon cancer (3.53 vs. 2.76) and breast cancer (3.23 vs. 2.73), all of these being statistically significant. Both breast and colon cancer, which have lower GIFs, are recognized to have a genetic component. Younger prostate cases had a higher GIF than older cases (GIF of 3.89 for $\leqslant$ 69 years vs. 3.76 for older cases).

Evidence that the increased risk to relatives in epidemiological studies is a genetic effect

The size of the relative risks from most case-control studies suggests a genetic effect. The relative risks of prostate cancer due to other factors, such as age at first marriage, are all about 1.5, which is the level risk from hormonal factors in breast cancer aetiology. All but one of the relative risk figures in the familial studies are higher than this, and all but two are higher than 2.0. The fact that an increased level of relatedness is present in the UPDB data even as distant as sixth- or seventh-degree relatives, may also suggest genetic effects, since such distant relatives might not even know each other. However, it is possible that, throughout Utah, Mormons would all have similar diets, and so one could still not exclude a dietary effect.

The best evidence that there is a genetic effect is the fact that the relative risk markedly increases as the age of the proband decreases[34] (Table 4.2), as the number of affecteds in the family increases (Table 4.3 and 4.4), or when both factors are taken together (Table 4.5). A relative risk of this size cannot be explained solely by an environmental effect.

The genetic model

Segregation analysis has only been performed in one data set using nuclear families. The results suggest that familial prostate cancer is due to a rare highly penetrant dominant gene (gene frequency 0.003) which causes 43% of cases by age 55, and 9% by age 80. The penetrance in carriers would be 88% by age 85[45].

Table 4.2 Relative odds for prostate cancer in brothers of prostate cancer cases by age

Age of patient	*Age of brother* *<65*	*65–79*	*≥80*
<65	5.97**	2.77*	2.29
65–79	2.77*	2.04**	2.52*
≥ 80	2.29	2.52*	1.14

* $p < 0.01$; ** $p < 0.001$. From Cannon *et al.* [29]

Table 4.3 Relative risks for prostate cancer in relatives of prostate cancer cases by degree of relationship

Affected relatives	*Relative risk (95% CI)*	
First-degree	2.0	(1.2–3.3)
Second-degree	1.7	(1.0–2.9)
Both first- and second-degree	8.8	(2.8–28.1)

From Steinberg *et al.* [35]

Table 4.4 Age-adjusted relative risk estimates for prostate cancer by number of additional affected family members

Affected relatives (besides proband)	*Odd ratio (95% CI)*	
1	2.2	(1.4–3.5)
2	4.9	(2.0–12.3)
3	10.9	(2.7–43.1)

From Steinberg *et al.*[35]

Table 4.5 Estimated risk ratios for prostate cancer in first-degree relatives of probands, by age at onset in proband and additional affected family members

	Risk ratio			
Age at onset of proband	*No additional relatives affected*		*One or more additional first-degree relatives affected*	
50	1.9	(1.2–2.8)	7.1	(3.7–13.6)
60	1.4	(1.1–1.7)	5.2	(3.1–8.7)
70	1.0*		3.8	(2.4–6.0)

* Reference group. Risk ratio is shown with 95% CI in brackets. From Carter *et al.*[45]

Until recently, all familial cancers were thought to be caused by tumour suppressor genes. Carcinogenesis in such cases arises following the Knudson two-hit hypothesis, where the first hit is inherited and loss of the remaining normal or wild-type allele results in tumour development[46]. However, it is now thought that at least one familial syndrome (MEN2) is caused by mutations in a dominant oncogene since loss of the normal allele does not occur at the predisposition locus in tumours[47]. Other familial cancers have been reported where mutation of one allele alone at the predisposition locus results in genomic instability and tumour formation[48,49] although there are now some reports of associated allele loss in these instances. The mechanism(s) of action of the prostate cancer predisposition gene is unknown.

Familial aggregation of prostate cancer with other cancers

A higher incidence of prostate cancer among male relatives of breast cancer patients has been reported[50–52]. Anderson and Badzioch[53] report a doubling of familial breast cancer risk when prostate cancer is present in the family history. Male carriers of the BRCA1 gene also have an increased risk of prostate cancer of about three-fold[54]. Carter *et al.*[55] showed a significant association of prostate cancer with brain tumours.

Prostate cancer is also now considered to be part of the extended definition of the Li-Fraumeni syndrome. A study of relatives of patients with soft-tissue sarcoma has shown that there is a 1.9-fold increased risk of prostate cancer in these relatives (95% CI 0.7–5.1)[56]. In Li-Fraumeni-like families, the incidence of germ-line mutations in the oncogene TP53 is about 10%[57], and, although families with TP53 germ-line mutations which contain cases of prostate cancer have been described[58], this gene still has to be studied as a candidate for the cause of large familial prostate cancer kindreds.

THE SEARCH FOR THE GENE(S) PREDISPOSING TO FAMILIAL PROSTATE CANCER

The study of familial prostate cancer is complicated by the fact that there may be a large number of sporadic cases in families since prostate cancer is common. In addition, screen-detected prostate cancer may behave differently from symptomatic disease: postmortem studies show that 15–30% of men have histological evidence of prostate cancer by the age of 50[5], but not all these histologically defined cancers progress to clinical disease. Men with a positive family history may be more likely to undergo screening, and this could detect histologically defined disease which would not progress.

To perform linkage analyses, several groups have been collecting nuclear families and have been trying to extend them to find further cases. Some of the most dramatic families are those from Utah. From the Utah family shown in Figure 4.1, it appears that male/male transmission of the disease can occur, so, unless there is a large number of sporadics in this family, it is unlikely that the susceptibility gene in this family is on the X chromosome. An ideal candidate would have been the androgen receptor gene which is on Xq but this is unlikely to be the susceptibility gene, at least in this family. Carter *et al.*[45] have shown the same phenomenon in some nuclear families. In others, maternal transmission excludes the Y chromosome as a site for the predisposing gene. To date, no susceptibility gene for prostate cancer has been located.

TUMOUR STUDIES

Cytogenetics

The amount of cytogenetic information on prostate cancer is sparse in comparison with other carcinomas, possibly due to overgrowth in culture of normal cells[59]. All studies have been performed in sporadic tumours. Cytogenetics of prostate tumours are difficult to perform but the reported studies to date show loss of the long arms of chromosomes 10[60–63] and 7[64] and loss of chromosomes 1, 2, 5 and Y[65]. Some studies have reported trisomy 7, 14, 20 and 22[65]. One patient with trisomy 4 has been reported, and one with a translocation from 5q to 7q[65]. Rearrangements involving chromosomes 2q, 7q and 10q are those most commonly observed[65].

Allele loss studies and tumour suppressor genes

Allele loss studies or loss of heterozygosity (LOH) indicate the sites of tumour suppressor genes since, in the tumour, the wild-type allele is lost, resulting in the

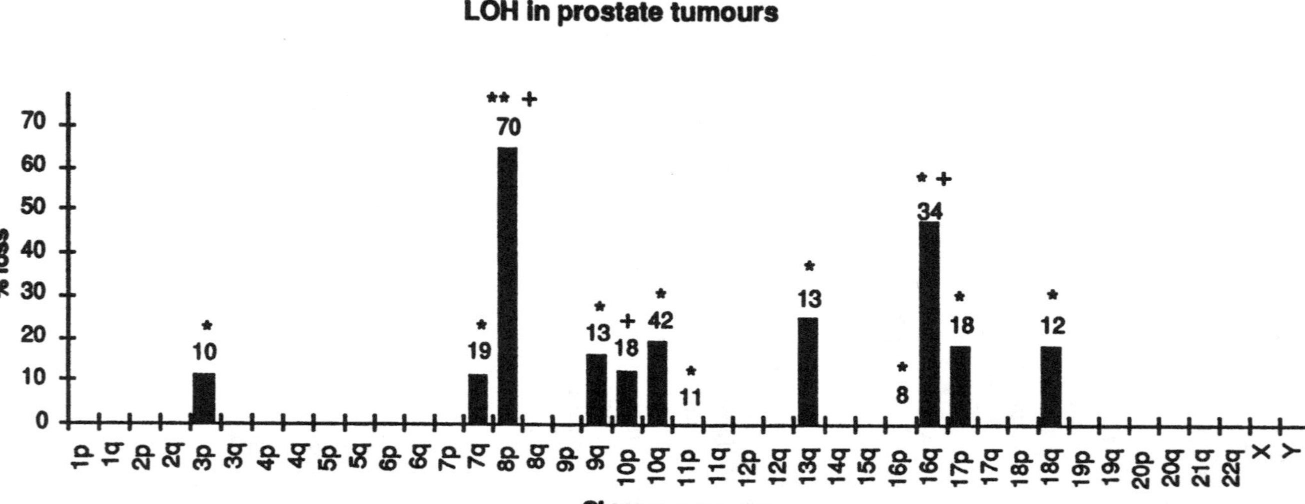

Figure 4.3 Results of loss of heterozygosity (LOH) studies in prostate tumours by chromosome arm. The numbers at the top of each bar are the numbers of informative tumours studied and the symbols refer to the reference source: *Reference 66; **Reference 68; +Reference 69

tumour suppressor gene exerting an unopposed effect. Individuals heterozygous for markers in the area of loss therefore have their heterozygous state reduced to homozygosity; hence the term LOH. The most likely candidates for locations of a tumour suppressor gene from LOH studies in prostate cancer are chromosomes 8p, 10q and 16q because the highest percentage of loss (30–50% of tumours) is in these regions[66,67]. LOH has also been seen in other regions (see Figure 4.3). In one study of 52 tumours, the loss at 8p was present in 63% of tumours studied[68]; and in a metastasis, a homozygous deletion of part of 8p (8p22) has been found. This deletion narrows the area of loss to a 14-cM interval[68] and is strongly suggestive of a tumour suppressor gene in this region. TP53 mutations are the most common genetic changes in many cancer types[70]; however, in prostate cancer, TP53 mutation is not very common in primary tumours. Mutations of TP53 were seen in 25% of 92 tumours in one study[71], but all the mutations were seen in metastatic tissue, and were a late event. Similar results have been obtained for the retinoblastoma gene[72] and the DNA polymerase β genes[73] where changes are more common in metastatic disease than in earlier disease.

Chromosome transfer studies using microcell-mediated chromosome transfer have shown that introduction of chromosomes 8 or 11 suppresses metastatic ability, but not tumorigenicity, in the highly metastatic Dunning rat AT3.1 prostatic cancer cell line[74,75]. Metastasis is also associated with loss of chromosome 2 (see below). Suppression of tumorigenicity of the human prostate cancer cell line DU 145 in nude mice[76] can be achieved by transfer of a portion of chromosome 12 (12pter–12q13). These would therefore be candidate areas for the sites of tumour suppressor genes.

DOMINANT ONCOGENES

All the reported mutations in dominant oncogenes in prostate cancer seem to be associated with disease progression rather than with the early stages of prostate cancer development. In MEN2, C cell hyperlasia predisposes to carcinoma, but it is unclear at present whether prostatic hypertrophy predisposes to carcinoma. These both argue against a dominant oncogene model for prostate cancer predisposition. Once the gene(s) are located, these issues will be resolved.

RAS

Mutations in the *RAS* oncogene are infrequent and are usually a late event in prostate cancer[77–79]. Overexpression of *RAS* does not correlate independently with decreased survival, but there is an inverse relation between *RAS* p21 expression determined using immunohistochemistry, tumour grade[80] and nodal status[81]. Treiger and Isaacs[82] have shown that expression of a mutated v-H-*RAS* oncogene can convert a tumorigenic non-metastatic Dunning rat prostatic cell line into a highly metastatic state. This is accompanied by decreased expression of fibronectin[83] and an increase in cell motility[84]. The acquisition of metastatic potential is accompanied by genomic instability. In particular, loss of chromosome 10 occurred in all of the transfectants, consistent with LOH studies which suggest that there is a tumour suppressor gene on chromosome 10[85]. When hybrids of the non-metastatic and metastatic lines are injected into rats, they form primary tumours, but do not metastasize[86], suggesting that a tumour suppressor gene(s), and not solely the mutated dominant oncogene v-H-*RAS*, is involved in the development of metastatic potential. The loss of metastatic ability in hybrids was shown not to be due to a product of the fusion process, because, when highly metastatic cells were fused with themselves, high metastatic ability was retained in the fused product.

The hybrid cells resulting from the fusion of metastasizing and non-metastasizing cells did not metastasize when injected into the flank of rats. However, when the primary tumours were passaged *in vivo*, they developed distant metastases in occasional animals, and this was accompanied by a loss of chromosome 2 in each of 8 cases[86]; in one of these cases, the loss of this chromosome was the only cytogenetic change. This suggests that a prostatic metastasis-suppressor gene is located on chromosome 2.

MYC

Increased levels of *MYC* transcripts have been found in high-grade prostate cancers[87].

BCL-2

BCL-2 overexpression has been associated with the over-riding of apoptosis. It has been shown by immunohistochemical and RNA studies to be overexpressed when prostate cancer progresses from androgen dependence to independence[88].

ADHESION MOLECULES, PROTEASES AND METASTASIS

Cadherins are a family of calcium-dependent cell adhesion molecules, and reduction in levels of these proteins is associated with decreased cell–cell adhesion and subsequent metastasis. Decreased expression of E-cadherin has been shown to be associated with disease progression in rat prostatic cancer[89]. Proteases are secreted as part of the metastatic process, and increased expression of metalloproteinase-7, types I and IV collagenase and stromelysin I have been reported in fresh prostate tumour by Northern analysis and *in-situ* hybridization[90].

CELL LINES AS MODELS

Three human prostate cancer cell lines developed from metastases are currently in wide use (DU145, LNCaP, PC-3)[91–93]. The phenotype of LNCaP is the closest to that of clinical prostate cancer because it is positive for acid phosphatase and prostate-specific antigen (PSA) and it is hormone sensitive[92]. It only grows when implanted in the prostate gland, but not in the skin, suggesting that stromal/tumour interactions may be important.

A variant with a mutation in the hormone-binding domain of the androgen receptor, LNCaPR, grows maximally without the presence of steroid hormones, but when exposed to them, then produces PSA (Muir, personal communication). Several sublines have been developed from PC-3 and LNCaP[94,95]. Other cell lines may be contaminated by normal tissue overgrowth, and their full characterization is awaited.

CLINICAL CONSIDERATIONS

Management of familial prostate cancer

There are a few epidemiological studies which provide data on the risks of developing prostate cancer according to the number of relatives affected in the family. This information can be used to advise individuals in prostate cancer families. Tables 4.4 and 4.5 show the relative risks according to the number of relatives affected and the age at diagnosis. For example, if there are two first-degree relatives affected with prostate cancer aged about 60 years, the relative risk in the unaffected related individual is about 5 at that age. The normal population risk is 0.5% by age 64 and 2% by age 74[96].

Since relatives of prostate cancer patients are at increased risk of the disease, the question arises whether they should be offered targeted screening. It has been shown that earlier diagnosis is associated with better survival[8], but screening for prostate cancer has yet to be proven to improve survival.

If a higher-risk population could be identified, in theory, prostate-specific antigen (PSA) screening should result in a higher yield of cancer cases detected per number screened. McWhorter *et al.*[97] have studied first-degree relatives of 17 sets of two brothers with prostate cancer. A total of 34 relatives were studied (sons and brothers aged 55–80). They underwent intensive screening with PSA, digital rectal examination (DRE), transrectal ultrasound (TRUS) and systematic as well as clinically directed core biopsies. Eight cancers were detected; only one was not visible on TRUS and was diagnosed by systematic biopsy only. It is often said that the problem with screening for prostate cancer is that it may detect cancer which will not become clinically relevant to the patient within their lifetime. However, this was not the case in this study. One of the 8 cancers detected was stage C disease, and so the other 7 subsequently underwent prostatectomy and lymph node dissection. Pathologically, their cancers were 3 stage B and 4 stage C. The overall cancer detection percentage was therefore 8/34 or 24% and all had clinically significant disease. Using a similar screening protocol in the general population, with the difference that biopsy was only performed if indicated, Catalona *et al.*[9] found only 36 cancers (2.2%) in a population of 1630 men aged 50–79. These limited data seem to support targeted prostatic cancer screening in relatives of cases, at least if two brothers have both been affected with the disease.

It is not known whether familial prostate cancer has a different prognosis from sporadic disease, as has been suggested in some studies of familial breast cancer[98].

Chemoprevention of prostate cancer in those at increased risk due to a genetic predisposition is an exciting new area in cancer prevention. Finasteride is a 5α reductase inhibitor previously used to treat benign prostatic hypertrophy and it is being piloted in a randomized controlled trial in the USA to assess whether it can reduce mortality from prostate cancer. Men at increased risk of the disease through age, and those with a positive family history, are randomized to finasteride or placebo[99].

SUMMARY

The characterization of genetic changes which predispose to prostate cancer formation or progression will enable the identification of individuals at risk of developing clinically significant disease to have early treatment at a stage when the disease is potentially curable, or to have preventative measures before the disease develops. The rapid developments in genetic research in prostate cancer are expected to make a significant contribution to these approaches in the next few years.

Acknowledgements

I am very grateful to Dr Lisa Cannon-Albright for Figures 4.1 and 4.2.

References

1. Office of Population Censuses and Surveys. London: HMSO; 1992.
2. Silverberg E, Lubera JA. Cancer statistics. CA. 1989;38:14–15.
3. Cancer facts and figures. American Cancer Society. 1992.
4. Coleman MP, Esteve J, Damiecki P, Arslan A, Renard H. Trends in cancer incidence and mortality. IARC. 1993:21. chapter 21.
5. Haas GP, Sakr W, Cassin B *et al.* The prevalence of prostate cancer in young black and white males. J Urol. 1992;147:290A.
6. McNeal JE, Redwine EA, Freiha FS, Stamey TA. Zonal distribution of prostatic carcinoma: correlation with histologic pattern and direction of spread. Am J Surg Pathol. 1988;12:897–906.
7. McNeal JE, Boswick DG. Intraductal dysplasia: a premalignant lesion of the prostate. Hum Pathol. 1986;17:64–71.
8. Hanks GE, Diamond JJ, Krall JM, Martz KL, Kramer S. A ten year follow-up of 682 patients treated for prostate cancer with radiation therapy in the United States. Int J Radiat Oncol Biol Phys. 1987;13:449–505.
9. Catalona WJ, Smith DS, Ratliff TL, Dodds KM, Coplen DE, Yuan JJJ, Petros JA, Andriole GL. Measurement of prostate-specific antigen in serum as a screening test for prostate cancer. N Engl J Med. 1991;324:1156–61.
10. Gustafsson O, Norming U, Almgard L-E, Fredriksson A, Gustavsson G, Harvig B, Nyman CR. Diagnostic methods in the detection of prostate cancer: a study of a randomly selected population of 2,400 men. J Urol. 1992;148:1827–31.
11. Office of Population Censuses and Surveys. London: HMSO; 1986.

12. Waterhouse J, Muir C, Shanmugaratnam K *et al.* In: Cancer incidence in five continents, Vol 6. Lyon, France: IARC, Publication 42;1982.
13. McWhorter WP, Schatztkin AG, Horm JW *et al.* Contribution of socioeconomic status to black/white differences in cancer incidence. Cancer. 1989;63:982–7.
14. Haenszel W. Cancer mortality among the foreign-born in the United States. J Natl Cancer Inst. 1988;40:43–68.
15. Zaridze DG, Boyle P. Cancer of the prostate: epidemiology and aetiology. Br J Urol. 1987;59:493–502.
16. Hill P, Wynder EL, Garnes H, Walker ARP. Environmental factors, hormonal status and prostatic cancer. Prev Med. 1980;90:657–66.
17. Meikle AW, Stringham JD, Bishop DT *et al.* Quantitating genetic and nongenetic factors influencing androgen production and clearance in men. J Clin Endocrinol Metab. 1988;67:104–9.
18. Armenian H, Lilienfeld A, Diamond E, Bron I. Epidemiologic characteristics of patients with prostatic neoplasms. Am J Epidemiol. 1975;102:47–54.
19. Steele R, Lees REM, Kraus AS, Rao C. Sexual factors in the epidemiology of cancer of the prostate. J Chron Dis. 1971;24:29–37.
20. Skegg DCG. Vasectomy and risk of cancers of prostate and testis. Eur J Cancer. 1993;29A(7):935–6.
21. King H, Diamond E, Lilienfeld A. Some epidemiological aspects of cancer of the prostate. J Chron Dis. 1963;16:117–53.
22. Schuman T, Mandel J, Blackard C, Bauer H, Scarlett J, McHugh R. Epidemiologic study of prostatic cancer: preliminary report. Cancer Treatment Rep. 1977;61:181–6.
23. Webber MM, Stonington OG, Lehman J. Virus in prostatic epithelium of man. Urology. 1973;1:561–7.
24. Ablin RJ. Serum antibody in patients with prostatic cancer. Br J Urol. 1976;48:355–61.
25. Richardson I. Prostatic cancer and social class. Br J Rev Soc Med. 1965;19:140–2.
26. Wynder F, Mabuchi K, Whitmore W. Epidemiology of cancer of the prostate. Cancer. 1971;28:344–60.
27. Kipling MD, Waterhouse JAH. Cadmium and prostatic carcinoma. Lancet. 1967;1:730–1.
28. McMichael AJ, Spirtas R, Gamble JF, Tousey PM. Mortality among rubber workers; relationship to specific jobs. J Occup Med. 1976;18:178–85.
29. Cannon LA, Bishop DT, Skolnick M, Hunt S, Lyon J, Smart C. Genetic epidemiology of prostate cancer in the Utah Mormon genealogy. Cancer Surveys. 1982;1:47–69.
30. Woolf CM. An investigation of the familial aspects of carcinoma of the prostate. Cancer. 1960;13:739–44.
31. Morganti G, Gianferrari L, Cresseri A, Arrigoni G, Lorati G. Recherches clinico-statistiques et genetiques sur les neoplasies de la prostate. Acta Genet Stat. 1959;6:304–5.
32. Krain LS. Some epidemiologic variables in prostatic carcinoma in California. Prev Med. 1974;3:154–9.
33. Fincham SM, Hill GB, Hanson J, Wijayasinghe C. Epidemiology of prostate cancer: a case control study. Prostate. 1990;17:189–206.
34. Meikle AW, Smith JA, West DW. Familial factors affecting prostatic cancer risk and plasma sex-steroid levels. Prostate. 1985;6:121–8.
35. Steinberg GS *et al.* Family history and the risk of prostate cancer. Prostate. 1990;17:337–47.
36. Spitz MR, Currier RD, Fueger JJ, Babaian J, Newell GR. Familial patterns of prostate cancer: a case-control analysis. J Urol. 1991;146:1305–7.
37. Ghadirian P, Cadotte M, Lacroix A, Perret C. Family aggregation of cancer of the prostate in Quebec: the tip of the iceberg. Prostate. 1991;19:43–52.
38. Cancer in Utah Report No. 3. 1967–77. Salt Lake City: Utah Cancer Registry; 1977.
39. Skolnick MH. The Utah genealogical data base: a resource for genetic epidemiology. In: Cairns J, Lyon JL, Skolnick MH, eds. Banbury Report No. 4: Cancer incidence in defined populations. New York: Cold Spring Harbor Laboratory; 1980:285–97.
40. Skolnick M, Bean L, May D, Arbon V, de Nevers K, Cartwright P. Mormon demographic history. I. Nuptiality and fertility of once-married couples. Popul Stud. 1978;32:5–19.
41. McLellan T, Jorde LB, Skolnick MH. Genetic distances between the Utah Mormons and related populations. Am J Hum Genet. 1984;36:836–7.
42. Jorde LB, Skolnick MH. Demographic and genetic application of computerized record linking: the Utah Mormon genealogy. Inf Sci Hum. 1981;56-57:105–117.

43. Malecot G. Les mathematiques de l'heredite. Masson et Cie. 1948; Paris.
44. Cannon-Albright LA, Thomas A, Goldgar DE *et al.* Familiality of cancer in Utah. Cancer Res. 1994;54:2378–85.
45. Carter BS, Beaty TH, Steinberg GD, Childs B, Walsh PC. Mendelian inheritance of familial prostate cancer. Proc Natl Acad Sci USA. 1992;89:3367–71.
46. Knudson AG. Hereditary cancer, oncogenes and antioncogenes. Cancer Res. 1985;45:1437–43.
47. Mulligan LM, Kwok JBJ, Healey CS *et al.* Germ-line mutations of the *RET* proto-oncogene in multiple endocrine neoplasia type 2A. Nature. 1993;363:458–60.
48. Fishel R, Lescoe MK, Rao MRS *et al.* The human mutator gene homolog MSH2 and its association with hereditary nonpolyposis colon cancer. Cell. 1993;75:1027–38.
49. Leach FS, Nicolaides NC, Papadopoulos N *et al.* Mutations of a MutS homolog in hereditary non-polyposis colorectal cancer. Cell. 1993;75:1215–25.
50. Macklin MT. The genetic basis of human mammary cancer. In: Proceedings of the second national cancer conference. New York: American Cancer Society; 1954;1074–87.
51. Thiessen E. Concerning a familial association between breast cancer and both prostatic and uterine malignancies. Cancer. 1974;34:1102–7.
52. Tulinius H, Egilsson V, Olafsdottir GH, Sigvaldason H. Risk of prostate, ovarian, and endometrial cancer among relatives of women with breast cancer. BMJ. 1992;305:855–7.
53. Anderson DE, Badzioch MD. Breast cancer risks in relatives of male breast cancer patients. JNCI. 1992;84:1114–7.
54. Ford D, Easton DF, Bishop DT, Narod SA, Goldgar DE and the Breast Cancer Linkage Consortium. Risks of cancer in BRCA1-mutation carriers. Lancet. 1994;343:692–5.
55. Carter BS, Bova GS, Beaty TH *et al.* Hereditary prostate cancer; epidemiologic and clinical features. J Urol. 1993;150:797–802.
56. Zahm SH, Blair A, Holmes FF, Boysen CD, Robel RJ, Fraumeni JF Jr. A case-control study of soft tissue sarcoma. Am J Epid. 1989;130:665–74.
57. Birch JM, Hartley AL, Tricker KJ *et al.* Prevalence and diversity of constitutional mutations in the p53 gene among 21 Li-Fraumeni families. Cancer Res. 1994;54:1298–304.
58. Eeles RA, Warren W, Knee G *et al.* Constitutional mutation in exon 8 of the p53 gene in a patient with multiple independent primary tumours: molecular and immunohistochemical findings. Oncogene. 1993;8:1269–76.
59. Sandberg AA. Chromosomal abormalities and related events in prostate cancer. Hum Pathol. 1992;23:368–80.
60. Gibas Z *et al.* Chromosome rearrangement in a metastatic adenocarcinoma of the prostate. Cancer Genet Cytogenet. 1984;11:399–404.
61. Atkin N, Baker M. Chromosome study of 5 cancers of the prostate. Hum Genet. 1985;70:359–64.
62. Lundgren R, Mandahl N, Heim S, Limon J, Henrikson H, Mitelman F. Cytogenetic analysis of 57 primary prostatic adenocarcinomas. Genes Chromosomes Cancer. 1992;4:16–24.
63. Arps S, Rodewald A, Schmalenberger B, Carl P, Bressel M, Kastendieck H. Cytogenetic survey of 32 cancers of the prostate. Cancer Genet Cytogenet. 1993;66:93–9.
64. Atkin NB, Baker MC. Chromosome 7q deletions: observations on 13 malignant tumors. Cancer Genet Cytogenet. 1993;67:123–5.
65. Brothman AR, Peehl DM, Patel AM, McNeal JE. Frequency and pattern of karyotypic abnormalities in human prostate cancer. Cancer Res. 1990;50:3795–803.
66. Carter BS, Ewing CM, Ward WS *et al.* Allelic loss of chromosomes 16q and 10q in human prostate cancer. Proc Natl Acad Sci USA. 1990;87:8751–5.
67. Collins VP, Kunimi K, Bergerheim U, Ekman P. Molecular genetics and human prostatic carcinoma. Acta Oncol. 1991;30:181–5.
68. Bova GS, Carter BS, Bussemakers MJG *et al.* Homozygous deletion and frequent allele loss of chromosome 8p22 loci in human prostate cancer. Cancer Res. 1993;53:3869–73.
69. Bergerheim USR, Kunimi K, Collins VP, Ekman P. Deletion mapping of chromosomes 8, 10 and 16 in human prostate carcinoma. Genes Chromosomes Cancer. 1991;3:215–20.
70. Hollstein MC, Sidransky D, Vogelstein B, Harris CC. p53 mutations in human cancers. Science. 1991;253:49–53.
71. Navone NM, Troncosco P, Pisters LL, *et al.* p53 protein accumulation and gene mutation in the progression of human prostate carcinoma. JNCI. 1993;85:1657–69.
72. Bookstein R, Rio P, Madreperla SA *et al.* Promoter deletion and loss of retinoblastoma gene expression in human prostate cancer. Proc Natl Acad Sci USA. 1990;87:7762–6.

73. Dobashi Y, Shuin T, Tsuruga H, Uemura H, Torigoe S, Kubota Y. DNA polymerase β gene mutation in human prostate cancer. Cancer Res. 1994;54:2827–9.
74. Ichikawa T, Niheii N, Suzuki H *et al.* Suppression of metastasis of rat prostatic cancer by introducing human chromosome 8. Cancer Res. 1994;54:2299–302.
75. Ichikawa T, Ichikawa Y, Dong J *et al.* Localization of metastasis suppressor gene(s) for prostatic cancer to the short arm of human chromosome 11. Cancer Res. 1992;52:3486–90.
76. Berube NG, Speevak MD, Chevrette M. Suppression of tumorigenicity of human prostate cancer cells by introduction of human chromosome del(12)(q13). Cancer Res. 1994;54:3077–81.
77. Peehl DM, Wehner N, Stamey TA. Activated Ki-ras oncogene in human prostatic adenocarcinoma. Prostate. 1987;10:281–9.
78. Carter BS, Epstein JI, Isaacs WB. *ras* gene mutations in human prostate cancer. Cancer Res. 1992;50:6830–2.
79. Sumiya H, Masai MN, Akimoto S, Yatani R, Shimazaki J. Histological examination of expression of *ras* p21 protein and R1881 binding protein in human prostatic cancer. Eur J Cancer. 1990;7:786–9.
80. Viola MV, Fromowitz F, Oravez S *et al.* Expression of *ras* oncogene p21 in prostate cancer. N Engl J Med. 1986;314:133–7.
81. Fan K. Heterogeneous subpopulations of human prostatic adenocarcinoma cells: potential usefulness of p21 as a predictor for bone metastasis. J Urol. 1988;139:318–22.
82. Treiger B, Isaacs J. Expression of a transfected v-H-ras oncogene in a Dunning rat prostate adenocarcinoma and the development of high metastatic ability. J Urol. 1988;140:1580–6.
83. Schalken JA, Ebeling SB, Issacs JT *et al.* Down modulation of fibronectin messenger RNA in metastasizing rat prostatic cancer cells revealed by differential hybridization analysis. Cancer Res. 1988;48:2042–6.
84. Partin AW, Isaacs JT, Treiger B, Coffey DS. Early cell motility changes associated with an increase in metastatic ability in rat prostatic cancer cells transfected with v-Harvey-ras oncogene. Cancer Res. 1988;48:6050–3.
85. Ichikawa T, Schalken JA, Ichikawa Y, Steinberg G, Isaacs JT. H-ras expression, genetic instability and acquisition of metastatic ability by rat prostatic cancer cells following v-H-ras oncogene transfection. Prostate. 1991;18:163–72.
86. Ichikawa T, Ichikawa Y, Isaacs JT. Genetic factors and suppression of metastatic ability of prostatic cancer. Cancer Res. 1991;51:3788–92.
87. Buttyan R, Sawczuk IS, Benson MC, Siegal JD, Olsson CA. Enhanced expression of the c-myc proto-oncogene in high grade human prostate cancers. Prostate. 1987;11:327–37.
88. McDonnell TJ, Troncoso P, Brisbay SM *et al.* Expression of the protooncogene *bcl*-2 in the prostate and its association with emergence of androgen-independent prostate cancer. Cancer Res. 1992;52:6940–4.
89. Bussemakers MJG, van Moorselaar RJA, Giroldi LA *et al.* Decreased expression of E-cadherin in the progression of rat prostatic cancer. Cancer Res. 1992;52:2916–22.
90. Pajouh MS, Nagole RB, Breathnach R, Finch JS, Brawer MK, Bowden GT. Expression of metalloproteinase genes in human prostate cancer. J Cancer Res Clin Oncol. 1991;117:114–50.
91. Stone KR, Mickey DD, Wunderli H, Mickey G, Paulson DF. Isolation of a human prostate carcinoma cell line (DU145). Int J Cancer. 1978;21:274–81.
92. Horoszewicz JS, Leong SS, Kawinski E *et al.* LNCaP model of human prostatic carcinoma. . Cancer Res. 1983;43:1809–18.
93. Kaighn ME, Narayan KS, Ohnuki Y, Lechner JF, Jones LW. Establishment and chracterization of a human prostatic carcinoma cell line (PC-3). Invest Urol. 1979;17:16–23.
94. Ware JL, Paulson DF, Mickey GH, Webb KS. Spontaneous metastasis of cells of the human prostate carcinoma cell line PC-3 in athymic nude mice. J Urol. 1982;128:1064.
95. Steenbrugge GJ, van Groen M, van Dongen JW *et al.* The human prostatic carcinoma cell line LNCaP and its derivatives. Urol Res. 1989;17:71.
96. Parkin DM, Muir CS, Whelan SL, Gao Y-T, Ferlay J, Powell J. Cancer incidence in five continents. IARC. 1993;6:971.
97. McWhorter WP, Hernandez AD, Meikle AW *et al.* A screening study of prostate cancer in high risk families. J Urol. 1992;148:826–8.
98. Lynch HT, Albano WA, Recabaren JA *et al.* Survival in hereditary breast and colon cancer. JAMA. 1981;246:1197.
99. Donodeo F. Prevention trial for prostate cancer piques public interest. JNCI. 1994;85:1801–2.

5
Lessons from developmental biology

E.T. Stuart and P. Gruss

INTRODUCTION

The mechanisms which underlie embryogenesis have puzzled many investigators in the past. The basic concept of embryogenesis is that a network of precisely regulated processes interact in such a fashion that specific populations of cells divide and differentiate and patterns are laid down over which organogenesis can proceed and result in the development of a normal embryo. In simple terms, the factors which control development processes involve the regulation of cell growth both in space and time.

Oncogenesis is the opposite – it is the end product of deregulated cell growth. It is now becoming clear that disruption of genes which direct development may lead to cancer. To varying extents, all genes involved in cell growth and differentiation contribute to development.

The ultimate control of developmental processes lies within the nucleus with the transcription of specific genes in a highly ordered temporal and spatial manner. However, the initiation of regulated transcription requires the cell to have knowledge of its location and surrounding environment and ultimately its destiny. Thus, proteins involved in the cell cycle e.g. p53, signal transduction mechanisms e.g. tyrosine kinases[1,2], the ras family[3] as well as nuclear proteins which actually determine the transcription of other genes e.g. PAX, HOX[4–8], FOS[9,10], must be considered when discussing the role of development-associated genes in cancer.

Although many genes show an interesting expression pattern during embryogenesis and have been shown to be involved in oncogenesis, a detailed discussion of their role in oncogenesis will not be presented here as the reader can refer to the many reviews already written on these topics for further details.

Thus far, most attention has been focused on identifying the genes which are involved in controlling developmental processes but there is a paucity of information concerning the genes which lie upstream or downstream of these genes. In this chapter, we will review the observations concerning some genes which are implicated in the control of development and discuss their oncogenic potential with regard to possible mechanisms of action.

PAIRED BOX (PAX) GENES ARE INVOLVED IN DIRECTING DEVELOPMENT AND ARE INVOLVED IN A NUMBER OF CANCERS

The paired box consists of a highly conserved DNA sequence of 384 base pairs[11–14] which was initially identified in *Drosophila* segmentation genes[15]. To date, *pa*ired bo*x* or PAX genes have been identified in the genomes of many different species, such as mouse[16,17], man[18], chicken[19], quail[20] and zebra fish[21–24]. Thus far, eight murine[25] and nine human PAX genes[26,27] have been isolated. PAX genes are grouped into four paralogous groups according to their structure and paired domain homology[25]. The first group consists of PAX 1 and PAX 9 which encode the paired domain and a conserved octapeptide sequence but lack a homeodomain. Group II PAX genes are represented by PAX 3 and 7, which, in addition to the paired domain and octapeptide sequence, encode a full homeodomain. PAX 2, 5 and 8 represent group III. Each encodes the paired domain and octapeptide but only a partial homeodomain. Group IV is represented by PAX 4 and 6 which encode the paired domain and homeodomain but lack the octapeptide.

PAX genes encode proteins which vary from 360–480 amino acids in length. Three α-helices have been shown to be present in the paired domain[15], the first of which is located at the amino terminal of the domain and the remaining two in close proximity to the carboxy terminal. The full homeodomain contains a helix-turn-helix[28].

PAX proteins act as nuclear transcription factors because they are localized in the nucleus[29] and are able to bind DNA *in vitro*[29–35]. The *Drosophila* paired protein (prd) can bind to a sequence in the even-skipped promoter e5[36,37]. The sequences bound by prd include the ATTA motif, which is recognized by the homeodomain, and sequences further downstream presumably recognized by the paired domain. Using this sequence, it has been demonstrated that PAX proteins have a large (20–24 base pair) recognition sequence. PAX proteins which contain the homeodomain and paired domain, e.g. PAX 3, also recognize the ATTA motif and a downstream motif characterized by the GTYMC core motif.

So far, relatively little is known concerning the regulators of PAX genes or target genes for PAX proteins. Functional target sequences for group III have been identified. PAX 5 was originally identified as a B-cell-specific transcription factor and potentially regulates the CD19 gene which encodes a B-cell-specific surface protein[38]. Its parallel in the sea-urchin, TSAP, regulates two pairs of non-allelic histone genes – H2A-2 and H2B-2[39]. PAX 8, which is expressed in the thyroid, binds to and regulates the thyroperoxidase and thyroglobulin genes[35].

PAX gene expression during development

In general, murine PAX genes are expressed during embryogenesis with a distinct spatiotemporal pattern beginning between day 8 and 9.5 postcoitus (pc). A common feature of PAX genes is that they are expressed in the central nervous system (CNS) and/or the paraxial mesoderm and its derivatives. PAX 2–8 are expressed in the developing and the adult CNS. PAX 1 is not expressed in the

CNS at any stage. For a definitive catalogue of PAX gene expression patterns during development of the murine nervous system, the reader should refer to Stoykova and Gruss[40].

PAX 3, PAX 6 and PAX 7, which contain a homeodomain, are expressed before the onset of differentiation (day 8–8.5 pc). In contrast, PAX genes which lack a homeobox (PAX 2, 5 and 8) begin to be expressed during neural differentiation (day 10 pc).

PAX genes are expressed in a number of different structures apart from the CNS. PAX 1 is expressed from day 9 pc in the segmented prevertebral column and later in the sternum and thymus[41]. PAX 2 is expressed transiently in the condensing mesenchyme of the developing kidney, its early epithelial derivatives and in the collecting duct epithelium[29,42]. PAX 2 is required for the earliest phase of mesenchyme-to-epithelium conversion during kidney development[43] and is repressed upon terminal differentiation of the renal tubule epithelium. PAX 2 is also expressed in the wolffian duct, the ureter and the developing eye and ear.

PAX 8 is expressed in the developing kidney but at a later stage than PAX 2, i.e. at more differentiated stages[44]. PAX 8 is also expressed in the thyroid[35] and in placenta[45].

PAX 5 is expressed in many tissues involved in B-cell differentiation, such as the spleen, lymph node and in the pre-B, pro-B and mature B cells. PAX 5 expression is also seen in the salivary gland, lung and adult testis[33].

Both PAX 3 and PAX 7 are expressed in the somites of day 9 and 10 pc embryos. Also, at this embryonic stage, PAX 3 is expressed in the undifferentiated mesenchyme of both fore- and hind-limb. At day 12 pc, the expanding myotome but not the dermatome still expresses PAX 7. At later stages, PAX 7 is still expressed in the myotome-derived intercostal muscles and the skeletal muscles of the trunk. In contrast, PAX 3 is not expressed in the mesoderm or its derivatives after day 11 pc. The expression of PAX 7 is related to myogenesis[46] and should exhibit a cell lineage-restricted expression similar to PAX 1 expression in sclerotome-derived cells. At day 13 pc, PAX 3 and PAX 7 are expressed in the nasal pits. The expression of PAX 6 extends to all structures of the developing eye and nose[47].

PAX genes and oncogenesis

Many nuclear transcription factors have been classified as proto-oncogenes and it has been suggested that PAX genes should also be considered proto-oncogenes[48]. There is an increasing amount of evidence to support this suggestion. Thus far, it has been demonstrated that murine PAX genes induce tumorigenesis in mice, and various members of the human PAX family have been shown to be inappropriately expressed in a number of diverse human cancers.

Overexpression of PAX genes in NIH3T3 and 208F fibroblasts is accompanied by uncontrolled cell growth *in vitro* and the growth of cells in foci demonstrates an ability to overcome contact inhibition. The cells are also able to grow in increasing concentrations of soft agar[48]. When injected into nude athymic mice, these cells have the ability to develop into solid tumours which are well-vascularized in contrast to tumours induced by homeobox genes – Hox-2.4 or Hox B8[7].

The oncogenic potential of murine PAX genes appears to be dependent on the presence of a functionally active paired box. The absence of the octapeptide motif (PAX 6), homeodomain (PAX 1) or only a partial homeodomain (PAX 2 and 8) does not affect the transforming potential. However, the undulated point mutation in the paired box which results in a protein deficient in DNA binding is sufficient to prevent transformation[48].

Wilms tumour – a paediatric renal carcinoma – is the most common malignancy in children, occurring with an incidence of approximately 1 in 10 000 of the population[49]. The tumour morphology is suggestive of a development malfunction[29]. It has been demonstrated that PAX 2 is required for mesenchyme-to-epithelium progression, and the presence of the PAX 2 protein has been demonstrated in primary Wilms tumours[29]. Similarly, PAX 8, which is also expressed in the developing kidney, has been demonstrated to be expressed in Wilms tumours[44].

The involvement of PAX 3 in cancer has been demonstrated with the recent observation that a frequent site for chromosomal rearrangement in paediatric alveolar rhabdomyosarcoma maps to the PAX 3 locus. The common translocation t(2;13)(q35;q14) in this type of rhabdomyosarcoma involves the PAX 3 locus and results in a portion of the PAX 3 coding region being translocated to chromosome 13q14[50]. A fusion protein is expressed which contains the wild-type PAX 3 DNA-binding domains with the novel portion fused to the 3′ end. Analysis of the novel gene sequence has shown that it encodes a forkhead gene termed FKHR[51] or ALV[52]. The complete forkhead domain is not present in the fusion protein and, since the activity of forkhead proteins is dependent on the presence of an intact forkhead domain[53], it would appear that the activity of the fusion protein is probably due to the PAX 3 DNA-binding domains which may or may not be modulated by the forkhead region of the fusion protein.

Due to the salient nature of PAX gene expression in the CNS, tumours of the human central nervous system should provide a suitable system in which to investigate whether PAX genes may be involved in the initiation or progression of such tumours. In general, astrocytic tumours account for 60% of all tumours of the human central system and are characterized by their almost inevitable tendency to progress to higher forms of malignancy. PAX 5 may be influential in the progression of astrocytomas to their most malignant and prognostically unfavourable form – glioblastoma multiforme[96].

Rearrangement of chromosome 9p and the incidence of the involvement of 9p13 – the location of the PAX 5 gene – suggests that PAX 5 may be involved in this type of tumour. PAX 5 is over- and inappropriately expressed in highly malignant astrocytomas. At present, the molecular basis for PAX 5 function in these tumours is not understood. PAX 5 is, however, expressed only in discrete cell populations within the tumour and is expressed with various oncogenes – Myc, Fos, Jun and the epidermal growth factor receptor – leading to the enticing possibility of PAX genes co-operating in a pathway which involves other transcription factors or signal transduction mechanisms.

Although few target genes have been identified to date, it is interesting to speculate on the identity of such target genes from the information available concerning PAX expression in embryogenesis, oncogenesis and mutants. The ability of PAX genes to induce transformation and tumours suggests that possible target genes have a role in coding for proteins which are involved in the regulation of the cell-cycle or components of signal transduction mechanisms. However, possible target genes could be either induced or suppressed. To date, PAX gene expression has been identified in undifferentiated cells and thus potentially induced genes may contribute to the undifferentiated state whereas suppressed genes may contribute to the differentiated state.

Therefore, it is apparent that our understanding of the oncogenic potential of PAX genes is expanding rapidly and thus another role for the PAX family is starting to unfold.

WNT – A FAMILY OF CELL SIGNALLING GLYCOPROTEINS REGULATING DEVELOPMENT – WAS ORIGINALLY IDENTIFIED AS AN ONCOGENE

The first member of the Wnt family was cloned from the mouse in an effort to identify cellular genes which are activated by insertion of proviral DNA in mammary tumours induced by the mouse mammary tumour virus (MMTV)[54]. Wnt genes encode proteins of 350–380 amino acids and have been identified in a number of different species, including man[55,56], mouse[54,57], zebra fish[58], *Drosophila*[59] and leech[60]. Wnt genes are highly conserved throughout evolution, suggesting that they play a key role in cellular processes.

The Wnt family of genes encode glycoproteins which display many of the characteristics of secreted growth factors, such as a hydrophobic signal peptide, a regulation site for signal peptidase, no additional transmembrane domains and glycosylation sites[61].

Wnt-1 expression during development

Wnt-1 is the best characterized of the family. It is expressed in the developing CNS, but restricted to the testis in the adult mouse[62]. Expression of Wnt-1 is first detected at day 8.5 pc soon after neural induction occurs, at the caudal limit of the future midbrain. On day 9.5 pc, expression extends from the midbrain through the hindbrain and along the full length of the neural tube in a continuous fashion along the dorsal midline with two exceptions: firstly, a circle of cells express Wnt-1 around the midbrain–hindbrain boundary, and secondly, expression is not detected in a region of the caudal midbrain[63]. This pattern continues up to at least day 14.5 pc.

It is likely that the protein in its mature form is secreted, and it is presumably involved in cell–cell signalling mechanisms and thus may regulate patterning in the developing CNS by influencing cellular differentiation. Using homologous recombination, McMahon and Bradley provided further evidence to support this hypothesis by 'knocking-out' the endogenous Wnt-1 gene. The absence of

Wnt-1 in homozygote mice results in the absence of the midbrain and the anterior portion of the hindbrain, leading to the absence of the cerebellum[62].

Wnt genes and carcinogenesis

The discovery of the involvement of Wnt genes in carcinogenesis has been a direct result of the method employed for their identification. In mammary carcinomas, there appears to be a repeated incidence of proviral insertion into the Wnt-1 locus (and, to a lesser extent, the Wnt-3 locus). The end result of these insertions is the activation of a normally silent gene. Indeed, the open reading frame is conserved in most cases. This deregulation of gene transcription confers the cell with a growth advantage, rendering it statistically more susceptible to clonal expansion, as proposed by Nowell[64,65]. Although Wnt genes are able to transform certain mammary cell lines *in vitro*, these cells are not able to form tumours in nude mice. However, transgenic mice which overexpress Wnt-1 are more susceptible to mammary carcinomas[61]. To date, the tumours induced by overexpression of Wnt- or MMTV-induced tumours provide the sole *in-vivo* evidence for the role of Wnt genes in mammary carcinomas.

WT1, A TUMOUR SUPPRESSOR GENE COMMONLY MUTATED IN PAEDIATRIC RENAL CANCERS

Nephroblastoma or Wilms tumour is the most common solid paediatric tumour and is also associated with aniridia, mental retardation and urogenital malfunctions – collectively termed the WAGR syndrome. Phenotypically, Wilms tumour is characterized by developmental abnormalities which result from the incomplete differentiation of mesenchymal stem cells into the normal epithelial components of the nephron[66].

WT1 is a good example of a developmentally expressed tumour suppressor gene. WT1 encodes a nuclear transcription factor which binds DNA via its four zinc fingers[67]. Elucidation of the role of the WT1 gene requires the identification of the upstream regulators of its transcription and of the downstream target genes. Thus far, some target genes have been proposed. The first suggested binding site for the WT1 protein was identified as being similar to that recognized by the early growth response-1 gene product (EGR-1)[67]. EGR-1, also known as Krox 24, is a serum-inducible nuclear protein which also contains zinc fingers and binds to the consensus sequence 5′-GGAGCGGGGGCG-3′. The identification of a consensus DNA-binding sequence aids the identification of potential target genes for the transcription factor and, thus far, this sequence has been identified in the genes which encode $TGF\beta_1$, CSF-1, EGR-1, PDGF-A chain, IGF-II, IGF-1 receptor and, interestingly, PAX 2[68]. WT1 is also capable of physically interacting with p53, which appears to be of importance for the proper functioning of WT1 in regulating transcription[69].

WT1 expression during development

WT1 is expressed in a developmentally regulated manner. In the mouse, WT1 expression is detected at day 12.5 pc and, in the human, at 49 days of gestation. During embryonic development, WT1 is expressed in the condensing metanephric blastema and podocytes of the developing kidney, in the mesothelial lining of all organs, the spleen, brain and spinal cord. Expression continues in the adult where WT1 is generally limited to the urogenital system, i.e. the kidney, ovary, testis and uterus[70,71].

WT1 and oncogenesis

The identification of WT1 as the gene most likely to be responsible for Wilms tumour was the result of cytogenetic studies which identified the rearranged locus involved in these tumours as 11p13. The 11p13 locus also harbours the PAX 6 gene; however, PAX 6 has not been implicated in this tumour type although it is involved in aniridia which itself is part of the WAGR syndrome[72]. The identification of the WT1 locus at 11p13 and its intragenic deletions leading to premature translational termination before zinc finger transcription in patients with Wilms tumour constitute the basis for the supposition of its involvement in this tumour type[73,74]. Although it is likely that a number of genes are involved in the genesis of Wilms tumour, such as PAX 2 and 8[29,75], loss of heterozygosity of the Wilms tumour suppressor gene locus appears to be one of the consistently observed features and thus is probably one of the primary factors required for Wilms tumour formation.

p53 IS INVOLVED IN MULTIPLE TYPES OF CANCER AND IS EXPRESSED IN A DEVELOPMENTALLY REGULATED MANNER

The p53 gene encodes a 393-amino-acid nuclear transcription factor[76] which is highly conserved throughout evolution[77] and demonstrates a developmentally restricted expression pattern[78]. The original suggestion that p53 should be classified as an oncogene was based on the fact that, although present in small amounts in normal cells, it was more abundant in transformed cells and tumours[79]. However, further analysis revealed that many of the initial findings were obtained while studying mutated forms of the protein which contribute to increased protein stability as well as negation of the wild-type DNA-binding functions. Wild-type p53 has a half-life of 15–30 minutes whereas the half-life of mutant forms is measured in hours. Many of the mutations are missense point mutations which result in altered protein formation[80]. Of interest is the observation that there are four common regions for point mutation in the p53 gene and three mutational hot-spots at residues 175, 248 and 273. These regions correspond to the areas most highly conserved in evolution[77].

In normal cells, p53 appears to be involved in cell-cycle regulation where it acts as a checkpoint for the cell to decide whether to continue with the cell cycle, stop and repair DNA damage or move into an apoptotic state. Expression of p53 is low in normal cells but increases in cells which enter into the cell cycle leading to arrest in the G_1 phase or induction of apoptosis. Indeed, p53 expression is increased in response to DNA damage induced by ultraviolet[81] or γ-irradiation[82].

The evident role of p53 in the cell cycle and cancer has led to a number of downstream target genes being identified, as well as identification of partners in protein–protein interaction. p53 is a sequence-specific transcription factor[83–85] which recognizes and binds to a motif consisting of two copies of the sequence 5′-PuPuPuCWWGPyPyPy-3′ separated by up to 13 base pairs[76]. This binding motif has been identified in a number of genes, including muscle creatine kinase[86], MDM2[85], GADD45[87], SV40 origin of replication[88,89] and, recently, WAF1[83], also known as CIP1[90], which encodes a protein which binds to cyclin complexes and inactivates cyclin-dependent kinases. Interestingly, MDM2 appears to act as a regulator of p53 activity because the MDM2 protein binds directly to the p53 protein and may therefore antagonize p53 binding to other promoters.

p53 expression during development

In early stages, i.e. days 8.5-10.5 pc, p53 is expressed in all tissues of the developing mouse embryo. Organogenesis and histogenesis start soon after and, by day 12.5 pc, expression of p53 is altered in a tissue-specific manner[78]. In the liver, p53 is highly expressed up to day 14.5 pc after which its expression declines rapidly to a basal level which continues throughout adult life. In the thymus and lung, p53 is highly expressed up to day 18.5 pc at which point it starts to decline. The kidney has high levels of p53 throughout embryogenesis although it is mainly restricted to the cortical areas with the more central medulla only weakly expressing. In the brain, expression of p53 is ubiquitous and high up to day 12.5 pc. From day 14.5 pc, expression becomes more limited with the forebrain and midbrain expressing highly put the developing hindbrain and spinal cord expressing weakly.

However, p53 is not essential for murine development. Mice lacking p53 generated by homologous recombination develop normally but are susceptible to developing cancer prematurely[91].

Involvement of p53 in cancer

It is estimated that p53 is mutated in approximately 50% of all human cancers although there is a preponderance in certain types, such as colon cancer, certain brain tumours and Li-Fraumeni syndrome[92,93]. However, in some cancers, p53 cannot be detected either in its wild-type or mutant form, e.g. small cell lung carcinoma[80]. Due to the extensive amount of literature already produced concerning p53 in cancer, the reader is advised to consult the following publications and references therein for specific information concerning p53 in cancer: References 76, 80, 92 and 94.

Mutation in p53 are a feature of many cancers and is frequently observed as an early event in the initation of oncogenesis. It is not surprising that it is involved in such a wide variety of cancers as its wild-type function is important in all cell types and is an integral component of normal cell function. Therefore, disruptions to its normal form would have wide-reaching implications for multiple cell types. However, the proteins which regulate p53 expression, either positively or negatively, are not yet understood. Although it has been suggested that p53 itself regulates its transcription[95] and that p53 levels are altered by (1) the adenovirus E1A gene product, (2) DNA damage and (3) genome instability[76], there is little evidence for other factors which may perform a similar role. Evidently the therapeutic value of an agent which could positively (when mutations are not present and the wild-type protein is not expressed) or negatively (when the mutant form is preferentially expressed in the tumour) regulate p53 expression would be advantageous.

CONCLUDING REMARKS

The inverse relationship of cell growth regulation during development and deregulated cell growth during oncogenesis is an area which is at present and will in the future provide an invaluable system through which we can gain a further understanding of both processes.

The identification of oncogenes and tumour suppressor genes constitutes the initial phase of understanding the molecular basis of cancer. However, as our understanding of these genes increases, it is likely that cooperating pathways will be identified between known genes and those awaiting discovery. Many of these genes will be involved in developmental processes and may therefore provide a therapeutic target through which one may be able to manipulate the cell's own machinery in an effort to restore the cellular state to a normal one.

Acknowledgements

The support of The Mildred Scheel Foundation and The Max-Planck Society is acknowledged.

References

1. Ullrich A, Schlessinger J. Signal transduction by receptors with tyrosine kinase activity. Cell. 1990;61:203–12.
2. Saltiel AR, Ohmichi M. Pleiotropic signaling from receptor tyrosine kinases. Curr Opin Neurobiol. 1993;3:352–9.
3. Boguski MS, McCormick F. Proteins regulating Ras and its relatives. Nature (London). 1993;366:643–54.
4. Perkins A, Kongsuwan K, Visvader V, Adams JM, Cory S. Homeobox gene expression plus autocrine growth factor production elicits myeloid leukemia. Proc Natl Acad Sci USA. 1990;87:8398–402.
5. Maulbecker CC, Gruss P. The oncogenic potential of deregulated homeobox genes. Cell Growth Differ. 1993;4:431–41.
6. Kongsuwan K, Allen J, Adams JM. Expression of Hox-2.4 homeobox gene directed by proviral insertion in a myeloid leukemia. Nucleic Acids Res. 1989;17(5):1881–92.

7. Blatt C, Aberdam D, Schwartz R, Sachs L. DNA rearrangement of a homeobox gene in myeloid leukaemic cells. EMBO J. 1988;7(13):4283–90.
8. Aberdam D, Negreanu V, Sachs L, Blatt C. The oncogenic potential of an activated Hox-2.4 homeobox gene in mouse fibroblasts. Mol Cell Biol. 1991;11(1):554–7.
9. Distel RJ, Spiegelman BM. Protooncogene c-fos as a transcription factor. Adv Cancer Res. 1990;55:37–55.
10. Angel P, Karin M. The role of Jun, Fos and the AP-1 complex in cell proliferation and transformation. Biochim Biophys Acta. 1991;1072:129–57.
11. Bopp D, Burri M, Baumgartner S, Frigerio G, Noll M. Conservation of a large protein domain in the segmentation gene *paired* and in functionally related genes of *Drosophila*. Cell. 1986;47:1033–40.
12. Baumgartner S, Bopp D, Burri M, Noll M. Structure of two genes at the *gooseberry* locus related to the *paired* gene and their spatial expression during *Drosophila* embryogenesis. Genes Dev. 1987;1(10):1247–67.
13. Dambly-Chaudère C, Jamet E, Burri M *et al.* The paired box gene *pox neuro*: a determinant of poly-innervated sense organs in *Drosophila.* Cell. 1992;69:159–72.
14. Frigerio G, Burri M, Bopp D, Baumgartner S, Noll M. Structure of the segmentation gene *paired* and the Drosophila *PRD* gene set as part of a gene network. Cell. 1986;47:735–46.
15. Noll M. Evolution and role of *Pax* genes. Curr Opin Genet Dev. 1993;3:595–605.
16. Dressler GR, Deutsch U, Balling R, Simon D, Guénet J-L, Gruss P. Murine genes with homology to *Drosophila* segmentation genes. Development. 1988;104 (Suppl):181–6.
17. Deutsch U, Dressler GR, Gruss P. Pax1, a member of a paired box homologous murine gene family, is expressed in segmented structures during development. Cell. 1988;53:617–25.
18. Burri M, Tromvoukis Y, Bopp D, Frigerio G, Noll M. Conservation of the paired domain in metazoans and its structure in three isolated human genes. EMBO J. 1989;8:1183–90.
19. Goulding MD, Lumsden A, Gruss P. Signals from the notochord and floor plate regulate the region-specific expression of two Pax genes in the developing spinal cord. Development. 1993;117:1001–16.
20. Martin P, Carriere C, Dozier C *et al.* Characterization of a paired box- and homeobox-containing quail gene (*Pax-QNR*) expressed in the neuroretina. Oncogene. 1992;7:1721–8.
21. Krauss S, Johansen T, Korzh V, Fjose A. Expression pattern of zebrafish *pax* genes suggests a role in early brain regionalisation. Nature (London). 1991:353:267–70.
21. Krauss S, Johansen T, Korzh V, Moens U, Ericson JU, Fjose A. Zebrafish *pax[zf-a]*: a paired box-containing gene expressed in the neural tube. EMBO J. 1991;10:3609–19.
23. Krauss S, Johansen T, Korzh V, Fjose A. Expression of the zebrafish paired box gene *par[zf-b]* during early neurogenesis. Development. 1991;113:1193–206.
24. Püschel AW, Gruss P, Westerfield M. Sequence and expression pattern of *pax-6* are highly conserved between zebrafish and mice. Development. 1992;114:643–51.
25. Walther C, Guénet J-L, Simon D *et al.* Pax: a murine multigene family of paired box containing genes. Genomics. 1991;11:424–34.
26. Pilz AJ, Povey S, Gruss P, Abbott CM. Mapping of the human homologs of the murine paired-box-containing genes. Mammalian Genome. 1993;4:78–82.
27. Stapelton P, Weith A, Urbanék P, Kozmik Z, Busslinger M. Chromosomal localization of seven *PAX* genes and cloning of a novel family member, *PAX-9*. Nature Genet. 1993;3:292–8.
28. Chalepakis G, Tremblay P, Gruss P. *Pax* genes, mutants and molecular function. Development. 1992;Suppl 16:61–7.
29. Dressler GR, Douglass EC. Pax-2 is a DNA-binding protein expressed in embryonic kidney and Wilms tumor. Proc Natl Acad Sci USA. 1992;89:1179–83.
30. Goulding MD, Chalepkis G, Deutsch U, Erselius JR, Gruss P. Pax-3, a novel murine DNA binding protein expressed during early neurogenesis. EMBO J. 1991;10:1135–47.
31. Chalepakis G, Fritsch R, Fickenscher H, Deutsch U, Goulding M, Gruss P. The molecular basis of the *undulated/Pax-1* mutation. Cell. 1991;66:873–84.
32. Chalepakis G, Goulding M, Read A, Strachan T, Gruss P. The molecular basis of *splotch* and Waardenburg *Pax-3* mutations. Proc Natl Acad Sci USA. 1994;91:3685–9.
33. Adams B, Dörfler P, Aguzzi A *et al.* Pax-5 encodes the transcription factor BSAP and is expressed in B lymphocytes, the developing CNS, and in adult testes. Genes Dev. 1992;6:1589–607.
34. Czerny T, Schaffner G, Busslinger M. DNA sequence recognition by Pax proteins: Bipartate structure of the paired domain and its binding site. Genes Dev. 1993;7:2048–61.

35. Zannini M, Francis-Lang H, Plachov D, Di Lauro R. Pax-8, a paired domain-containing protein, binds to a sequence overlapping the recognition site of a homeodomain and activates transcription from two thyroid-specific promoters. Mol Cell Biol. 1992;12:4230–41.
36. Treisman J, Gönczy P, Vashishita M, Harris E, Desplan C. A single amino acid can determine the DNA binding specificity of homeodomain proteins. Cell. 1989;59:553–62.
37. Treisman J, Harris E, Desplan C. The paired box encodes a second DNA-binding domain in the paired homeo domain protein. Genes Dev. 1991;5:594–604.
38. Kozmik Z, Wang S, Dörfler P, Adams B, Busslinger M. The promoter of the CD19 gene is a target for the B-cell-specific transcription factor BSAP. Mol Cell Biol. 1992;12:2662–72.
39. Barberis A, Superti-Furga G, Vitelli L, Kemler I, Busslinger M. Developmental and tissue-specific regulation of a novel transcription factor of the sea urchin. Genes Dev. 1989;3:663–75.
40. Stoykova A, Gruss P. Roles of Pax-genes in developing and adult brain as suggested by expression patterns. J Neurosci. 1994;14(3):1395–412.
41. Deutsch U, Dressler GR, Gruss P. Pax1, a member of a paired box homologous murine gene family, is expressed in segmented structures during development. Cell. 1988;53:617–25.
42. Dressler GR, Deutsch U, Chowdhury K, Nornes HO, Gruss P. *Pax2*, a new murine paired-box-containing gene and its expression in the developing excretory system. Development. 1990;109:787–95.
43. Phelps DE, Dressler GR. Aberrant expression of *Pax-2* in *Danforth's Short Tail (Sd)* mice. Dev Biol. 1993;157:251–8.
44. Poleev A, Fickenscher H, Mundlos S *et al.* *PAX8*, a human paired box gene: isolation and expression in developing thyroid, kidney and Wilms' tumor. Development. 1992;116:611–23.
45. Kozmik Z, Kurzbauer R, Dörfler P, Busslinger M. Alternative splicing of *Pax-8* gene transcripts is developmentally regulated and generates isoforms with different transactivation properties. Mol Cell Biol. 1993;13(10):6024–35.
46. Jostes B, Walther C, Gruss P. The murine paired box gene, *Pax7*, is expressed specifically during the development of the nervous and muscular system. Mech Dev. 1991;33:27–38.
47. Walther C, Gruss P. Pax-6, a murine paired box gene, is expressed in the developing CNS. Development. 1991;113:1435–49.
48. Maulbecker CC, Gruss P. The oncogenic potential of Pax genes. EMBO J. 1993;12(6):2361–97.
49. Hastie ND. Wilms' tumor gene and function. Curr Opin Genet Dev. 1993;3:408–13.
50. Barr FG, Galili N, Holick J, Biegel JA, Rovera G, Emanuel BS. Rearrangement of the PAX3 paired box gene in the pediatric solid tumor alveolar rhabdomyosarcoma. Nature Genet. 1993;3:113–17.
51. Galili N, Davis RJ, Fredericks WJ *et al.* Fusion of a fork head domain gene to *PAX3* in the solid tumour alveolar rhabdomyosarcoma. Nature Genet. 1993;5:230–5.
52. Shapiro DN, Sublett JE, Li B, Downing JR, Naeve CW. Fusion of *PAX3* to a member of the forkhead family of transcription factors in human alveolar rhabdomyosarcoma. Cancer Res. 1993;53:5108–12.
53. Lai E, Prezioso VR, Smith E, Litvin O, Costa RH, Darnell JE. HNF-3A, a hepatocyte-enriched transcription factor of novel structure is regulated transcriptionally. Genes Dev. 1990;4:1427–36.
54. Nusse R, Varmus HE. Many tumors induced by the mouse mammary tumor virus contain a provirus integrated in the same region of the host genome. Cell. 1982;31:99–109.
55. Van't Veer LJ, Geurts van Kessel A, van Heerikhuizen H, van Ooyen A, Nusse R. Molecular cloning and chromosomal assignment of the human homolog of int-1, a mouse gene implicated in mammary tumorigenesis. Mol Cell Biol. 1984;4:2532–4.
56. Wainwright BJ, Scambler PJ, Stanier P *et al.* Isolation of a human gene with protein sequence similarity to human and murine *int-1* and the *Drosophila* segment polarity mutant *wingless*. EMBO J. 1988;7:1743–8.
57. Gavin BJ, McMahon JA, McMahon AP. Expression of multiple novel *Wnt-1/int-1*-related genes during fetal and adult mouse development. Genes Dev. 1990;35:43–54.
58. Molven A, Njolstad P, Fjose A. Genomic structure and restricted neural expression of the zebrafish *wnt-1 (int-1)* gene. EMBO J. 1991;10:799–807.
59. Rijsewijk F, Schuermann M, Wagenaar E, Parren P, Weigel D, Nusse R. The *Drosophila* homolog of the mouse mammary oncogene *int-1* is identical to the segment polarity gene *wingless*. Cell. 1987;50:649–57.
60. Kostriken R, Weisblat D. Expression of a Wnt gene in embryonic epithelium of the leech. Dev Biol. 1992;151:225–41.

61. Nusse R, Varmus HE. *Wnt* genes. Cell. 1992;69:1073–87.
62. McMahon AP, Bradley A. The *Wnt-1 (int-1)* proto-oncogene is required for development of a large region of the mouse brain. Cell. 1990;62:1073–85.
63. Wilkinson DG, Bailes JA, McMahon AP. Expression of the proto-oncogene *int-1* is restricted to specific neural cells in the developing mouse embryo. Cell. 1987;50:79–88.
64. Nowell P. The clonal evolution of tumor cell populations. Science. 1976;194:23–8.
65. Nowell P. Mechanisms of tumor progression. Cancer Res. 1986;46:2203–7.
66. Hastie ND. Wilms' tumour gene and function. Curr Opin Genet Dev. 1993;3:408–13.
67. Rauscher FJ, Morris JF, Tournay OE, Cook DM, Curran T. Binding of the Wilms' tumor locus zinc finger protein to the EGR-1 consensus sequence. Science. 1990;250:1259–62.
68. Rauscher FJ. The WT1 Wilms tumor gene product: a developmentally regulated transcription factor in the kidney that functions as a tumor suppressor. FASEB J. 1993;7:896–903.
69. Maheswaran S, Park S, Bernard A *et al.* Interaction between the p53 and Wilms tumor (WT1) gene products: physical association and functional cooperation. Proc Natl Acad Sci USA. 1992;90:5100–4.
70. Pritchard-Jones K, Fleming S, Davidson D *et al.* The candidate Wilms' tumour gene is involved in genitourinary development. Nature (London). 1990;346:194–7.
71. Pelletier J, Schalling M, Buckler AJ, Haber DA, Housman D. Expression of the Wilms' tumor gene WT1 in the murine urogenital system. Genes Dev. 1991;5:1345–56.
72. Ton CCT, Hirvonen H, Miwa H *et al.* Positional cloning of a paired box- and homeobox-containing gene from the aniridia region. Cell. 1991;67:1059–74.
73. Pelletier J, Bruening W, Li FP, Haber DA, Glaser T, Housman DE. WT1 mutations contribute to abnormal genital system development and hereditary Wilms' tumor. Nature (London). 1991;353:431–4.
74. Haber DA, Buckler AJ, Glaser T *et al.* An internal deletion within an 11p13 zinc finger gene contributes to the development of Wilms' tumor. Cell. 1990;61:1257–69.
75. Poleev A, Fickenscher H, Mundlos S *et al. PAX8*, a human paired box gene: isolation and expression in developing thyroid, kidney and Wilms' tumor. Development. 1992;116:611–23.
76. Zambetti GP, Levine AJ. A comparison of the biological activities of wild-type and mutant p53. FASEB J. 1993;7:855–65.
77. Soussi T, Caron de Fromentel C, May P. Structural aspects of the p53 protein in relation to gene evolution. Oncogene. 1990;5:945–52.
78. Schmid P, Lorenz A, Hameister H, Montenarh M. Expression of p53 during mouse embryogenesis. Development. 1991;113:857–65.
79. Crawford LV, Pim DC, Lamb P. The cellular protein p53 in human tumors. Mol Biol Med. 1984;2:261–72.
80. Levine AJ, Momand J, Finlay CA. The p53 tumor supressor gene. Nature (London). 1991;351:453–6.
81. Maltzman W, Czyzyk L. UV irradiation stimulates levels of p53 cellular tumor antigen in non-transformed mouse cells. Mol Cell Biol. 1984;4:1689–94.
82. Kastan MB, Onyinye O, Sidransky D, Vogelstein B, Craig R. Participation of p53 in the cellular response to DNA damage. Cancer Res. 1991;51:6304–11.
83. El-Deiry WS, Tokino T, Velculesco VE *et al. WAF1*, a potential mediator of p53 tumor supression. Cell. 1993;75:817–25.
84. Kern SE, Kinzler KW, Bruskin A *et al.* Identification of p53 as a sequence-specific DNA-binding protein. Science. 1991;252:1708–11.
85. Barak Y, Juven T, Haffner R, Oren M. mdm2 expression is induced by wild type p53 activity. EMBO J. 1993;12(2):461–8.
86. Zambetti GP, Bargonetti J, Walker K, Prives C, Levine AJ. Wild-type p53 mediates positive regulation of gene expression through a specific DNA sequence element. Genes Dev. 1992;6:1143–52.
87. Kastan MB, Zhan Q, El-Deir WS *et al.* A mammalian cell cycle checkpoint pathway utilizing p53 and GADD45 is defective in ataxia–telangiectasia. Cell. 1992;71:587–97.
88. Ludlow JW. Interactions between SV40 large-tumor antigen and the growth supressor proteins pRB and p53. FASEB J. 1993;7:866–71.
89. Bargonetti J, Friedman PN, Kern SE, Pietenpol JA, Ogelstein B, Prives C. Wild-type but not mutant p53 immunopurified proteins bind to sequences adjacent to the SV40 origin of replication. Cell. 1991;65:1083–91.

90. Harper JW, Adam GR, Wei N, Keyomarsi K, Elledge SJ. The p21 Cdk-interacting protein Cip1 is a potent inhibitor of G1 cyclin-dependent kinases. Cell. 1993;75:805–16.
91. Donehower LA, Harvey M, Slagle BL *et al.* Mice deficient for p53 are developmentally normal but susceptible to spontaneous tumours. Nature (London). 1992;356:215–21.
92. Malkin D, Li FP, Strong LC *et al.* Germ line p53 mutations in a familial syndrome of breast cancer, sarcomas and other neoplasms. Science. 1990;250:1233–8.
93. Stanbridge EJ. Human tumor supressor genes. Ann Rev Genet. 1990;24:615–57.
94. Nigro JM, Baker SJ, Preisinger AC *et al.* Mutations in the p53 gene occur in diverse human tumour types. Nature (London). 1989;342:705–9.
95. Deffie A, Wu H, Reinke V, Lozano G. The tumor suppressor p53 regulates its own transcription. Mol Cell Biol. 1993;13(6):3415–23.
96. Stuart ET, Kioussi C, Aguzzi A, Gruss P. PAX5 expression correlates with increasing malignancy in human astrocytomas. Clin Cancer Res. 1995;1:207–14.

6
Animal models for the study of genetic susceptibility to cancer

M.N. Gould

INTRODUCTION

Many human cancers have a genetic component in their aetiology. In recent years, many specific genetic defects involved in cancer causation have been described. However, most remain to be discovered. The majority of known cancer genes have not yet been sufficiently characterized to be able to define their role in the multistage process of carcinogenesis. In order to both identify new cancer genes and to better define the function of known cancer genes, the use of appropriate model systems is crucial. While cell culture models are of value in this process, few exist in which the multistage process of carcinogenesis in specific tissues can be fully characterized. Thus, much attention is currently focused on developing rodent models of human cancer.

Animal models for the study of cancer genetics can be divided into two broad categories. The first group of models is used to identify novel cancer genes. This group of models focuses on spontaneous genetic variation and induced mutations in specific rodent populations that confer either an increased or decreased risk of cancer development. The second group of rodent models includes those engineered to study the function of known cancer genes. Examples in this second group of models include both transgenic and 'knock-out' rodent models. Models in the first group are also useful for functional studies once the genetic basis for altered cancer susceptibility is defined.

RODENT MODELS FOR THE STUDY OF INHERITED DIFFERENCES IN SUSCEPTIBILITY TO CANCER

Most studies of differential susceptibility to cancer have been conducted in either rats or mice. In several early studies, many rat and mouse outbred types and inbred strains were allowed to live out their life span and then, upon necropsy, all tumors were identified and catalogued. Interestingly, a wide range of susceptibilities to the development of organ-specific cancers was found[1–7].

While differences in susceptibility of outbred rat types to various cancers were documented, detailed genetic studies were facilitated by the description of differential susceptibilities in inbred rodent strains. Most rodent models of cancer susceptibility have been confined to organ sites of common human malignancies, including mammary gland[8], lung[9], kidney[10], liver[11] and pituitary[12]. Several examples of these organ-specific models will be given to illustrate both their usefulness and approaches to their analysis. No attempt will be made to catalogue all existing models.

Breast cancer

Both mouse and rat strains vary in susceptibility to mammary cancer. Mouse strains vary considerably in their likelihood of developing spontaneous mammary cancer; however, for the most part, these strains are relatively resistant to chemically induced cancers. Strains of laboratory mice (*Mus musculus*), such as C3H, DBA and BALB/cf will develop mammary cancer in over 70% of females in life-time studies. In contrast, BALB/c, C57BC, AR and DBA/2f are resistant to spontaneous mammary carcinomas. Some strains, including 020 and C3Hf/He, are intermediate between these in susceptibility[13].

In general, strains with high susceptibility to mammary cancer which is passed from one generation to the next carry a Bittner-type mammary virus (MMTV-S). Resistant strains are usually virus free, while intermediate strains carry a variant of MMTV[13]. Thus, this example illustrates that what at first appeared to be genetically controlled susceptibility to cancer could be explained by a viral aetiology.

In contrast to the mouse, rat mammary cancer does not have a viral aetiology[8], making it a simpler model for the study of inherited susceptibility. Strains of the laboratory rat (*Rattus norvegicus*) vary in their life-time risk of developing mammary cancer. Strains vary from the Copenhagen (Cop) rat, in which a zero incidence of spontaneous mammary carcinomas has been reported, to the Fisher (F-344) rat, with a rate of spontaneous mammary carcinomas of 8%[8]. An analysis of strain-specific incidence of spontaneous mammary cancer has suggested that the aetiology of these cancers is abscopal (that is, due to factors acting at a distance from the mammary gland). This aetiology probably involves an increased serum level of the mammary mitogenic hormone, prolactin, which originates from a genetic predisposition to pituitary hyperplasia and neoplasia of the pituitary[8,12].

In contrast to an indirect or abscopal genetic control mechanism for strain-specific susceptibility to spontaneous mammary cancer in the rat, susceptibility to carcinogen-induced mammary cancer is under direct or scopal genetic control. Rat strains vary in their susceptibility to the induction of mammary cancer by chemical carcinogens, such as DMBA or NMU. Strains such as Cop[14] or Wistar–Kyoto (Wky)[15] are almost completely resistant to carcinogen-induced mammary cancer, while strains such as Wistar–Furth (WF) are highly susceptible to mammary cancer following carcinogen administration[15]. Strains such as F-344 have an intermediate susceptibility[16]. Genetic analysis suggests that the increased susceptibility to induced mammary cancer in WF rats is controlled as a dominant trait[16]. Similarly, resistance to mammary cancer in the Cop rat is also a dominant genetic trait[17]. Rat strains such as F-344 that have an intermediate susceptibility to chemically-induced cancer lack genes for both the susceptibility and resistance traits[16]. Interestingly, the resistance trait carried by the Wky and Cop rat is epistatic over the susceptibility trait carried by the WF rat strain[15].

In order to determine whether these inherited susceptibility and resistance traits were controlled by gene activity within the mammary parenchyma (i.e. a direct genetic control), chimeric rats were constructed and tested. The site of gene action of the mammary cancer susceptibility trait in the WF strain was tested by grafting WF or F-344 (non-susceptible) mammary gland into (WF × F344) F1 rats. Since this F1 is of high susceptibility to mammary carcinogenesis, it would be expected that, if susceptibility was abscopally controlled, ectopic WF and F-344 glands in F1 hosts would be equally and highly susceptible to carcinogen-induced mammary carcinogenesis. In contrast, if susceptibility was controlled by genes acting within the mammary parenchyma, the ectopic grafts of WF mammary gland in F1 rats would develop more cancers than those of F-344 mammary grafts in similar F1 rats. The latter scenario was observed in ectopic sites in these F1 rats, suggesting that the increased heritable susceptibility to carcinogen-induced mammary cancer in WF rats was under dominant genetic and scopal control[16].

The site of action of the mammary cancer resistance gene in Cop rats was also investigated using a similar approach. Mammary tissue from susceptible WF rats was grafted into either resistant (WF × Cop) F1 or mammary tumour susceptible (WF × F344) F1 rats. Following grafting, the host F1 rats were given the mammary carcinogen DMBA. A similar frequency of mammary carcinomas developed in WF ectopic mammary gland in both the susceptible and resistant F1 hosts. This suggested that the resistance trait was also controlled within the mammary parenchyma. The Cop mammary carcinoma resistance trait is thus also a dominant genetic and scopal trait[17].

In order to understand better both the function of a gene in a rodent species and its relevance to human disease, it is important to establish its chromosomal location. Both the mouse and rat genetic maps are sufficiently dense to make mapping of genes controlling the susceptibility to specific cancers achievable. Currently, many mapping strategies used in these rodent species are based on Type II loci which consist of polymorphic regions of DNA. The most popular markers for mapping are microsatellite markers which include various specific nucleotide repeats such as di- or tetra nucleotide repeats. Other Type II markers include minisatellite and RFLP markers. The current mouse map contains approximately 4000 Type II markers[18], while the rat map contains approximately 300 but is rapidly becoming more dense[19]. Thus, the mouse map has markers that, on average, are separated by 1 cM (cMorgan) while the rat map is an order of magnitude less dense in Type II markers.

As discussed above, the Cop rat possesses a dominant genetic trait which causes it to be resistant to both spontaneous and chemically induced mammary cancer. In order to map this gene, a cosegregation approach was used in which the inheritance of the resistance trait was compared with the inheritance of many Type II markers, including both micro- and minisatellite markers. Genetic mapping for this resistance phenotype in the Cop rat was done in a (WF × Cop) F1 × WF backcross. Females of this backcross were exposed to the mammary carcinogen, DMBA. The phenotype of each rat was established 18 weeks post carcinogen administration by quantifying the number of mammary carcinomas per rat. DNA samples from each rat were also collected for genetic analyses. Sufficient numbers of informative genetic markers were available to cover approximately 75% of the genome of this backcross. A marker located on rat chromosome 2 was found to show linkage (LOD score = 4) to the resistance phenotype. A combination of genetic mapping and FISH analysis suggested that a gene, termed Mcs-1, was located on rat chromosome 2 near its centromere[20]. Further fine-mapping studies are required to identify the homologous region of Mcs-1 in the human genome.

This is an example of the genetic identification of a new breast cancer-related gene. The use of animal models to identify breast cancer genes is especially valuable because of the difficulty of mapping breast cancer genes by linkage analysis in humans. This difficulty in humans is due to the very high prevalence of breast cancer in most populations which makes it very difficult to distinguish between inherited and sporadic breast cancer in a pedigree.

Colon cancer

As was the case for mammary cancer, rodent strains vary in their propensity to develop both spontaneous and induced colon cancer. A description of animal genetic models for colon cancer allows the opportunity to contrast naturally occurring variant strains with those that were purposely, but randomly, induced.

Mouse strains vary widely in their susceptibility to chemically induced colon cancer. Using a backcross to a resistant strain, colon cancer was found in 40 of 122 dimethylhydrazine-treated mice. DNA from each phenotyped backcross mouse was characterized using polymorphic microsatellite markers which covered the entire genome at 5–30 cM chromosomal intervals. Multiple loci were found to be involved in specifying the phenotype of susceptibility to colon tumours. Jacoby *et al.*[21] reported linkage of this phenotype to a locus designated *Ccs-1*, which is located on mouse chromosome 12 between microsatellite markers D12 Mit5 and D12 and Mit6. Unlike the rat, excellent comparative maps exist between mice and humans. Using this resource, Jacoby *et al.* suggested that the human homologue for *Ccs-1* is located on human chromosome 14q near the *fos* gene[21].

While *Ccs-1* is carried by a standard mouse strain, not all genes that could alter susceptibility to colon cancer are represented in the current genetic pool of inbred mouse strains. Reasons for this include the fact that homozygosity of certain cancer genes are likely to be developmentally lethal. Thus, in order to obtain rodent models for many mutant cancer genes, mutant rodents must be actively sought. These rodent mutants may occur spontaneously and, if identified early enough, may be propagated as heterozygotes with extreme effort. Alternatively, mice may be treated with physical or chemical mutagens to increase the likelihood for the development of rare mutations that facilitate cancer development. An example of the latter approach provided an important genetic mouse model for the study of the aetiology of colon cancer.

A mouse model for colon cancer has recently been identified by Moser *et al.*[22]. Male C57BL/6J (B6) mice were treated with the mutagen ENU to cause germ-line mutation. Mutagenized male B6 mice were crossed with AKR females and the offspring of this cross were screened for inherited mutations. A pedigree was identified that carried a fully penetrant dominant mutation that caused heterozygote carrier mice rapidly to develop multiple independent colon adenomas. This mutant is termed Min for multiple intestinal neoplasia[22]. The Min mutation was mapped on mouse chromosome 18 and is tightly linked to the mouse *Apc* gene, a homologue of the human *APC* gene located on human chromosome 5q21-22. Su *et al.*[23] showed that Min mice carry a non-sense mutation in exon 15 of the *Apc* gene. This class of mutations is commonly found in human *APC* in families in which adenomatous polyposis coli is inherited. Thus, this mutation arising following germ-line mutagenesis provided the first rodent model of *APC*. It has been valuable in defining the genetic aetiology and biology of this disease. This example illustrates the utility of supplementing naturally occurring genetic susceptibility cancer models with models based on random germ-line mutagenesis.

The availability of such a penetrant mutation as Apc-Min for colon cancer also provides a murine genetic model to explore the subtle variations that are often seen in a human cancer genetic syndrome. Families inheriting mutant alleles of *APC* display variations in phenotype that cannot be accounted for by differences in the inherited mutant allele. The first indication that the Min mutation could be useful to explore modifying genes that interact with the mutant *Apc* gene came from the observations of Moser *et al.*[24] which indicated that, when Min was placed on a different genetic background, the yield of colon tumours varied greatly. For example, when Min was on a B6 background, an average of 29 intestinal adenomas developed. In contrast, only 5 tumours developed in B6 × AKR background.

The above observation provided the framework for the identification of a locus which could modify the biological consequences of Min. Progeny of (AKR × B6-Min) × B6 backcross were genotyped using microsatellite probes distributed throughout the genome. A marker on the distal portion of mouse chromosome 4 was linked to the frequency of intestinal tumours developing in Min/+ mice. This genetically identified locus was named *Mom-1*. Animals with the AKR allele of *Mom-1* had, on average, 10 fewer tumours than animals that were homozygous for the B6 allele of *Mom-1*. Further genetic analyses suggested the possibility of additional modifier genes in the AKR mouse[25].

The above is an example of an important use of animal models in the study of cancer genetics. This is one of the first well-documented genetic characterizations of a polygenic cancer trait. The study of polygenic traits provides a new approach in cancer genetics to investigate gene function by identifying loci which modify the penetrance of mutant genes.

The study of the Min mouse also illustrates an additional utility of animal genetic models. Characterization of *APC* mutant alleles in cancers in humans has thus far only implicated neoplasms of the gastrointestinal tract as being associated with this genotype. The Min murine model has extended the search for new organ sites at which the *APC* mutation may be involved in carcinogenesis. Mice carrying the Min mutation (Min/+) both develop spontaneous mammary carcinomas and are highly susceptible to chemically induced mammary cancers[26]. Furthermore, the propensity of Min/+ mice to develop mammary cancer is modifiable by genetic background[26]. Whether the same or different modifier genes interact with the Min allele in the genesis of mammary and intestinal cancers is as yet unknown. Thus, a murine model of a well-documented human cancer syndrome gene has extended the study of this gene beyond the human target organs currently being examined.

ENGINEERED CANCER GENETIC MODELS

As discussed above, natural and randomly-induced variations in rodent strains are valuable for both identifying new cancer genes and for studying the function of known cancer genes. These variant strains are now complemented by new biotechnically engineered rodent strains that either express a specifically introduced gene or lack the expression of a normally expressed gene. The former strains are termed transgenic and have been constructed in mice and rats for oncological investigations. The latter strains are termed 'knock-outs' and are so far restricted to murine strains.

Transgenic rodents

Transgenic rodents have been valuable in studying the aetiology and biology of cancer. Not only has this technology been useful to assess the role of specific genes, such as oncogenes, and growth factors in the carcinogenic process, but is now starting to provide strategies to identify new cancer-related genes. Listing of oncogenes and growth factors that have been inserted into transgenic rodents is outside the focus of this review and they have been tabulated elsewhere[27]. Examples of this technology will be discussed here in order to illustrate the utility and limitations of this class of cancer genetic models.

Most recent uses of transgenic models to define the role of oncogenes in the carcinogenic process have targeted expression of oncogenes and growth factors to specific tissues. This has generally been accomplished by the use of organ-specific promoters to drive targeted genes. For example, the Keratin-10 promoter has been used to drive *ras* in mouse-skin causing papillomas[28]. The albumin promoter has been used in the liver to direct genes associated with the hepatitis P virus to induce liver carcinomas[29] while the insulin gene promoter region has been used to target T antigen to the pancreas, resulting in pancreatic carcinoma[30]. Mammary carcinomas have been induced by directing a large variety of oncogenes and growth factors to the mammary gland using the regulatory region of the MMTV[31] or whey acidic protein (WAP)[32]. These and related studies have clearly demonstrated the utility of the transgenic model for characterizing the role of specific oncogenes in the aetiology of cancer in specific organs.

It must, however, also be stressed that these transgenic models have limitations in experimental oncology. Cancer is a clonal disease in which cancers develop from an individual cell surrounded by genetically normal tissue. In the transgenic model, cancer develops from a single cell with an activated oncogenic transgene surrounded by genetically similar cells. Additionally, the quantitative regulation of gene expression in transgenic tissues is limited by the availability of organ-specific promoters. This makes matching tissue protein levels from transgenes to physiological levels difficult. Also, several organ-specific promoters, such as MMTV and WAP, require hormonal stimulation for expression. The same hormones that drive these genes can independently modulate carcinogenesis in the target organ. This latter situation confounds the interpretation of the transgene's role in cancer aetiology.

Finally, in most studies, only a limited number of independent transgenic strains are produced and characterized. Often differences in cancer incidence in seemingly similar strains are reported. For example, the MMTV-*neu* mouse, first reported by Muller *et al.* had such a high frequency of mammary tumours that the authors suggested that, when activated, *neu* transformed by a single-step mechanism[33]. When very similar mice were produced by a second group of investigators, a much lower number of cancers per mouse developed, challenging the initial conclusion of a single-step mechanism of *neu* transformation[34]. This discrepancy was probably due to a positional-integration effect due to the limited number of strains under study. In spite of all of these limitations, if used with appropriate caution, the transgenic model can be very useful to characterize oncogene activity in an organ-specific *in vivo* setting.

For a limited number of organ sites, an alternative 'transgenic' model can be used to complement the classical transgenic model while overcoming certain of the above listed limitations. This model uses replication-defective retroviral vectors to deliver transgenes to either neonatal or adult rodents. An example of this technology as applied to mammary carcinogenesis will be discussed.

In this alternative model, the c-DNA for an oncogene or growth factor is subcloned into a retroviral ('gene-therapy') vector which is then packaged into a replication-defective virus. This virus is concentrated to give titres up to 10^8 cfu/ml and is then used to transfer the gene of interest into a specific tissue. The tissue to be target must be physically accessible and have receptors for the virus. It must also be capable of cell division for permanent integration of the gene under study. An ideal tissue for this approach is the adult mammary gland. Here, the concentrated virus is infused into the milk lumen of the gland and is taken up through amphotrophic receptors found on the luminal surface of the mammary epithelial cells. Integration is encouraged by inducing mammary cell division by pharmacologically raising the circulating level of the mammary mitogen prolactin. This method allows one, not only to target the cell type to be genetically supplemented, but also to control the percentage of altered cells in a tissue by adjusting the virus titre that is infused. In addition, since organ specificity is achieved physically, a much larger array of promoters can be used to better model tissue-specific physiological conditions. Importantly, for the most part DNA integration following virus uptake is random. Thus, each infected cell has a unique integration site, reducing the confounding effect of integration position on the function of the gene under study.

This *in-situ* gene-transfer method has so far been used to target two oncogenes, *ras*[35] and *neu*[36], to the adult rat mammary gland. Transfer of both genes resulted in the development of metastatic mammary carcinomas. *Neu* transfer to a mammary cell was, however, approximately 250 times more likely to yield a carcinoma than was *ras*. Tumours arising from the activity of both oncogenes gave monoclonal tumours that required events in addition to oncogene insertion for their development. The latter conclusions can not always be determined in classical transgenic models.

Recently several groups have combined the use of classical transgenic models with retroviral models. For example, if transgenic mice carrying C-*Myc* with haemopoietic targeting are infected with retrovirus carrying activated *ras* or *raf*, the incidence of B-lymphoid tumorigenesis is increased[37]. This combination of gene transfer technologies is also being used to identify new cancer genes. In this approach, transgenic mice carrying a specific oncogene are infected with retrovirus which does not carry an oncogene, but relies on integrating in the vicinity of an undefined gene that could cooperate with the transgene following its activation by the insertion of a retrovirus in its vicinity. This method allows the tagging and identification of new candidate cancer genes[27].

Knock-out mice

Transgenic models provide an excellent tool to study dominant oncogenes or overexpressed growth factors. However, it is now clear that many important genetic lesions in malignant tumours involve the loss of genetic information. In order to model this loss in animal cancer models, it is necessary to inactivate one or both copies of specific target genes. While this can sometimes be accomplished by random germ-line mutagenesis as described above for the *Apc* gene, this approach is far from efficient if a specific gene, such as p53, is being targeted. Fortunately, an alternative more-specific technology is now available to establish animal models that lack specific gene function.

The products of this technology are referred to as 'knock-out' mice. As generally used, the researcher first manipulates an embryonic stem cell (ES) to mutate or delete specific genes. This manipulation is based on introducing into a cell constructs that contain both homologous and non-homologous or mutant regions of a targeted gene. This sequence then replaces a region of the wild-type gene through homologous recombination. Following selection of a cell line in which the desired recombination event occurred, the cell is used to generate knock-out mice. In order to produce such mice, ES cells are injected into blastocysts which are then implanted into pseudopregnant mothers. This procedure results in the production of chimeric mice with some having germ cells derived from the altered ES cell[38]. Such mice are then founders for mice strains that are heterozygous for a specific gene deletion or mutation. Homozygotes can also be produced, either through selective breeding or via *in-vitro* manipulation of the ES clone prior to blastocyst injection. It should, however, be stressed that it is often not possible to produce homozygous knock-out of many cancer-related genes which are required for normal development. This is unfortunate since it would be very enlightening to be able to observe the biology of the target tissue which completely lacked a suppressor gene-encoded protein.

Fortunately, a new technology is beginning to emerge that will provide methods to selectively inactivate genes in specific target tissues. Such technology could then be used to totally delete a gene in a specific organ while sparing the other organs and possibly avoiding prenatal or neonatal death. Thus far, this new technology has not been used to inactivate cancer-specific genes. In the first published report of its use, Gu *et al.* deleted the DNA polymerase B gene in just the T cells of mice[39]. The method used takes advantage of a recombinase enzyme from bacteriophage P1 termed Cre. Cre acts by first aligning short DNA sequences termed loxP that naturally occur in phage. Next, this recombinase removes the DNA between these loxP sequences. In order to selectively knock-out a gene in a specific mouse tissue, this enzymology is combined with standard ES and transgenic technologies. ES cells are produced so that the targeted gene remains intact, but is flanked by loxP sequences. Mice derived from these ES cells have normal gene function and are thus developmentally normal. Using such a mouse strain, it is possible to remove the flanked target gene in any specific tissue by targeting expression of Cre recombinase to that tissue. In practice, this is accomplished by mating the mouse with the loxP flanked target gene to a transgenic mouse in which Cre is targeted to a specific tissue by its promoter region. In the future, Cre may also be delivered by alternative means, such as by retroviral vectors.

This new technology to produce organ-specific knock-outs should rapidly increase the usefulness of knock-out mice in cancer genetic research. For example, it may allow the production of homozygous knock-outs of *Apc* in the intestine or mammary gland which is not now achievable. In spite of the limitations of the conventional knock-out technology, there have been certain gene targets that have been totally knocked-out allowing the study of important cancer genes, such as p53.

Donehower *et al.* were able to successfully use the classical non-specific ES technology to produce mice that were total deficient in p53 expression[40]. This fact alone was quite important in that it showed that the p53 was not necessary for the completion of the developmental process in mice. In addition, it was shown that these p53 null mice developed a variety of cancers by the time they were 6 months old. Many of these tumours were lymphomas[41]. As was the case for the Apc-Min mouse, the genetic background on which the mutation was placed was also important for phenotypes resulting from the p53 null mutation. For example, when p53 null was placed into 129 mouse strain, which normally has a low incidence of lymphoma, lymphomas readily appeared. In addition, tumours to which 129 mice are normally susceptible, such as teratocarcinomas, appeared at greater frequencies with shorter latencies[41].

Such mice can also be used to study multistage chemical carcinogenesis. For example, Kemp *et al.* showed that p53 loss was associated with the later progression step in skin carcinogenesis in which papillomas progressed to advanced carcinomas[42].

SUMMARY AND CONCLUSIONS

The mouse and rat are the two most often used animal models for cancer investigations. Both species have overlapping utilities; however, both also have unique characteristics for modeling organ-specific cancers. It is thus important that genetic models of both species be established and used in a complementary manner. Currently the mouse is both the best genetically characterized species and has best had procedures for genetic engineering adapted to it. Fortunately, great progress is being made both in genetically characterizing the rat and in adapting genetic engineering methods for use in this species. The mouse and rat genetic maps are now sufficiently dense for most mapping studies. In addition, methods are now routinely available to produce both mouse and rat transgenic strains. Unfortunately, at the present time, the 'knock-out' technology is only available for the mouse. Work, however, is proceeding to develop ES cells for the rat in order to adapt this key technology to this species.

Identification of genetic loci which control susceptibility to cancer is not only important in studying cancer aetiology, but is important in both cancer risk assessment and in experimental therapeutics. Animal models are invaluable in rapidly identifying new independent and interacting loci that are involved in cancer aetiology. The use of inbred rodent models with short generation times allows efficient identification of simple genetic and polygenic traits which are difficult or impossible to study in higher species. While many cancer genes that will be identified in rodents have important human counterparts, others may not. Genes that do not have human homologues that are involved in rodent cancer aetiology may still be valuable for addressing cancer in man. For example, if a rodent gene is found that prevents a certain cancer, the product of that gene may be a novel drug discovery target. In other words, it may be possible to produce a pharmacological agent that will mimic the activity of the rodent gene in humans. Such a drug might be used to treat or prevent a specific type of human cancer.

In addition to uncovering new cancer genes, animal models are the key in defining mechanisms by which identified cancer syndrome genes participate in cancer aetiology, biology and therapy. The use of transgenic models to study dominant oncogene function has made important contributions to our understanding of the role of these genes in the multistage process of carcinogenesis. These models are also now being used to screen potential cancer chemopreventive agents and to develop new approaches to cancer therapy.

These transgenic models are complemented by knock-out murine models for similar studies of recessive cancer genes. These models have thus far been limited in that, unlike the case for transgenic models, organ specificity is not available with current knock-out technologies. This situation is soon to be remedied with the advent of new organ-specific knock-out technology. These new methods will greatly expand the utility of animal models for cancer study.

Finally, it should be stated that while the current emphasis in cancer genetics is shifting to the direct study of cells and DNA obtained from human pedigree members and tumour biopsies, these approaches have important limitations. The study of family pedigrees is limited to the identification of major genetic factors, especially in prevalent cancers, such as those of the female breast. In addition, the study of macromolecules from cancers yields more descriptive than mechanistic information. Finally the study of genetic alterations in tissue cultured human cells may not always reflect *in-vivo* realities. Animal models have played and will continue to play a key role in the study of the genetics of cancer.

Acknowledgements

Work in the author's laboratory on the genetics of cancer in rodent models is supported by NIH PHS grants CA28954 and CA44387.

References

1. Burek JD, Hollander CV. Incidence patterns of spontaneous tumors in BN/Bi rats. J Natl Cancer Inst. 1977;58:99–105.
2. Sass B, Rabstein LS, Madison R, Nims RM, Peters RL, Kelloff GJ. Incidence of spontaneous neoplasms in F344 rats throughout the natural life-span. J Natl Cancer Inst. 1975;54:1449–56.
3. Davis RK, Stevenson GT, Busch KA. Tumor incidence in normal Sprague–Dawley female rats. J Natl Cancer Inst. 1955;15:194–7.
4. Thompson SW, Huseby RA, Fox MA, Davis CL, Hunt RD. Spontaneous tumors in the Sprague–Dawley rat. J Natl Cancer Inst. 1961;27:1037–57.
5. Maekawa A, Odashima S. Spontaneous tumors in ACI/N rats. J Natl Cancer Inst. 1975;55:1437–45.
6. Dunning WF, Curtis MR. The respective roles of longevity and genetic specificity in the occurrence of spontaneous tumors in the hybrids between two inbred lines of rats. Cancer Res. 1945;5:62–81.
7. Crain RC. Spontaneous tumors in the Rochester strain of the Wistar rat. Am J Pathol. 1958;34:311–23.
8. Gould MN, Wang B, Moore CJ. Modulation of mammary carcinogenesis by enhancer and suppressor genes. In: Colburn NJ, ed. Genes and signal transduction in multistage carcinogenesis. New York: Marcel Decker, Inc.; 1989:19–38.
9. Chen B, Johanson L, Wiest JS, Anderson MW, You M. The second intron of the K-*ras* gene contains regulatory elements associated with mouse lung tumor susceptibility. Proc Natl Acad Sci USA. 1994;91(4):1589–93.
10. Yeung RS, Buetow KH, Testa JR, Knudson AG Jr. Susceptibility to renal carcinoma in the Eker rat involves a tumor suppressor gene on chromosome 10. Proc Natl Acad Sci USA. 1993;90(17):8038–42.
11. Buchmann A, Bauer-Hofmann R, Mahr J, Drinkwater NR, Luz A, Schwarz M. Mutational activation of the c-Ha-*ras* gene in liver tumors of different rodent strains: Correlation with susceptibility to hepatocarcinogenesis. Proc Natl Acad Sci USA. 1991;88(3):911–5.
12. Wiklund J, Rutledge J, Gorski J. A genetic model for the inheritance of pituitary tumor susceptibility in F344 rats. Endocrinology. 1981;109:1708–14.
13. Medina D. Mammary tumors. In: Foster JH, Small JD, Fox JG, eds. The mouse in biomedical research, Vol 4. New York: Academic Press; 1982:373–96.
14. Dunning WF, Curtis MR, Segaloff A. Strain differences in response to diethylstilbestrol and the induction of mammary gland and bladder cancer in the rat. Cancer Res. 1947;7:511–21.
15. Haag JD, Newton MA, Gould MN. Mammary carcinoma suppressor and susceptibility genes in the Wistar–Kyoto rat. Carcinogenesis. 1992;13(10):1933–5.
16. Gould MN. Inheritance and site of expression of genes controlling susceptibility to mammary cancer in an inbred rat model. Cancer Res. 1986;46:1199–202.
17. Isaacs JT. Genetic control of resistance to chemically induced mammary adenocarcinogenesis in the rat. Cancer Res. 1986;46:3958–63.
18. Dietrich WF, Miller JC, Steen FG *et al.* A genetic map of the mouse with 4,006 simple sequence high polymorphisms. Nature Genet. 1994;7 Suppl:220–45.
19. Serikawa T, Kuramoto T, Hilbert P *et al.* Rat gene mapping using PCR-analyzed microsatellites. Genetics. 1992;131:701–21.

20. Hsu L-C, Kennan WS, Shepel L *et al.* Genetic identification of Mcs-1, a rat mammary carcinoma suppressor gene. Cancer Res. 1994;54:2765–70.
21. Jacoby R, Hohman, Marshall *et al.* The use of microsatellite markers to map colon susceptibility genes in the mouse. Genomics. 1994;22:381–7.
22. Moser AR, Pitot HC, Dover WF. A dominant mutation that predisposes to multiple intestinal neoplasia in the mouse. Science. 1990;247:322–4.
23. Su LK, Kinzler KW, Vogelstein B *et al.* A germline mutation of murine homolog of the APC gene causes multiple intestinal neoplasia. Science. 1992;256:668–70.
24. Moser AR, Dove WF, Roth KA, Gordon JI. The *Min* (multiple intestinal neoplasia) mutation: its effect on gut epithelial cell differentiation and interaction with a modifier system. J Cell Biol. 1992;116:1517–26.
25. Dietrich WF, Lander ES, Smith JS *et al.* Genetic identification of Mom-1, a major modifier locus affecting *min*-induced intestinal neoplasia in the mouse. Cell. 1993;75:631–9.
26. Moser AR, Mattes EM, Dove WF, Lindstrom MJ, Haag JD, Gould MN. *Min*, a mutation in the murine Apc gene, predisposes to mammary carcinomas and focal alveolar hyperplasias. Proc Natl Acad Sci USA. 1993;90:8977–81.
27. Fowlis DJ, Balmain A. Oncogenes and tumour suppressor genes in transgenic mouse models of neoplasia. Eur J Cancer. 1993;29(4):638–45.
28. Bailleul B, Surani MA, White S *et al.* Skin hyperkeratosis and papilloma formation in transgenic mice expressing a *ras* oncogene from a suprabasal keratin promoter. Cell. 1990;62:697–708.
29. Chisari FV, Klopchin K, Moriyama T *et al.* Molecular pathogenesis of hepatocellular carcinoma in hepatitis B virus transgenic mice. Cell. 1989;59:1145–56.
30. Hanahan D. Heritable formation of pancreatic β-cell tumours in transgenic mice expressing recombinant insulin/simian virus 40 oncogenes. Nature. 1991;315:115–22.
31. Sinn E, Muller W, Pattengale P, Tepler I, Wallace R, Leder P. Co-expression of MMTV/v-Ha-*ras* and MMTV/c-*myc* genes in transgenic mice. Synergistic action of oncogenes *in vivo*. Cell. 1987;49:465–75.
32. Langdon WY, Harris AW, Cory S. Acceleration of B-lymphoid tumorigenesis in Eμ-*myc* transgenic mice by v-H-*ras* and v-*raf* but not v-*abl*. Oncogene Res. 1989;4:253–8.
33. Muller WJ, Sinn E, Pattengale PK, Wallace R, Leder P. Single-step induction of mammary adenocarcinoma in transgenic mice bearing the activated c-*neu* oncogene. Cell. 1988;54:105–15.
34. Bouchard L, Lamarre L, Tremblay PJ, Jolicoeur P. Stochastic appearance of mammary tumors in transgenic mice carrying the MMTV/c-*neu* oncogene. Cell. 1989;57:931–6.
35. Wang B, Kennan WS, Yasukawa-Barnes J, Lindstrom MJ, Gould MN. Carcinoma induction following direct *in situ* transfer of v-Ha-*ras* into rat mammary epithelial cells using replication-defective retrovirus vectors. Cancer Res. 1991;51:2642–8.
36. Wang B, Kennan WS, Yasukawa-Barnes J, Lindstrom MJ, Gould MN. Frequent induction of mammary carcinomas following *neu* oncogene transfer into *in situ* mammary epithelial cells of susceptible and resistant strains of rats. Cancer Res. 1991;51:5649–54.
37. Langdon WY, Harris AW, Cory S. Acceleration of B-lymphoid tumorigenesis in Eμ-*myc* transgenic mice by v-H-*ras* and v-*raf* but not v-*abl*. Oncogene Res. 1989;4:253–8.
38. Capecchi MR. The new mouse genetics: Altering the genome by gene targeting. Trends Genet. 1989;5:70–6.
39. Gu H, Marth JD, Orban PC, Mossmann H, Rajewsky K. Deletion of a DNA polymerase β gene segment in T cells using cell type-specific gene targeting. Science. 1994;265:103–6.
40. Donehower LA, Harvey M, Slagle BL *et al.* Mice deficient for p53 are developmentally normal but susceptible to spontaneous tumours. Nature. 1992;356:215–21.
41. Harvey M, McArthur MJ, Montgomery CA Jr, Bradley A, Donehower LA. Genetic background alters the spectrum of tumors that develop in p53-deficient mice. FASEB J. 1993;7(10):938–43.
42. Kemp CJ, Donehower LA, Bradley A, Balmain A. Reduction of p53 gene dosage does not increase initiation or promotion but enhances malignant progression of chemically induced skin tumors. Cell. 1993;74(5):813–22.

7
Animal models to look for polygenic effects in cancer predisposition

T.A. Dragani and M.A. Pierotti

RODENT INBRED STRAINS GENETICALLY SUSCEPTIBLE TO DIFFERENT TYPES OF TUMOURS

Most inbred strains of laboratory rodents derive from the wild *Mus musculus musculus* and *Mus musculus domesticus* that were trapped at the beginning of the century. Although some intermixing between strains has occurred, and some stains are derived one from the other, phylogenetic analysis has shown that laboratory inbred strains differ genetically from each other[1]. Therefore, the laboratory inbred strains may be a sufficiently wide representation of the distribution and frequency of different alleles, including those related to cancer predisposition, of the wild-type murine population from which they were derived.

A recent listing of 430 murine inbred strains was reported[2]. We found in this listing 38 different strains with a spontaneous incidence of a particular tumour type higher than 10% (Table 7.1). These strains could be considered as genetically susceptible to this tumour type, even if to varying degrees. There are strains with a high genetic predisposition to develop lymphomas/leukaemias, mammary, liver, ovary, pituitary, stomach and renal tumours. In most cases, genetic susceptibility is limited to a single tumour type. This figure, however, is a significant underestimation of reality, because only a minority of the strains reported in the listing[2] have been checked for their incidence of spontaneous tumours. In addition, it is worth mentioning that another way to assess the susceptibility of mice to tumour development is to treat them with chemical carcinogens. Indeed, in all cases that have been studied, a high incidence of spontaneous tumours is parallelled by a high susceptibility to the development of the same tumour type by chemical carcinogen administration[3,4].

By using chemical carcinogens, murine strains susceptible and resistant to sarcoma development were identified[5,6]. Genetic susceptibility and resistance to carcinogen-induced intestinal tumour development have also been described in mouse strains[7,8].

The possibility that genes which give a predisposition to developing tumours are relatively frequent is also suggested by the results of Bangrazi *et al.*[9]. They

Table 7.1 Inbred murine strains with more than a 10% incidence of spontaneous tumours at defined sites, as listed in Reference 2

*Tumour type**	*Strain*
Fibrosarcoma	AB
Haemangio–endothelioma	HR/De
Intestine	$C57BL/6J^{Min\dagger}$
Leukaemia–lymphoma**	AB; ACR; AKR; BALB/c; C57BL/10; C57L; C58; FB; HRS; NZO; P/J; PBA; PL; RF; RFM; RW; SAMR1; SJL
Liver	CBA; CE; C3H; VY
Lung	A; ACR; A2G; BALB/c; BN/a; BN/b; CCD57BR; MA; PBA; RFM; SWR; TM; T739; XVII
Ovary	CE; C3H; RIII
Ovary–teratoma	LT
Pituitary	C57BR/cd; C57L; NZB
Renal	BALB/c/Cd
Stomach	I; TM
Testicular teratoma	129

* mammary tumors were not included, because their incidence may vary in the same strain, depending on the MMTV infection;
† see Reference 25;
** including: reticulum cell sarcoma, reticulum tissue neoplasm, lymphatic leukaemia, haematopoietic tumour, histiocytic neoplasm

showed that, starting from eight different laboratory inbred strains of mice, and crossing them together mix the different genotypes, they were able to select two lines, one highly susceptible and the other one highly resistant to skin tumorigenesis.

Genetic predisposition and resistance to tumour development is not limited to mice, but is also observed in rats for mammary[10–13], intestine[14,15], gastric[16,17], liver[18] and renal[19] tumours and in hamsters for tumours of endocrine glands[20].

From these data, we can conclude that it is relatively easy to select inbred strains predisposed to particular tumour types and, therefore, that the frequency of alleles which give a predisposition to cancer must be relatively high in wild populations of rodents. These alleles can be selected and revealed by the inbreeding process. Whereas, in an outbred population, because of genetic heterogeneity, it cannot be proved if an individual animal developed a cancer by chance or because it was genetically predisposed, in inbred strains, the genetic effect can be demonstrated. Therefore, inbred strains predisposed to tumour development may provide a unique experimental system of analysis of genes which predispose to cancer.

In this review, we do not consider the murine models of genetic susceptibility to lymphoma and mammary tumours associated with viral infection, since they have been reviewed in great detail already[21–24].

EXPERIMENTAL EVIDENCE FOR MULTIPLE GENES INVOLVED IN GENETIC SUSCEPTIBILITY TO DIFFERENT FORMS OF CANCER

Recently, an interesting mutant strain of mouse (*Min*) with a high spontaneous incidence of multiple intestinal neoplasms has been isolated[25]. The *Min* mutation has been mapped to proximal chromosome 18, in a region homologous to human chromosome 5q21-q22, where the APC and MCC genes have been mapped[26]. The mutation responsible for multiple intestinal neoplasia in *Min* mice has been identified as a non-sense mutation in the *Apc* gene, the murine homologue of the human *APC* gene, whose germ-line mutations are responsible for familial adenomatous polyposis (FAP)[27]. Therefore, the *Min* mouse provides an experimental model for a human cancer syndrome (FAP). However, the occurrence of intestinal tumours in *Min* mice is modified by its genetic background, and a locus that suppresses *Min*-induced intestinal neoplasia has been mapped to mouse distal chromosome 4, and named *Mom-1* (Table 7.2)[28].

It has been suggested that another locus, named *Scc-1* and located on chromosome 2, controls carcinogen-induced colon tumours in recombinant congenic mouse strains[29].

Plasmacytomas, i.e. tumours of mature B cells, can be induced in mice by ip administration of paraffin oils or pristane. Genetically susceptible and resistant strains to plasmacytomagenesis have been identified, and different loci were found associated with resistance to plasmacytoma induction and mapped on chromosomes 1 and 4 (Table 7.2)[30,31]

Murine models of genetic predisposition and resistance to carcinogen- and radiation-induced lymphomas have been recently described. The analysis of different samples (F2, backcross, recombinant inbred) with a limited number of genetic markers showed that a locus on chromosome 7 (near *Hbb*) and a locus on chromosome 4 (in a region between *Ifa* and *b*) are involved in carcinogen- and radiation-induced lymphomas, respectively. The authors also indicated the possible existence of other loci which affect lymphoma development (Table 7.2)[32,33].

Genetic susceptibility to skin carcinogenesis appears to be controlled by multiple genes, as shown by different groups in different crosses. However, these genes have not yet been mapped[9,34].

GENETIC SUSCEPTIBILITY TO LUNG CARCINOGENESIS

Some inbred murine strains have a high genetic predisposition to lung tumour development. Lung tumours develop spontaneously late in life and are also easily induced by chemical carcinogens[3,4,35,36].

The A/J strain is genetically susceptible to lung carcinogenesis, whereas the C57BL/6J, C3H/He and other strains are resistant. The F1 hybrids of susceptible and resistant strains are usually susceptible[3,4,35,36]. Genetic studies of susceptibility to lung carcinogenesis have shown that three genes, called pulmonary adenoma susceptibility or Pas genes, control the multiplicity (i.e. the number of macroscopically identified lung tumours per mouse) of urethan-induced lung tumours in recombinant inbred (RI) mice derived from a cross of the A/J and the

Table 7.2 Mapped loci affecting genetic predisposition to certain tumour types in mice

Locus	*Chromosome*	*Closest genetic marker (s)*	*Target organ or tumour type*	*Cross*	*LOD score*	*Variance explained (%)*	*Reference*
Hcs-1	7	*Mtv-1*	Liver	AC3F2	3.2	16.9	53
Hcs-2	8	*D8Mit35*	Liver	AC3F2	3.2	21.5	53
Hcs-3	12	*Igh-V*	Liver	AC3F2	2.8	13.9	53
Hcs-4	2	*D2Mit25*	Liver	(C3S)B6	3.7	14.8	55
Hcs-5	5	*D5Mit6*	Liver	(C3S)B6	2.3	9.4	55
Hcs-6	19	*D19Mit27*	Liver	(C3S)B6	2.8	11.5	55
Lyr	4	*b/Ifa*	Lymphoma	CXS RI	—	—	33
Min	18	*Apc*	Colon	B6X (AKRXB6-Min)	—	—	26
				B6X (CASTXB6-Min)	—	—	—
Mom-1	4	*D4Mit13/D4Mit16*	Colon	B6X (AKRXB6-Min)	4.7	35	28
		D4Mit13/D4Mit54		B6X (MAXB6-Min)	10.9	68	—
		D4Mit54/D4Mit16		B6X (CASTXB6-Min)	2.5	25	—
Pas-1	6	*Kras2*	Lung	AC3F2	9.4	44.5	42
Pct^{r1}	4	*Ifa/D4Rck41*	Plasmacytoma	BALB/c.DBA/2 congenic	—	—	31
Pct^{r2}	4	*Tnfr-1/Pkcz*	Plasmacytoma	BALB/c.DBA/2 congenic	—	—	31
Scc-1	2	CD44	Colon	Balb/c-STS recombinant congenic	—	—	29
Unnamed	1	*Fcgr2*	Plasmacytoma	BALB/cX (BALB/cXDBA/2N)	≈ 2.2	—	30
Unnamed	7	*c/Hbb*	Lymphoma	AKRX (AKRXC57L/J)	—	—	32

C57BL/6J strains[37]. One of these genes has been previously associated with the *Kras-2* locus on chromosome 6[38]. Several studies have indicated that the H-2 locus, or genes close to H-2, affect lung tumour susceptibility in mice[39–41].

We have studied the segregation of lung tumour susceptibility in an F2 cross of the susceptible A/J and the resistant C3H/He mouse strains. We used quantitative factors, measuring the number (N), volume (V) and total lung tumour volume (N×V) as indices of susceptibility to lung carcinogenesis[4]. We identified a genomic region important in determining quantitative variation in lung tumour susceptibility (measured as N×V) on chromosome 6. The distal markers on chromosome 6, *D6Mit10, Raf-1, D6Mit13 (Prp), Kras-2 (D6Mit1-4)* and *D6Int1*, covering a region of 35 cM, were all significantly associated ($p<0.01$) with the expression of the phenotype. By using interval mapping techniques (MAPMAKER-QTL), a single quantitative trait locus (QTL) appears to be found near *Kras-2*. The locus we have identified represents a major lung tumour susceptibility factor, due to its high LOD score and percentage of variability explained, and, therefore, we named it *Pas-1*[42] (Table 7.2).

In our cross, we did not find any other association between other chromosomal regions and lung tumour susceptibility. It is possible that additional genes involved in lung tumour development lie in genomic regions that we have not covered by genetic markers. Phylogenetic relationships indicate that the A/J and the C3H/He strains we used in our previous analysis are closely related[1]. As a consequence, we had difficulties in finding polymorphisms between the two strains and we did not succeed in saturating the whole genome with the available genetic markers. The difficulty in finding markers between the A/J and the C3H/He strains could be overcome by the use of phylogenetically distant strains, such as the *Mus spretus* or *Mus castaneus*[43,44], to be crossed with the A/J (lung tumour susceptible) strain. Interspecific crosses have been used successfully to improve the degree of polymorphism in plants[45,46] where QTLs were mapped at a resolution as high as 3 cM. Since this is also true in mice, we could expect a good saturation of the genome with the available molecular markers, following interspecific crosses.

Therefore, we repeated the lung carcinogenesis experiment in an interspecific test-cross population, obtained by crossing the A/J strain with *M. spretus*, and then crossing the resulting F1 mice with C57BL/6J mice. The interspecific (A/J × *M. spretus*) × C57BL/6J mice were treated and analysed in the same way as the previous AC3F2 mice. We were able to confirm the mapping of *Pas-1* on distal chromosome 6, around *Kras-2*. In addition, we obtained evidence for the existence of lung tumour suppressor loci deriving from the *M. spretus* strain (data not shown). The complete analysis of the genome in this interspecific sample will allow the mapping of these loci.

Analysis of homology between mice and humans in the chromosome 6 region containing the lung tumour-susceptibility gene(s) showed that the murine *Raf-1* region corresponds to a human 3p region. Interestingly, the 3p region is frequently deleted in human lung tumours, and it has been suggested that an oncosuppressor gene is found in this region[47]. A longer region of homology in mouse chromosome 6, spanning from *D6Mit13 (Prp)* to *Kras-2*, corresponds to human 12p. Our results showed that *Pas-1* gene is probably localized near *Kras-2*, i.e. in a mouse chromosomal region corresponding to human 12p12.

Murine lung tumours appear to represent the experimental counterpart of human lung adenocarcinomas, since these two tumour types show common molecular features, e.g. KRAS mutations, expression of the SP-A gene[48,49]. Therefore, the mapping of a gene responsible for genetic susceptibility to lung carcinogenesis on mouse chromosome 6 (near *Kras-2*) would suggest that genetic markers localized in the corresponding human chromosomal region (12p12) should be studied for possible linkage with lung adenocarcinoma development.

MURINE HEPATOCARCINOGENESIS AS AN EXPERIMENTAL MODEL OF MULTIPLE TUMOUR SUSCEPTIBILITY GENES

A well-documented experimental model of hepatocellular carcinoma (HCC) is the murine inbred strain C3H which presents a high spontaneous incidence of HCCs (up to 70% incidence in a life-time experiment)[3]. Although this strain exhibits such a high incidence of spontaneous HCCs, it does not show any sign of liver cirrhosis or liver dysfunction that could be associated with a genetic susceptibility.

Genetic susceptibility to liver carcinogenesis is not a discrete trait but refers to relative quantitative values. We and others have previously reported that genes affecting susceptibility to murine hepatocarcinogenesis control the progression (tumour size) but not the frequency (tumour number) of carcinogen-induced liver tumours[4,50,51]. The genes responsible for the susceptibility to murine liver carcinogenesis were called *Hcs*[52].

We investigated the segregation of liver tumour susceptibility in the same F2 population obtained from the cross between the strains C3H/He and A/J (resistant to liver carcinogenesis). The percentage of liver volume occupied by nodules (V%) was used as a quantitative index of susceptibility to liver carcinogenesis. This index differs from one parental strain to the other[4] by a factor of more than 100, thus making the dissection of genes affecting the character possible.

Three genomic regions important in determining quantitative variation in liver tumour susceptibility were identified on chromosomes 7, 8 and 12. We named these loci *Hcs-1, Hcs-2,* and *Hcs-3* respectively[53] (Table 7.2). *Hcs-1* (chromosome 7) and *Hcs-2* (chromosome 8) derived from the C3H/He strain, and the *Hcs-3* was unexpectedly associated with the A/J allele.

Our results showed that the three *Hcs* loci we found accounted together for up to 40% of the variability of susceptibility for liver tumour development, as measured by the V% index. We cannot exclude that chromosomal regions not covered by any of our 91 markers contain additional *Hcs* loci. Additional *Hcs* loci may also be found in murine strains other than those we used in our study.

To improve the saturation of the genome with genetic markers, we decided to repeat the linkage analysis in an interspecific test cross. Thus, we crossed the liver tumor-susceptible C3H/He strain with the *M. spretus* strain, to obtain an F1 interspecific hybrid displaying polymorphisms at any genetic locus[43]. Since we had no information on the susceptibility of the *M. spretus* strain to hepatocarcinogenesis, we made the cross between the (C3H/He × *M. spretus*) F1 mice and the C57BL/6J strain, which is resistant to hepatocarcinogenesis but whose F1 hybrids with the C3H/He strain are genetically susceptible[3,54]. The resultant test-cross individuals were analysed to detect segregation between susceptibility to hepatocarcinogenesis and a set of molecular markers.

The interspecific mapping panel of 106 individuals was genotyped at 222 loci. Markers were randomly distributed throughout the 19 autosomes and the X chromosome. We obtained a genetic linkage map spanning 1473 cM with an average distance between markers of 6.6 cM, and a 98% coverage of the mouse genome, compared with a length of 1492 cM in the GBASE map.

The linkage analysis between the indices of liver tumour susceptibility and the 222 genetic markers indicated that 3 chromosomal regions contain *Hcs* loci. We named these *Hcs-4* to *Hcs-6* (Table 7.2). A genomic region important in determining the quantitative variation in liver tumour susceptibility was identified on the distal part of chromosome 2. The region included between the markers *D2Mit26* and *D2Mit74*, spanning 18 cM, was significantly associated with the liver tumour-susceptibility phenotype (peak LOD score of 3.7 at *D2Mit25*, variance explained 14%). We named the locus on chromosome 2, *Hcs-4*, on the basis of our previous positioning of other three *Hcs* loci[53,55].

A central region of chromosome 5, around *D5Mit6*, contained the *Hcs-5* locus, and a distal region of chromosome 19 was also significantly associated with susceptibility to liver tumour development. We named this locus *Hcs-6*. The *D19Mit27* marker had the best association with the tumour susceptibility indexes.

We found an increase in tumour susceptibility derived from inheritance of the C3H/He allele at *Hcs* loci on chromosomes 2 and 5, and from inheritance of the *M. spretus* allele at the *Hcs* locus on chromosome 19. However, this kind of analysis cannot distinguish whether the strain whose genomic region is associated with susceptibility carries a susceptibility gene or whether the effect is due to the presence of a resistance gene contributed by the other strain.

To sum up, we found that in our interspecific cross, three loci can control liver tumour development. The total number of tumours was not significantly correlated with any of the other indices and showed no significant linkage with any of the 222 genetic markers, indicating that it is not genetically determined, as previously suggested[4,50].

Interestingly, the loci controlling liver tumour development that we previously mapped in the AC3F2 cross, i.e. the loci on chromosomes 7, 8 and 12, were not detected in the present cross. Since the locus on chromosome 12 derived from the A/J parental strain, absent in the present cross, we did not expect to confirm this locus in the (C3S)B6 mice. However, the loci on chromosomes 7 and 8 in the AC3F2 mice derived from the C3H/He parent, but were not confirmed in the present analysis. Moreover, we tested back the genetic markers of the chromosomal regions containing *Hcs* loci of the (C3S)B6 cross in the AC3F2 mice. The corresponding regions in the AC3F2 sample did not contain *Hcs* loci (data not shown).

A possible explanation for the discrepancies in the positioning of *Hcs* loci in the two samples may be the different parental strains used in the two crosses. Indeed, if both parental alleles contain the same *Hcs* locus, no differences can be detected in the phenotype of the test sample, since linkage analysis can only detect *Hcs* loci when they are retained in just one of the two segregating alleles. In this work, the use of *M. spretus* as one of the parents allowed us to identify new regions involved in the determination of susceptibility to hepatocarcinogenesis.

The comparison of our previous result in AC3F2 mice[53] and the present data indicate that multiple genetic loci control liver tumour development in mice. This would represent a new genetic model for tumour predisposition. It is also possible that we have not yet detected all the loci involved. The phenotype of genetic susceptibility to liver tumour development results from the interaction of multiple genetic factors that, individually, provide a relatively low contribution, not sufficient to elicit the tumour-susceptible phenotype (variance explained between 10% and 15%). A threshold for gene dosage might operate to predispose to hepatocellular tumour development in any given mouse strain.

FUTURE PERSPECTIVES IN THE ANALYSIS AND IDENTIFICATION OF GENETIC FACTORS ASSOCIATED WITH INHERITED PREDISPOSITION TO CARCINOGENESIS IN MURINE MODELS AND THEIR POSSIBLE APPLICATIONS FOR HUMANS

The importance of mapping tumour susceptibility genes in mice is not limited to the understanding of an experimental pathogenetic mechanism, but may be applicable to human pathology. Indeed, in humans, the identification of cancer-predisposing genes and of the related carriers is very difficult unless the cancer genes are highly penetrative and give rise to inherited cancer syndromes[56–58]. However, a large portion of the mouse genome shows conserved syntenies with the human genome and comparative genetic maps between mice and humans have been used to predict the location of human and murine disease genes on the basis of their mapping in the other species[59].

In the case of lung tumour susceptibility, a single locus seems to play a major role in determining genetic predisposition. Therefore, it might be possible to transfer the experimental findings to the corresponding human tumours (lung adenocarcinomas) and to look for associations between particular haplotypes and the risk of lung adenocarcinoma development. The human chromosomal region corresponding to the murine region where *Pas-1* maps is the human chromosome 12p, around KRAS2. However, our recent results, in other murine populations, suggest that genes other than *Pas-1* may be involved in susceptibility and resistance to lung carcinogenesis in mice. It is possible that these other genes are also involved in human lung tumour development, and therefore, association studies in humans may be weakened, due to the possible contribution of multiple genes to lung tumour risk.

At present, two major points have emerged in the description of genetic susceptibility to murine hepatocarcinogenesis, i.e. susceptibility affects liver tumour growth, not tumour frequency, and it is controlled by multiple genes[4,50,53,55].

If the situation described for the genetic predisposition to liver tumours is also true for other tumour types and for species other than mice, we can speculate that, in humans, the interaction of multiple genetic factors could determine individual genetic susceptibility to the development of particular tumour types. This model is compatible with both a very high risk of cancer development in genetically predisposed individuals and a very low penetrance of the character in their progeny. Indeed, in the progeny of genetically susceptible individuals (1) the segregation of different multiple genetic loci affecting tumour development, (2) the interaction of inherited tumour-predisposing loci with tumour-resistance loci, and (3) the interaction of genetic loci with the environment, would either dilute the number of predisposing loci or disrupt the necessary interactions between loci, leading to a very small increase in the risk factor in the siblings and in the progeny of cancer patients. In humans, a slight (about 2-fold) increase in cancer risk has indeed been described in relatives of patients with different types of cancer, including lung and liver tumours[58,60–62].

The mouse liver tumour system is important for the risk assessment of potential carcinogenicity of chemicals to humans, since the genetically susceptible B6C3F1 mouse is used in the bioassay of chemicals for their carcinogenicity under the National Toxicology Program in the USA. The understanding of the mechanisms responsible for the genetic susceptibility to hepatocarcinogenesis of the C3H/He strain, and the analysis of their relevance for the pathology of human HCCs, may provide a strong scientific basis for judging the results of the carcinogenicity bioassays[63].

Our data[53,55] indicate that cloning by reverse genetics of each individual locus affecting predisposition to liver tumour development is almost impossible today. This is due both to the relatively large regions of linkage and to the relatively small effects of each individual locus. Only if one or several final biochemical products were produced by the interaction of *Hcs* genes, could we identify and isolate these products and test them as markers of genetic predisposition in humans.

Recent results indicate that genetic heterogeneity may play an important role in familial predisposition to some forms of cancer in humans, as has been reported recently for familial predisposition to melanoma, non-polyposis colon cancer and breast cancer[64–70]. At present, these findings simply indicate that different genes may confer genetic predisposition to the same tumour type. However, it seems to be clear that the segregation of multiple genes predisposing to the same form of cancer in the same individual would lead to a very high genetic risk of developing a particular tumour type.

In conclusion, the inbred strains genetically predisposed to the development of different types of cancer may offer a unique opportunity to investigate the genetic components associated with the pathogenesis of these tumours. The results obtained in the experimental systems could then be tested in the corresponding human situation, and it could be possible that the study of cancer genetics in experimental animals will provide insights into the understanding of the genetic bases of human cancer.

Acknowledgements

This work was supported in part by grants from PF CNR 'ACRO' and Associazione Italiana Ricerca Cancro.

References

1. Atchley WR, Fitch WM. Gene trees and the origins of inbred strains of mice. Science. 1991;254:554–558.
2. Festing MFW. Origins and characteristics of inbred strains of mice. Mouse Genome. 1993;91:393–509.
3. Della Porta G, Capitano J, Parmi L, Colnaghi MI. Urethan carcinogenesis in newborn, suckling, and adult mice of C57BL, C3H, BC3F1, C3Hf and SWR strains. Tumori. 1967;53:81–102.
4. Dragani TA, Manenti G, Della Porta G. Quantitative analysis of genetic susceptibility to liver and lung carcinogenesis in mice. Cancer Res. 1991;51:6299–6303.
5. Turusov VS, Lanko NS, Krutovskikh VA, Parfenov YD. Strain differences in susceptibility of female mice to 1,2-dimethyl-hydrazine. Carcinogenesis. 1982;3:603–608.
6. Turusov VS, Chemeris GY, Parfenov YD. Pararenal angiosarcoma induced in male mice by 1,2-dimethylhydrazine – a model for studying the role of androgens in chemical carcinogenesis. Carcinogenesis. 1985;6:325–331.
7. Deschner EE, Long FC, Hakissia M, Herrmann SL. Differential susceptibility of AKR, C57BL/6J, and CF1 mice to 1,2-dimethylhydrazine-induced colonic tumor formation predicted by proliferative characteristics of colonic epithelial cells. J Natl Cancer Inst. 1983;70:279–282.
8. Diwan BA, Meier H, Blackman KE. Genetic differences in the induction of colorectal tumors by 1,2-dimethylhydrazine in inbred mice. J Natl Cancer Inst. 1977;59:455–458.
9. Bangrazi C, Mouton D, Neveu T *et al.* Genetics of chemical carcinogenesis. 1. Bidirectional selective breeding of susceptible and resistant lines of mice to two-stage skin carcinogenesis. Carcinogenesis. 1990;11:1711–1719.
10. Haag JD, Newton MA, Gould MN. Mammary carcinoma suppressor and susceptibility genes in the Wistar-Kyoto rat. Carcinogenesis. 1992;13:1933–1995.
11. Isaacs JT. Genetic control of resistance to chemically induced mammary adenocarcinogenesis in the rat. Cancer Res. 1986;46:3958–3963.
12. Melhem MF, Kunz HW, Gill III TJ. A major histocompatibility complex-linked locus in the rat critically influences resistance to diethylnitrosamine carcinogenesis. Proc Natl Acad Sci USA. 1993;90:1967–1971.
13. Zhang R, Haag JD, Gould MN. Site of expression and biological function of the rat mammary carcinoma suppressor gene. Carcinogenesis. 1989;11:1765–1770.
14. Berman JJ, Rice JM, Wenk ML, Roller PP. Intestinal tumors induced by a single intraperitoneal injection of methyl(acetoxymethyl) nitrosamine in three strains of rats. Cancer Res. 1979;39:1462–1466.
15. Takizawa S, Watanabe H, Naito Y, Terada Y, Fujii I. Hirose F. Strain differences in susceptibility of rat colon to 1,2-dimethylhydrazine carcinogenesis. Gann. 1978;69:719–722.
16. Ohgaki H, Kawachi T, Matsukura N, Morino K, Miyamoto M, Sugimura T. Genetic control of susceptibility of rats to gastric carcinoma. Cancer Res. 1983;43:3663–3667.
17. Tatematsu M, Aoki T, Inoue T, Mutai M, Furihata C, Ito N. Coefficient induction of pepsinogen 1-decreased pyloric glands and gastric cancers in five different strains of rats treated with N-methyl-N′-nitro-N-nitrosoguanidine. Carcinogenesis. 1988;9:495–498.
18. Masuda R, Yoshida MC, Sasaki M, Dempo K, Mori M. High susceptibility to hepatocellular carcinoma development in LEC rats with hereditary hepatitis. Jpn J Cancer Res. 1988;79:828–835.
19. Eker R, Mossige J. A dominant gene for renal adenomas and adenocarcinomas in the rat. Nature. 1961;189:858–859.
20. Pour P, Althoff J, Salmasi S, Stepan K. Spontaneous tumors and common diseases in three types of hamsters. J Natl Cancer Inst. 1979;63:797–811.
21. Hilgers J, Bentvelzen P. Interaction between viral and genetic factors in murine mammary cancer. Adv Cancer Res. 1978;26:143.
22. Lilly F, Pincus T. Genetic control of murine viral leukemogenesis. Adv Cancer Res. 1973;17:231.
23. Nandi S, McGrath CM. Mammary neoplasia in mice. Adv Cancer Res. 1973;17:353.
24. Rowe WP, Hartley JW, Bremner T. Genetic mapping of a murine leukemia virus-inducing locus of AKR mice. Science. 1972;178:860.
25. Moser AR, Pitot HC, Dove W. A dominant mutation that predisposes to multiple intestinal neoplasia in the mouse. Science. 1990;247:322–324.

26. Luongo C, Gould KA, Su L-K, *et al.* Mapping of multiple intestinal neoplasia (Min) to proximal chromosome 18 of the mouse. Genomics. 1993;15:3–8.
27. Su L-K, Kinzler KW, Vogelstein B, *et al.* Multiple intestinal neoplasia caused by a mutation in the murine homolog of the APC gene. Science. 1992;256:668–670.
28. Dietrich WF, Lander ES, Smith JS, *et al.* Genetic identification of Mom-1, a major modifier locus affecting Min-induced intestinal neoplasia in the mouse. Cell. 1993;75:631–639.
29. Moen CJA, Snoek M, Hart AAM, Demant P. *Scc-1*, a novel colon cancer susceptibility gene in the mouse: Linkage to CD44(Ly-24, Pgp-1) on chromosome 2. Oncogene. 1992;7:563–566.
30. Mock BA, Krall MM, Dosik JK. Genetic mapping of tumor susceptibility genes in mouse plasmacytomagenesis. Proc Natl Acad Sci USA. 1993;90:9499–9503.
31. Potter M, Mushinski EB, Wax JS, Hartley J, Mock BA. Identification of two genes on chromosome 4 that determine resistance to plasmacytoma induction in mice. Cancer Res. 1994;54:969–975.
32. Angel JM, Morizot DC, Richie ER. Localization of a novel chromosome 7 locus that suppresses development of *N*-methyl-*N*-nitrosurea-induced murine thymic lymphomas. Mol Carcinog. 1993;7:151–156.
33. Okumoto M, Nishikawa R, Imai S, Hilgers J. Genetic analysis of resistance to radiation lymphomagenesis with recombinant inbred strains of mice. Cancer Res. 1990;50:3848–3850.
34. Naito M, Chenicek KJ, Naito Y, Di Giovanni J. Susceptibility to phorbol ester skin tumor promotion in (C57BL/6 × DBA/2) F1 mice is inherited as an incomplete dominant trait: Evidence for multi-locus involvement. Carcinogenesis. 1988;9:639–645.
35. Malkinson AM. (1989) The genetic basis of susceptibility to lung tumors in mice. Toxicology. 1989;54:241–271.
36. Shimkin MB, Stoner GD. Lung tumors in mice: Application to carcinogenesis bioassay. Adv Cancer Res. 1975;21:1–58.
37. Malkinson AM, Nesbitt MN, Skamene E. Susceptibility to urethan-induced pulmonary adenomas between A/J and C57BL/6J mice: Use of AXB and BXA recombinant inbred lines indicating a three-locus genetic model. J Natl Cancer Inst. 1987;75:971–974.
38. Ryan J, Barker PE, Nesbitt MN, Ruddle FH. KRAS2 as a genetic marker for lung tumor susceptibility in inbred mice. J Natl Cancer Inst. 1987;79:1351–1357.
39. Miyashita N, Moriwaki K. H-2-controlled genetic susceptibility to pulmonary adenomas induced by urethane and 4-nitroquinoline 1-oxide in A/Wy congenic strains. Jpn J Cancer Res. 1987;78:494–498.
40. Miyashita N, Moriwaki K, Migita S. The H-2 class II genes and the susceptibility to the development of pulmonary adenoma in mice. Immunogenetics. 1989;29:14–18.
41. Oomen LC, van der Valk MA, Demant P. MHC and non-MHC genes in lung tumor susceptibility in the mouse: Implications for the study of the different lung tumor types and their cell of origin. Exp Lung Res. 1991;17:283–304.
42. Gariboldi M, Manenti G, Canzian F, *et al.* A major susceptibility locus to murine lung carcinogenesis maps on chromosome 6. Nature Genet. 1993;3:132–136.
43. Avner P, Amar L, Dandolo L, Guenet JL. Genetic analysis of the mouse using interspecific crosses. Trends Genet. 1988;4:18–23.
44. Dietrich W, Katz H, Lincoln SE, *et al.* A genetic map of the mouse suitable for typing intraspecific crosses. Genetics. 1992;131:423–447.
45. Paterson AH, Damon S, Hewitt JD, *et al.* Mendelian factors underlying quantitative traits in tomato: Comparison across species, generations, and environments. Genetics. 1991;127:181–197.
46. Weller JI, Soller M, Brody T. Linkage analysis of quantitative traits in an interspecific cross of tomato (*Lycopersicon esculentum* × *Lycopersicon pimpinellifolium*) by means of genetic markers. Genetics. 1988;118:329–339.
47. Birrer MJ, Minna JD. (1989) Genetic changes in the pathogenesis of lung cancer. Ann Rev Med. 1989;40:305–317.
48. Malkinson AM. Primary lung tumors in mice: An experimental manipulable model of human adenocarcinoma. Cancer Res (Suppl). 1992;52:2670s–2676s.
49. Re FC, Manenti G, Borrello MG, *et al.* Multiple molecular alterations in mouse lung tumors. Mol Carcinog. 1992;5:155–160.
50. Dragani TA, Manenti G, Della Porta G. Genetic susceptibility to murine hepatocarcinogenesis is associated with high growth rate of NDEA-initiated hepatocytes. J Cancer Res Clin Oncol. 1987;113:223–229.

51. Hanigan MH, Kemp CJ, Ginsler JJ, Drinkwater NR. Rapid growth of preneoplastic lesions in hepatocarcinogen-sensitive C3H/HeJ male mice relative to C57BL/6J male mice. Carcinogenesis. 1988;9:885–890.
52. Drinkwater NR, Ginsler J. Genetic control of hepatocarcinogenesis in C57BL/6J and C3H/HeJ. Carcinogenesis. 1986;7:1701–1707.
53. Gariboldi M, Manenti G, Canzian F, *et al.* Chromosome mapping of murine susceptibility loci to liver carcinogenesis. Cancer Res. 1993;53:209–211.
54. Dragani TA, Manenti G, Gariboldi M, Falvella FS, Pierotti MA, Della Porta G. Genetics of hepatocarcinogenesis in mouse and man. In: Zervos C, ed. Oncogenes and transgenic correlates of cancer risk assessment. NATO ASI Series A, Life Sciences, Vol 232. London, UK: Plenum Publ. Co.; 1992:71–90.
55. Manenti G, Binelli G, Gariboldi M, *et al.* Multiple loci affect genetic predisposition to hepatocarcinogenesis in mice. Genomics. 1994;23:118–24.
56. Peto J. Genetic predisposition to cancer. In: Cancer incidence in defined populations (Bambury Report 4). Cairns J, Lyon JL, Skolnick M, eds. Cold Spring Harbor Laboratory Press;1980:203–213.
57. Pierotti MA, Dragani TA. Genetics and cancer. Curr Opin Oncol. 1992;4:127–133.
58. Ponder BAJ. Inherited predisposition to cancer. Trends Genet. 1990;6:213–218.
59. Copeland NG, Jenkins NA, Gilbert DJ, *et al.* A genetic linkage map of the mouse: Current applications and future prospects. Science. 1993;262:57–66.
60. Fernandez E, La Vecchia C, D'Avanzo B, Negri E, Franceschi S. Family history and the risk of liver, gallbladder, and pancreatic cancer. Cancer Epidemiol Biomarkers Prev. 1994;3:209–212.
61. Ooi WL, Elston RC, Chen VW, Bailey-Wilson JE, Rothschild H. Increased familial risk for lung cancer. J Natl Cancer Inst. 1986;76:217–222.
62. Sellers TA, Potter JD, Bailey-Wilson JE, Rich SS, Rothschild H, Elston RC. Lung cancer detection and prevention: Evidence for an interaction between smoking and genetic predisposition. Cancer Res. 1992;52:2694s–2697s.
63. Della Porta G, Dragani TA. (1990) Long-term assays for carcinogenicity. Teratogenesis Carcinog Mutagen. 1990;10:137–145.
64. Bronner CE, Baker SM, Morrison PT, *et al.* Mutation in the DNA mismatch repair gene homologue *hMLH1* is associated with hereditary non-polyposis colon cancer. Nature. 1994;368:258–261.
65. Easton DF, Bishop DT, Ford D, *et al.* Genetic linkage analysis in familial breast and ovarian cancer: Results from 214 families. Am J Hum Genet. 1993;52:678–701.
66. Fishel R, Lescoe MK, Rao MRS, *et al.* The human mutator gene homolog *MSH2* and its association with hereditary nonpolyposis colon cancer. Cell. 1993;75:1027–1038.
67. Goldstein AM, Dracopoli NC, Engelstein M, Fraser MC, Clark WH, Tucker MA. Linkage of cutaneous malignant melanoma/dysplastic nevi to chromosome 9p, and evidence for genetic heterogeneity. Am J Hum Genet. 1994;54:489–496.
68. Leach FS, Nicolaides NC, Papadopoulos N, *et al.* Mutations of a *mutS* homolog in hereditary nonpolyposis colorectal cancer. Cell. 1993;75:1215–1225.
69. Nancarrow DJ, Walker GJ, Weber JL, Walters MK, Palmer JM, Hayward NK. (1992) Linkage mapping of melanoma (MLM) using 172 microsatellite markers. Genomics. 1992;14:939–947.
70. Papadopoulos N, Nicolaides NC, Wei Y-F, *et al.* Mutation of a *mutL* homolog in hereditary colon cancer. Science. 1994;263:1625–1629.

8
Human repair deficiencies and predisposition to cancer

M. Hall, P.G. Norris and R.T. Johnson

INTRODUCTION

The maintenance of genetic stability is essential to the viability of multicellular organisms. However, at the cellular level, the integrity of the genome is constantly challenged. Structural alterations continually appear in DNA, either spontaneously or as a result of environmental insult. Endogenously, base sequence modifications occur at a steady rate as byproducts of DNA metabolic transactions which habitually erode the accuracy of the encoded information. Organisms have, therefore, evolved a wide range of molecular mechanisms to cope with the requirement for cell survival by removing DNA damage and at the same time protecting the cell from the accumulation of deleterious mutations. These are the processes of DNA repair[1]. The proteins performing the functions of DNA repair are also encoded by the very DNA they protect and therefore mutations arising in genes coding for DNA repair proteins may inactivate or alter the repair processes themselves. The absence of DNA repair may prove fatal for individual cells in the face of DNA damage but, more importantly, is likely to be disastrous for a multicellular organism, where the unchecked accumulation of mutations may lead to accelerated tumorigenesis. From a human perspective, individuals with hereditary defects in DNA repair mechanisms may harbour an increased risk of cancer in their lifetime.

The link between deficiencies in DNA damage processing and mutagenesis was first established in *Escherichia coli*, where repair-deficient mutants were found to accumulate large numbers of mutations after exposure to DNA-damaging agents. However, direct correlation between enhanced carcinogenesis and DNA repair deficiencies had to await the discovery by James Cleaver that cells from sufferers of the skin cancer-prone disease, xeroderma pigmentosum, lacked a mechanism for the repair of UV light-induced DNA lesions[2]. The importance of DNA repair mechanisms in protecting against malignancy has been underlined by the recent finding that defects in the repair of replication errors (mismatch repair) are found in some cases of non-polyposis colorectal cancer and that patients with hereditary non-polyposis colorectal cancer (HNPCC) carry defective alleles for mismatch repair genes[3]. At present, a small number of hereditary diseases predisposing to malignancy has been associated with abnormalities in the processing of DNA damage and these are listed in Table 8.1. In this chapter, we shall give a brief overview of repair mechanisms and then focus on the diseases listed.

AN OVERVIEW OF REPAIR MECHANISMS

Both prokaryote and eukaryote cells possess several largely distinct DNA damage processing pathways[1]. Most of our current understanding of DNA repair mechanisms has been elucidated in prokaryotic organisms but, with our rapidly expanding knowledge of eukaryotic repair, it is becoming increasingly apparent that the same basic models and frequently the same types of protein are at the heart of DNA repair in all cells. Furthermore, whilst the role of many proteins is solely to carry out repair functions, other proteins which play a crucial role in repair processes are also involved with other DNA transactions in the cell. The integration of DNA repair with other DNA processing systems leads to versatility, a prerequisite for repair systems which must deal with diverse DNA lesions occurring at any point in the cell cycle. The various DNA-damage processing pathways are illustrated schematically in Figure 8.1.

Some repair proteins are designed to remove specific lesions. Pyrimidine dimers are bulky DNA lesions involving the chemical bonding of adjacent

Table 8.1 Human syndromes with DNA repair abnormalities and a predisposition to cancer

Syndrome	*Clinical features*	*Cancer proneness*	*Cellular characteristics*
Xeroderma pigmentosum (XP)	Sun-sensitive Neurological abnormalities Ocular defects	+++ skin cancer	7 complementation groups, UV hypersensitive, UV hypermutable, defective in early stage of nucleotide excision repair (NER)
XP variant	As for classical XP groups	++ skin cancer	UV hypersensitive, UV hypermutable, normal NER but defective replication after UV
Ataxia telangiectasia	Progressive ataxia telangiectasia Ionizing-radiation sensitive	++ lymphomas/ leukaemia	Hypersensitive to ionizing radiation, radioresistant DNA synthesis, elevated chromosome rearrangements
Bloom syndrome	Sun-sensitive Retarded growth Narrow face	+++ early onset all cancers	Elevated spontaneous sister chromatid exchanges, hypermutable, elevated chromosome rearrangements
Hereditary non-polyposis colon cancer (HNPCC)	Early diagnosis Colon cancer, no florid polyposis	+++ colon cancer	Defective in mismatch repair, instability of simple repeat sequences
Fanconi anaemia	Small size Bone marrow failure Anaemia	+/− myeloid leukaemia	Spontaneous chromatid aberrations, hypersensitivity to DNA crosslinking agents

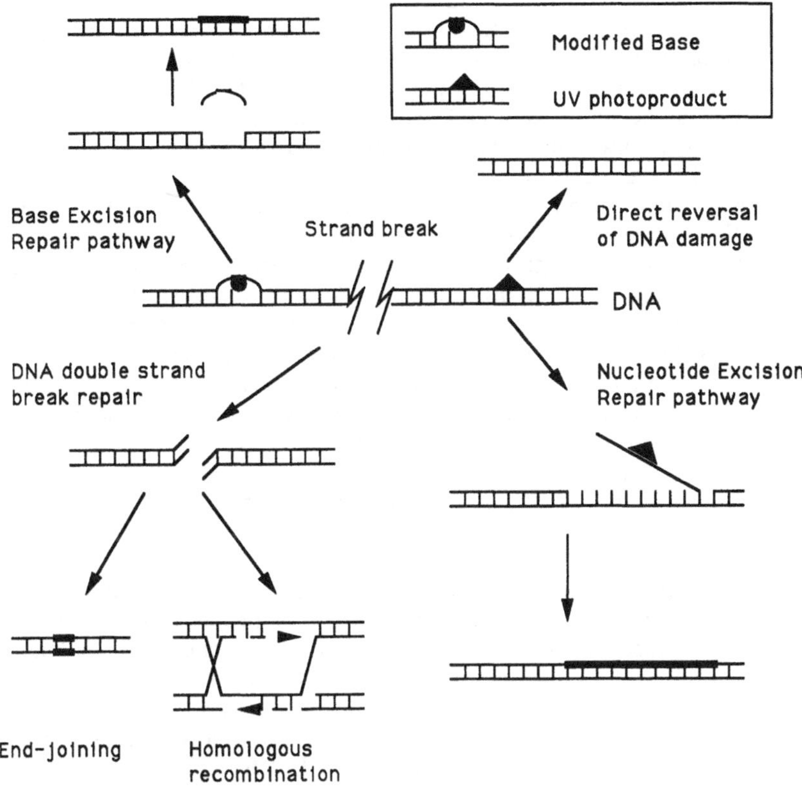

Figure 8.1 Cellular pathways of DNA damage processing

thymine or cytosine bases to form cyclobutane rings using the energy from ultraviolet light. Such dimers distort the DNA helix and inhibit both transcription and replication. The DNA repair enzyme, photolyase, found in many plant and animal species but not in man, can recognize and bind to the UV-induced cyclobutane dimers and using energy from the visible light spectrum directly cleaves the chemical linkage between adjacent bases[4]. A particularly mutagenic lesion is formed by the action of simple alkylating agents present in trace amounts in many foodstuffs. This lesion, O^6 methylguanine, is produced by the addition of a methyl group to the oxygen atom at position 6 of guanine bases. The methyl is removed by a 'suicide' enzyme called DNA alkyltransferase, which catalyses the transfer of the methyl groups from the modified DNA base to itself, thereby becoming irreversibly inactivated[5].

Other repair systems are more versatile and can deal with a number of different DNA lesions. These tend to involve complexes of proteins acting in concert with each other and sometimes with other DNA metabolic processes. The nucleotide excision repair (NER) pathway is perhaps the most versatile and can remove a wide variety of lesions which cause large structural distortions in the DNA, including UV photoproducts and adducts caused by chemical carcinogens as well as by chemotherapeutic agents such as *cis*-platin[6]. Proteins of the NER pathway operate to monitor the DNA and recognize structural distortions in the helix. The DNA strand carrying the lesion is incised on both sides close to the damaged base(s) by endonuclease action and the intervening double helical DNA (with damaged bases) is unwound by a helicase and discarded. Repair synthesis fills the resultant single-strand gap by copying the undamaged complementary strand to form a repair patch which is then ligated to the parental DNA by a DNA ligase to complete the process. We will examine the NER pathway in more detail later.

Two of the most damaging agents in living cells are oxygen and water. Spontaneous oxidation and hydrolysis of DNA bases would produce intolerable instability in a DNA molecule if it were not for the base excision repair pathway[7], the first step of which is the creation of an abasic site. These sites, which have lost a purine or pyrimidine base whilst leaving the phosphodiester DNA backbone intact, can result from spontaneous hydrolysis of the base-sugar glycosyl bond or from direct cleavage by a DNA glycosylase enzyme which recognizes the modified base. The DNA glycosylases exist as a family of proteins, with each member recognizing and initiating repair of a different type of base adduct. The abasic sites are, in turn, recognized by AP endonuclease enzymes, which cut the DNA backbone precisely 5′ to the baseless nucleotide. The sugar phosphate moiety is removed by the action of another enzyme, this time a phosphodiesterase, which cuts the DNA 3′ to the baseless site. Similar to NER, a polymerase fills in the single nucleotide gap and a ligase seals the remaining nick to restore the integrity of the DNA molecule.

DNA double-strand breaks (DSBs) represent a serious threat to genome integrity. A single DSB can be cytotoxic or cause aberrant segregation of mammalian chromosomes during mitosis/meiosis[8]. Eukaryotic cells have several efficient ways of repairing DSBs, including recombination with a homologous duplex[9] or simple ligation of the broken ends[10]. Other less well understood mechanisms are involved in filling the daughter strand gaps or discontinuities created when replication forks collide with sites of bulky lesions in the template. In prokaryotes, this process, termed post-replication recovery (PRR), may occur via the recombination mechanism of template switching or via translesion synthesis; in eukaryotes, gap filling by translesion synthesis probably predominates and may be error prone[11].

Finally, in addition to exogenous DNA-damaging agents, DNA replication itself creates lesions which require correction. High-fidelity replication of the chromosome is necessary to preserve the informational integrity of the DNA. However, while DNA replication is a largely accurate process, it is not infallible, and, after proofreading, there remains an estimated error rate of 1 misincorporated nucleotide per million base pairs of replicated DNA[12]. In a human genome of 3 billion base pairs, this error rate will result in 3000 mistakes per cell generation – sufficient to corrupt the informational content of our DNA beyond recognition over a short period, bearing in mind that an adult human is composed of between 10^{12} and 10^{13} cells. Clearly, a post-replication scanning and correction mechanism is desirable and consists of the DNA mismatch correction system, which is present in all cells so far studied and, like other basic DNA repair systems, has been highly conserved during evolution[13]. The proteins of mismatch repair can recognize DNA base pair mismatches as well as sites of replication slippage where the replication machinery has skipped past a few bases at regions of simple repeat sequence. The mismatch repair proteins bind to the DNA in the mispaired region and initiate excision of the mismatched base(s) before synthesizing the repair patch. We will consider the process of mismatch repair in some detail later.

XERODERMA PIGMENTOSUM AND NUCLEOTIDE EXCISION REPAIR

Clinical features

Xeroderma pigmentosum (XP) is a relatively rare inherited disease (1 in 250 000 live births) found in all races world wide. XP patients are genetically heterogeneous, more common clinical characteristics including sunlight sensitivity, cutaneous pigmentary anomalies, a high incidence of skin cancer, and sometimes progressive neurological deterioration.

Onset of clinical features is usually between 1 and 2 years of age[14], most often with ultraviolet sensitivity. Approximately 50% of patients experience exaggerated sun burning, sometimes with blistering after minimal sun exposure; this often takes days to weeks to resolve. Freckling also frequently occurs by the age of 2 years, particularly affecting sun-exposed areas but also in the mucous membranes and palms and soles. Progressive dryness, telangiectasia, atrophy and scarring are also common.

For patients younger than 20 years of age, the incidence of basal and squamous cell carcinomas of the skin is nearly 5000 times greater than that of the general United States population and the incidence of melanoma is 2000 times greater[14]. The median age for first skin cancer is 8 years, nearly 50 years younger than usual. These skin cancers, especially squamous and basal cell carcinomas, arise predominantly on sites exposed to the sun. Other reported skin tumours include actinic keratoses, keratoacanthomas, fibromas, angiomas and fibrosarcomas. There is also some evidence for an increased instance (12 times above average) of internal malignancies in XP patients[15]. Neoplasms of the brain (especially a rare sarcoma of the meninges) and of the oral cavity are more common in XP patients under the age of 40, but increased representation of the more common lethal internal cancers, such as lymphoma and female genital tract and endocrine system neoplasms, has not been reported.

Ocular abnormalities commonly occur and are generally confined to those areas exposed to ultraviolet radiation, including the eyelids, conjuctiva and cornea. Approximately one tenth of subjects develop neoplasms of the conjunctiva, cornea or eyelids. About one in five patients develop neurological disorders that begin in infancy and occasionally the second decade, owing to progressive loss of neurons from the cerebral cortex, but sometimes also the cerebellum, medulla and spinal cord[16,17]. Neurological abnormalities may be mild or severe and include hypo- or areflexia, sensorineural deafness, abnormal speech, seizures, abnormal motor activity and mental retardation. In the most extreme cases, severe and progressive neurological features are combined with microcephaly, dwarfism and immature sexual development[18].

Table 8.2 Clinical features of different XP complementation groups

Complementation group	*Unscheduled DNA synthesis (%)*	*Cutaneous features*	*Predominant skin cancer*	*Neurological features*
A	<5	+++	SCC	++
B	10	CS		+
C	10–47	++/+++	BCC/SCC	–
D	25–60	++	LMM	+/–
E	40–60	+	BCC	–
F	<10	++		+
G	2	++		+
Variant	10	+	BCC	–

CS: Cockayne syndrome; SCC: squamous cell carcinoma; BCC: basal cell carcinoma; LMM: lentigo maligna melanoma

Approximately 75% of XP patients have 'classical' XP associated with a defect in DNA nucleotide excision repair. The remaining 25% constitute patients with an XP 'variant'. These have a deficiency in an ill-characterized post-replicative repair process and are free of neurological disease. They present clinically either in a form indistinguishable from classical XP or with late onset of pigmentation, neoplasms and occasional photosensitivity. In classical XP, cell fusion studies have identified seven complementation groups, designated A–G. There exists considerable variability in the clinical features typical of each complementation group and the clinical severity of these features correlates only roughly with the magnitude of the DNA repair defect (Table 8.2). The most common complementation groups are A, C and D; group A is particularly common in Japan, probably as a result of a founder mutation, while group C is most prevalent in Europe and North America. Although most patients within each complementation group have broadly similar clinical characteristics, it is becomingly increasingly clear that different alterations in the genes responsible for the individual complementation groups are associated with some differences in clinical features.

Molecular genetics of XP

UV hypersensitivity is the hallmark of defective nucleotide excision repair (NER) and the seven 'classical' complementation groups of xeroderma pigmentosum are now known to represent defects in separate genes acting at an early stage in the NER pathway[19]. This pathway is responsible for the removal of bulky adducts, including the two major UV-induced lesions; pyrimidine cyclobutane dimers and (6-4) photoproducts (Figure 8.2). The lack of repair of UV lesions by XP cells can be demonstrated by measuring unscheduled DNA synthesis (UDS or repair synthesis) in normal and XP fibroblasts. Normal human fibroblasts exhibit levels of UDS proportional to the UV dose given. XP cells almost all demonstrate a striking reduction in repair synthesis after UV, the degree of residual repair varying with complementation group and usually corre-

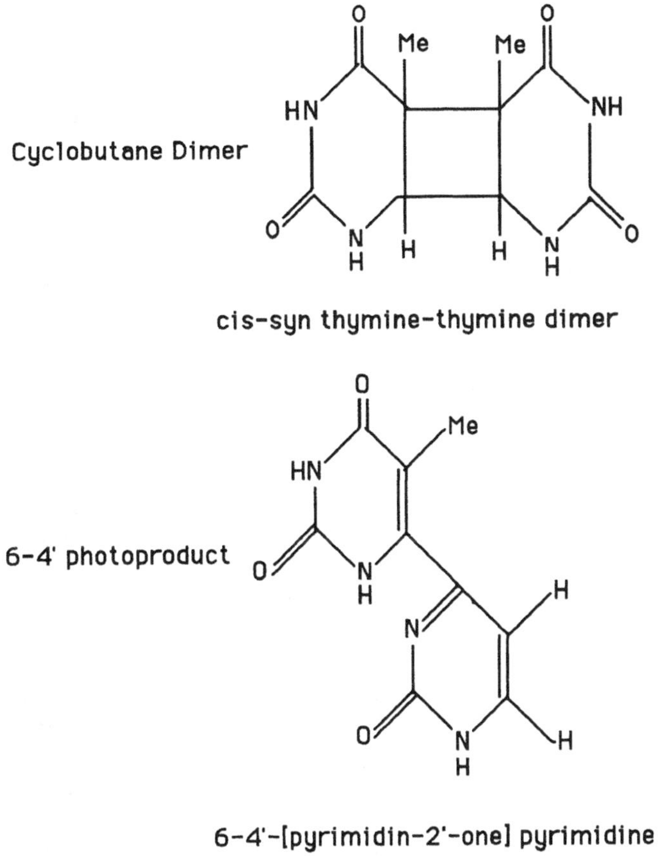

Cyclobutane Dimer

cis-syn thymine-thymine dimer

6-4' photoproduct

6-4'-[pyrimidin-2'-one] pyrimidine

Figure 8.2 The structure of the two main UV photoproducts, pyrimidine cyclobutane dimers and (6-4) photoproducts, both formed between adjacent thymine bases

lating with the severity of clinical symptoms[20]. Since all cells from XP patients demonstrate the same repair deficiency, prenatal diagnosis of XP in families at risk is made possible by assaying isolated amniotic cells for UV-induced UDS[21].

We have previously outlined the five steps of NER: DNA-damage recognition, incision of the damaged strand either side of the lesion, removal of a short region of DNA containing the lesion, repair replication using the undamaged strand as a template, and ligation. Figure 8.3 illustrates this process using *E. coli* as a model organism in which NER has been intensively investigated[6]. While the gene products involved differ between *E. coli* and humans, the basic mechanism of NER has been conserved throughout evolution and provides a strong foundation for the investigation of this process in higher organisms, most importantly in humans. However, looking at the deceptive simplicity of the *E. coli* NER reaction, it remains surprising to discover that biochemical and genetic studies implicate more than 20 gene products in the analogous eukaryotic repair

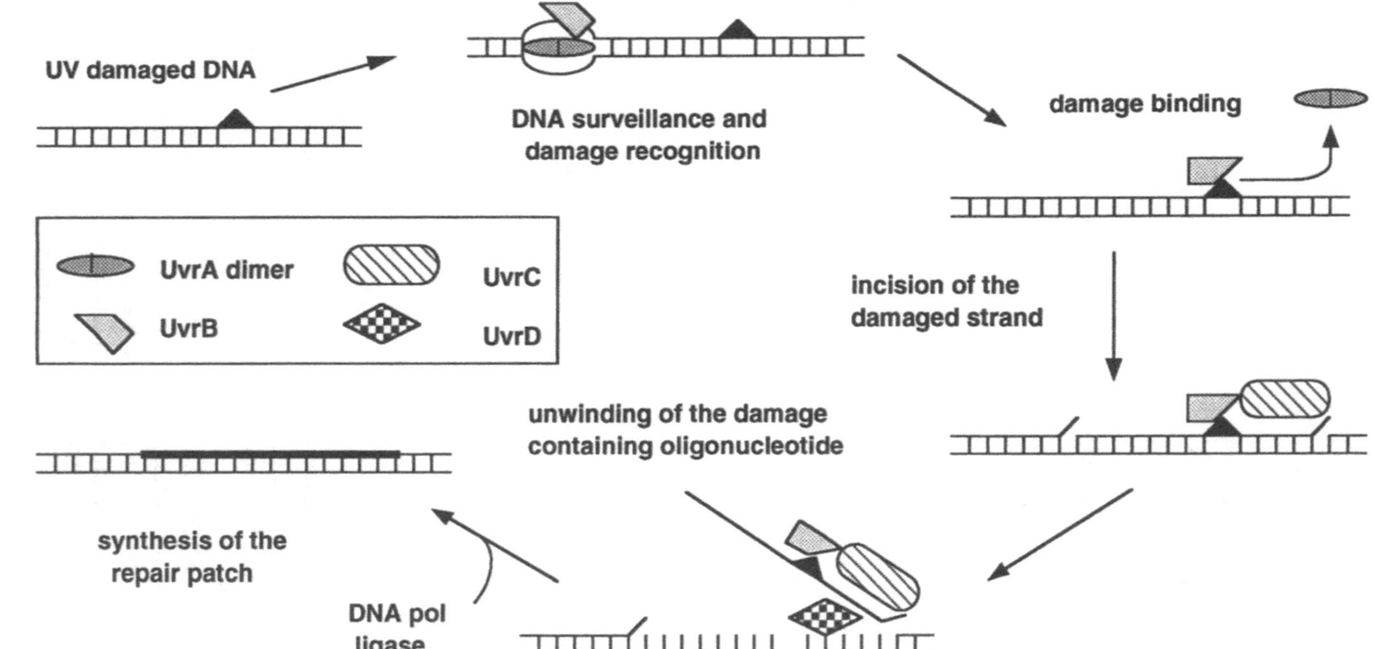

Figure 8.3 Nucleotide excision repair (NER) in *E. coli*. NER in *E. coli* is performed by the UvrA-D proteins as well as DNA polymerase I and DNA ligase. The weak helicase activity of the UvrA dimer complexed to a molecule of UvrB allows translocation along the DNA, scanning for helix-distorting lesions. When the $UvrA_2B$ surveillance complex encounters damage, the UvrB protein binds the DNA and the UvrA dimer dissociates. The dissociation of UvrA proteins allows UvrC to bind to UvrB to form a complex which incises the damaged DNA strand either side of the lesion. The UvrD helicase then unwinds and releases the damaged oligonucleotide, and DNA polymerase I and DNA ligase synthesize the repair patch. Other proteins, including photolyase and the transcription coupling factor, mfd, are also involved in NER in *E. coli* but are not shown

reaction[22]. As in *E. coli*, the late steps of NER in human cells require DNA polymerase, a DNA ligase and, in addition, eukaryotic replication accessory factors, such as proliferating cell nuclear antigen (PCNA)[23] and human single-strand binding (hSSB) protein[24]. Together these enzymes synthesize and ligate the repair patch. The early steps of NER in eukaryotes are significantly more complex, probably because the DNA is packaged in chromatin, and it is in these early steps that XP cells are deficient and on which much recent work has focused. The early steps are required for surveillance of the DNA for helix-distorting lesions and for incision at sites of damage. Fine tuning of the repair process is also provided in both *E. coli* and man by the existence of two subpathways of NER. One is responsible for the rapid repair of the transcribed strand of actively expressed genes (transcription-coupled repair) and the other for the slower and less-efficient repair of the bulk untranscribed DNA (overall genome repair)[25,26] (Figure 8.4). Preferential repair of transcribed DNA can be seen either as a clear priority for a cell where transcription by RNA polymerase II is inhibited by the presence of helix-distorting lesions in the template DNA, or as

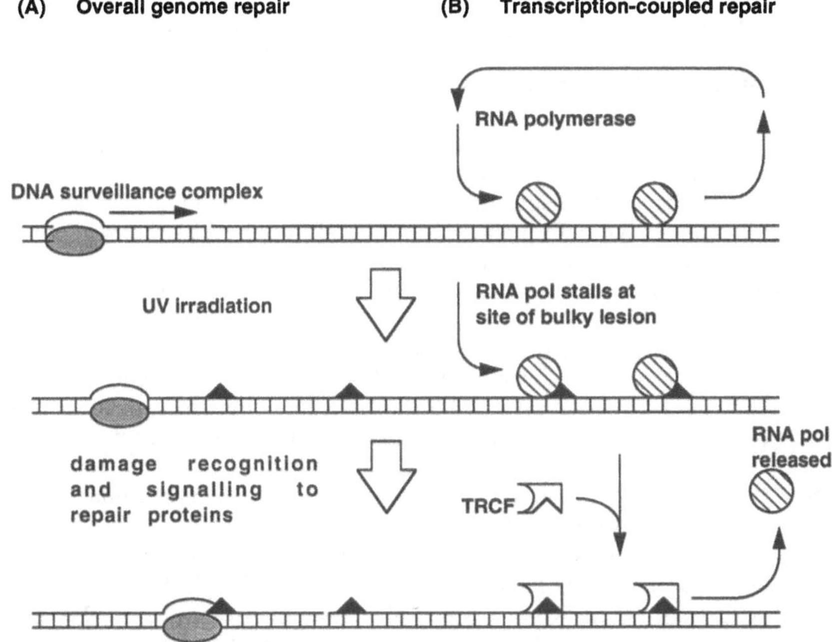

Figure 8.4 The two subpathways for nucleotide excision repair (NER): (A) Overall genome repair, which operates on both the transcribed and non-transcribed DNA, relies on mechanisms of DNA surveillance to recognize DNA damage and initiate repair; (B) Transcription-coupled repair operates to remove certain bulky lesions (e.g. pyrimidine cyclobutane dimers) more rapidly from the transcribed strand of the active DNA only. This subpathway of repair relies on RNA polymerases stalled at sites of bulky lesions to indicate the presence of DNA damage. Stalled polymerases are recognized by transcription–repair coupling factors (TRCFs) which release the stalled RNA polymerase from the DNA and bind at the site of damage, initiating repair by directly recruiting further repair enzymes

an inevitable consequence of the fact that the transcription complex already has in place several elements of the NER system (see below).

The seven complementation groups of NER each correspond to a gene participating at an early stage of NER. This is confirmed by the rescue to near-normal unscheduled DNA synthesis of all seven complementation groups by the introduction of bacteriophage T4 UV endonuclease V into permeabilized cells. This enzyme specifically recognizes cyclobutane pyrimidine dimers and incises the damaged strand[27]. In addition to the classical XP groups, patients suffering from the rarer human disorder, Cockayne syndrome (CS) are also defective in an early stage of NER and two complementation groups have been described (CSA and CSB). In addition, some individuals with XP may also show symptoms of CS, and, though diagnosis has often been difficult, combined XP/CS occurs in XP complementation groups B, D and G. Patients with CS are clinically characterized by acute sun sensitivity, cachectic dwarfism, pigmentary retinal degeneration, and progressive demyelinating neurological defects[28]. Cellular sensitivity of CS cells to UV is associated with a specific defect in the repair of the actively transcribing DNA and therefore CS cells may lack factors coupling repair to transcription[29]. Remarkably, although CS cells show increased frequencies of UV-induced mutations[30], CS patients do not suffer from an increased risk of skin or other cancers. A further genetically complex human NER defect has been identified in cells from patients with the extremely rare human disorder, PIBIDS (also referred to as trichthiodystrophy or TTD). PIBIDS is an acronym for a complex syndrome comprising **P**hotosensitivity, **I**cthyosis, **B**rittle hair, **I**mpaired intelligence, **D**ecreased fertility and **S**hort stature. Whilst cells from some PIBIDS patients also display decreased unscheduled DNA synthesis (15% of normal) similar to XP cells, and commonly fall into the XPD complementation group, PIBIDS patients are otherwise more similar to CS individuals: growth and neural impairment, photosensitivity in 50% of cases but no increase in skin cancer[31].

Other eukaryotes have also proved vital in the process of identifying NER genes. A set of laboratory-derived rodent cells, selected for their enhanced sensitivity to UV light, has been assigned to 11 different complementation groups. It was anticipated that the UV-sensitive rodent mutant cells would provide XP group homologies corresponding to defects in human NER genes. This hope has been borne out in part. Human genes which correct the rodent mutants are known as ERCC (excision repair cross-complementing rodent repair deficiencies) genes, followed by the number of the complementation group. To date, the following human genes have been isolated: ERCC1, 2, 3, 5 and 6. All except ERCC-1 correct an XP or CS complementation group (Table 8.3). Due to the extensive degree of evolutionary conservation of NER, lower eukaryotes also possess functional homologues of XP and ERCC genes; for example genes from the yeast RAD3 epistasis group, mutants of which are characterized by UV sensitivity and repair deficiency, are frequently homologous to higher eukaryote NER genes (Table 8.3). Tanaka and colleagues directly cloned the first XP gene (XPA) in 1989[32], and since then, with the help of rodent and yeast NER mutants, the genes or proteins responsible for the defect in six of the seven complementation groups of XP and one of the CS groups have been identified.

Table 8.3 Cloned XP and ERCC genes involved in nucleotide excision repair (NER)

Syndrome	*Gene*	*Chromosomal location*	*Protein size/aa (kDa)*	*Yeast homologues*	*Protein properties*
XPA	XPA	9q34	273	RAD14	Binds ss and UV-irradiated dsDNA. Zn^{2+} finger motif
XPB (XPB/CS)	XPB (ERCC3)	2q21	782	RAD25/SSL2	Putative DNA helicase. Part of TFIH transcription factor
XPC	XPC	—	823	RAD4?	Associated with TFIH in a complex with the human homologue of RAD23
XPD (XPD/CS PIBIDS)	XPD (ERCC2)	19q 13.2	760	RAD3	DNA helicase. Part of the TFIH basal transcription complex
XPE	—	—	(125 kDa)	—	Binds UV-irradiated DNA
XPF	XPF (ERCC4?)	—	—	RAD1?	Complexed with ERCC1 and ERCC11. DNA nuclease?
XPG (XPG/CS)	XPG (ERCC5)	13q32-33	1186	RAD2	DNA nuclease?
CSB	CSB (ERCC6)	10q11-21	1493	—	DNA helicase. Involved in transcription–repair coupling
	(ERCC 1)	19q13.2	297	RAD10	Complexed with ERCC11/XPF. DNA nuclease

XPA and XPE: damage recognition and photoproduct binding?

Cells from XPA and XPE patients appear to lack proteins involved in DNA binding and damage recognition respectively. The XPA gene was directly cloned by genomic complementation of repair-defective XPA cells[32] and was found to encode a 40–42-kDa protein capable of binding to both single-stranded and UV-irradiated double-stranded DNA, with a preference for binding to the UV lesions on DS DNA[33,34]. Mutations in the endogenous XPA gene have been reported for XPA patients; most are homozygous for a splicing mutation at intron III and develop severe skin manifestations from early infancy as well as severe progressive neurological abnormalities, whereas patients heterozygous for this mutation generally have milder cutaneous and neurological features[35]. A 125-kDa protein which specifically binds DNA-containing UV photoproducts has been isolated from crude extracts of mammalian cells and was found to be absent in cells derived from some, but not all, XPE patients, suggesting that defects in this protein may underlie XPE[36]. In those XPE cell extracts where the 125-kDa factor is present, the XPE phenotype may still arise from mutations in the same protein, but which affect a function other than DNA binding. Such functions may include protein–protein interactions associated with the recruitment of other repair enzymes to the newly discovered lesion.

XPB, XPD and XPC: DNA surveillance?

The genes responsible for both XPB and XPD were isolated by correction of the repair defect in mutant rodent cells from ERCC complementation groups 3 and 2 respectively[37,38]. Both genes share significant homology with the two superfamilies of genes encoding the DNA and RNA helicases of both prokaryotes and eukaryotes, and both the XPB and XPD proteins are now known to possess ATP-dependent helicase activity[39]. In a ground-breaking discovery, Egly and colleagues[40] have shown that the ERCC3/XPB helicase is a component of the TFIIH (BTF2) basic transcription factor required for initiation of all class II gene transcription in eukaryotes and that microinjection of purified TFIIH could complement not only the repair defect in ERCC3/XPB mutants, but also that in ERCC2/XPD mutant cells[40]. Using an *in-vitro* excision repair assay, this work has now been extended to show that highly purified TFIIH (BTF2) complex can complement three different cell extracts deficient in NER: XPB/ERCC3, XPC and XPD/ERCC2. Co-elution of the TFIIH transcription activity with activities complementing XPB and XPD extracts was absolute, whereas, in the final purification step, the XPC complementing activity was separated from the TFIIH transcription activity. This indicates that XPB/ERCC3 and XPD/ERCC2 are integral components of TFIIH and that the XPC complementing activity is closely associated with TFIIH but is not essential for transcription initiation by TFIIH[41]. It is now thought likely that the TFIIH complex performs a dual role in both RNA polymerase II transcription and in NER in eukaryotic cells. Considering the helicase activity of XPB/ERCC3 and XPD/ERCC2, this role undoubtedly involves the local melting of the DNA duplex. This is required during transcription to allow further proteins (particularly RNA polymerase II) greater access to the DNA; in NER, a similar function can be envisaged[42]. Helicase activities in NER might be involved in the scanning of native DNA for lesions, or they might function to unwind the DNA at sites of damage to allow access by an incision nuclease or to displace the oligonucleotide which contains the damage. The XPC complementing activity is not required for transcription but is associated with the TFIIH complex for overall genome NER. This view is supported by the fact that null mutants of XPB/ERCC3 and XPD/ERCC2 have not been isolated, probably because they result in lethality due to a transcriptional deficiency while, by contrast, XPC null mutants have been found in XPC patients[43]. The yeast homologues of XPB and XPD genes, RAD25 and RAD3 respectively, also comprise a complex required for transcription and repair in yeast and are homozygous lethal[44].

Purification of the XPC complementing activity using a cell-free system yielded a protein complex which alone could complement the repair defect in XPC cell extracts. The complex contains the previously identified XPC gene product (125 kDa) together with a 58-kDa protein homologous to the yeast RAD23 protein (named HHR23B)[45]. While sequence analysis provided few clues as to function, one speculation might be that the XPC–HHR23B complex is required to uncouple the TFIIH complex (containing the XPB/CS and XPD helicases) from the basal transcription apparatus, thus allowing it to function in overall genome repair. Examination of the XPC gene at the nucleotide level in five XPC patients indicated unique mutations in each case, the severity of the mutation correlating well with the degree of repair deficiency and the clinical severity of the disease[43].

A dual role for the XPB and XPD proteins in NER and transcription explains the wide diversity of clinical symptoms arising from mutations in these genes. All of the three known XPB patients possess the rare combination of XP and Cockayne syndrome and show phenotypes atypical of other XPs, such as a severe growth defect and variable neurological abnormalities caused by the demyelination of neurons. While a complete absence of XPB gene product is fatal during embryogenesis, different mutations in an expressed XPB gene might have subtle effects on transcription, giving rise to the variable clinical symptoms as well as impaired NER leading to photosensitivity and, in some cases, to elevated skin malignancy. Certainly, the XPB/ERCC3 polypeptide is the largest subunit of TFIIH and is known to interact with at least one other component of the basal transcription apparatus, namely TFIIE, which modulates helicase activity of TFIIH. In this light, it has been suggested that the XPB group represents, at least in part, a transcription defect syndrome[46]. In a similar way, the wide diversity of observed mutations in the XPD/ERCC2 gene can give rise to the highly cancer-prone XPD phenotype alone or to the combinations of XPD and CS or XPD and PIBIDS.

XPG: DNA nuclease?

The XPG-correcting cDNA was accidentally isolated when serum from a patient suffering from the autoimmune disorder, systemic lupus erythematosus, unexpectedly reacted against a 1196-amino-acid protein with significant homology to the yeast NER protein RAD2[47]. Expression of the human cDNA related to the RAD2 gene specifically complements the repair defect in XPG cells, indicating that it is the gene defective in XPG. RAD2 encodes a DNA nuclease activity the function of which in NER is still unknown.

XPF: incision complex?

The first of the human NER genes to be cloned was the ERCC1 gene, which specifically corrects the repair deficiency in the group 1 rodent mutants but does not correct any known form of human DNA repair syndrome[48]. Despite this, the ERCC1 gene is essential for NER, and rodent cells lacking functional ERCC1 are hypersensitive to ultraviolet light and to other bulky adduct inducing agents. Recently, it was shown by two groups of researchers that a 100-kDa protein complex, purified from human HeLa cells and containing the 33-kDa ERCC1 gene product, was capable, not only of complementing the repair defect in rodent group 1 mutants in an NER assay *in vitro*, but also of complementing the defect in rodent groups 4 and 11 and in XPF cell extracts[49,50]. This implies the existence of a protein complex containing the XPF gene product associated with the ERCC1, ERCC4 and/or the ERCC11 gene products in mammalian cells. It is likely that, when the XPF gene is cloned, it will prove identical to either the ERCC4 or ERCC11 genes, which will simplify the story a little. Clues as to the function of this repair complex come from the strong homology of ERCC1 to the yeast RAD10 gene product. In yeast, the RAD10 and RAD1 gene products form a complex with endonuclease activity required for both NER and for the removal of non-homologous sequences during mitotic recombination[51]. Thus, incision of the damaged DNA strand is the predicted function of the ERCC1, XPF and ERCC4/ERCC11 protein complex.

Xeroderma pigmentosum and human nucleotide excision repair

Based on the known and predicted activities of the mammalian NER genes and by analogy with the NER pathway in prokaryotes, the following picture of the involvement of the XP genes in human NER can be drawn up (Figure 8.5): the TFIIH complex, in part comprising the XPB and XPD helicases, unwinds duplex DNA, scanning it for helix-distorting lesions. XPA and XPE proteins recognize and perhaps bind to the lesions, and may act to initiate the NER process. Local unwinding of the DNA at the site of damage creates a structure recognized by the XPF, ERCC1, ERCC4/ERCC11 complex, which performs the dual incision either side of the lesion. The damaged oligonucleotide is removed, either by further helicase activity or through displacement by a DNA polymerase, which is recruited together with the replication proteins, hSSB (human single-strand binding protein) and PCNA (proliferating cell nuclear antigen), to synthesize the repair patch. In addition, the gene for Cockayne syndrome B (CSB) has been cloned and found to encode a putative helicase protein, the role of which appears to couple RNA transcription to repair[52]. The XPC–HHR23B

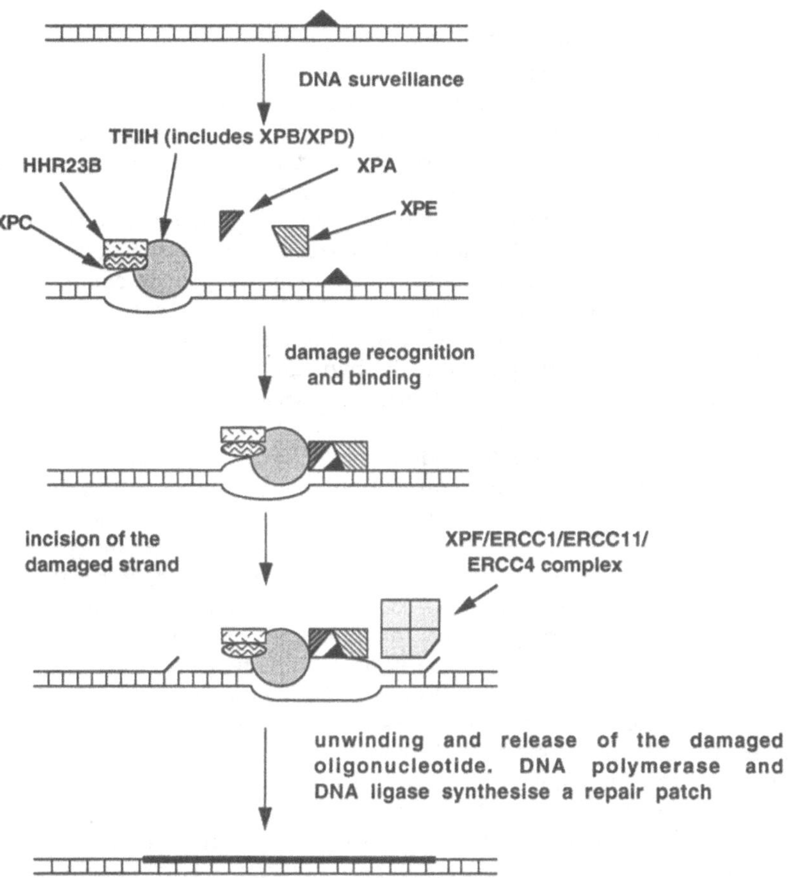

Figure 8.5 Nucleotide excision repair in human cells, indicating the presumed role of the XP/ERCC gene products (see text for further details)

complex in some way facilitates the repair of the bulk genome and the non-transcribed strand of active genes.

Xeroderma pigmentosum and predisposition to cancer

Now that almost all the genes responsible for the seven xeroderma pigmentosum complementation groups have been cloned and the NER pathway in which they, and the genes defective in Cockayne syndrome act, is being elucidated, the link between XP and cancer can be considered further. Two of the most common DNA lesions induced by 254-nm UV irradiation are the cyclobutane pyrimidine dimer (CPD) and the (6-4) photoproduct (Figure 8.2), and they are induced in a ratio of around 3:1 respectively[53,54]. While both types of lesion are mutagenic in human cells if unrepaired[55], their relative contributions to mutagenesis remain unclear with substantial bodies of evidence to support a greater role for either lesion. However, there is general agreement that GC to AT transitions are the predominant mutations arising after UV irradiation. This is probably due to the preferential insertion of an A opposite a non-instructive lesion (such as an unrepaired UV photoproduct) during replicative DNA synthesis[56], and CC to TT double mutations are regarded as a hallmark of UV-induced lesions. To demonstrate a link between the lack of repair of UV photoproducts in XP cells and the elevated risk of cancer in XP patients, it is necessary to show that the unrepaired UV lesions in XP cells give rise to mutations in the growth-controlling genes associated with skin or other tumours.

Reduction in DNA repair in XP cells is associated with an increase in the UV-induced mutation frequency at the hypoxanthine–guanine phosphoribosyl transferase (HPRT) locus in fibroblasts, following either 254-nm or UVB radiation[30], and also an increased mutation frequency in circulating T lymphocytes cultured directly from affected individuals[57]. The UV-induced mutation spectrum of XP cells also appears to differ from that of normal cells. UV-irradiated shuttle vectors replicated in normal human cells show 65% C to T transitions compared with 90% in XP cells[58,59]. Recent studies highlighting the role of unrepaired UV lesions in skin carcinogenesis have compared the mutation spectra in endogenous genes from skin tumours of normal and XP patients. Higher frequencies of *ras* oncogene modifications have been found in XP skin tumours compared with those from normal individuals, together with a strong correlation between UV-specific lesions and p53 mutations in XP skin tumours. One study found that, out of 40 XP skin tumours examined (mainly basal cell and squamous cell carcinomas), 17 had at least one point mutation in the p53 gene[60]. All the mutations were located at potential pyrimidine dimer sites, i.e. CC dinucleotides, and 61% of these were tandem CC to TT transitions characteristic of UV-induced lesions. Only 13% of p53 mutations found in non-XP skin tumours were CC to TT transitions. These insights convincingly demonstrate the importance of unrepaired UV damage in the activation or loss of important growth-controlling genes in skin tumours of XP patients. However, since p53 is not mutated in all skin tumours of normal or XP patients, further studies are required to ascertain the mutation spectra of a wider range of tumour-suppressor genes as well as oncogenes and their likely association with ultraviolet radiation in the aetiology of skin tumours.

Sunlight as a complex carcinogen

In the development of skin cancer, it is important to remember that sunlight is a complex carcinogen comprising, at the earth's surface, wavelengths from the visible to the UVB region, and, while action spectra for cell killing and mutation induction indicate strong associations with UVA and UVB radiations[61,62], the induction of at least some cancers, including melanoma, may also be associated with longer wavelengths of UVA (320–400 nm) and even visible light[62]. These longer wavelengths create DNA damage indirectly via the free radicals generated following absorption of light energy by cellular chromophores. The DNA damage caused by free radicals (base damage, strand breaks)[63] more closely resembles that caused by ionizing radiation than by shorter UVB and C wavelengths, and the level of damage produced is critically dependent on the effectiveness of cellular free radical scavenging pathways[64]. In this context, it is therefore important to note that the activity of catalase, a key enzyme which protects against reactive oxygen species, is significantly reduced in fibroblasts from XP individuals[65]. The aetiology of elevated skin cancer in XP may, thus, be more complex than was initially envisaged.

Xeroderma pigmentosum heterozygotes and cancer

Studies in the US have indicated that individuals heterozygous for XP genes may be slightly predisposed to skin cancer[66]. However, no excess of skin cancer has been reported for similar studies in the UK[67] and, in neither case was an increase in mortality from cancer observed in relatives of XP patients. Furthermore, while cells from XP heterozygotes demonstrate normal UV sensitivity, there is evidence for a reduced efficiency of excision repair in at least some XP heterozygote cells[68,69]. In another study, the V_{max} value for incision in XPA heterozygotes following UV irradiation was found to be roughly half that of normal cells[70]. Since the increased incidence of skin cancer in the US amongst XP heterozygotes is confined mainly to the southern States[66], this may be explained by supposing that, as a result of gene dosage, some XP heterozygotes do possess suboptimal excision repair capacity, which is only associated with increased skin cancer in areas where high sunlight exposure is sufficient to saturate the limited repair capacity.

The paradox of Cockayne syndrome and cancer predisposition

Given their defective NER, the question which remains is why CS patients do not suffer from an excess of skin cancer. In CS, the lack of a subpathway of NER required for preferential repair of transcribed DNA might be expected to lead to more frequent mutations in active genes. Indeed, an elevated frequency of HPRT mutants in T lymphocytes has been reported for CS patients, but studies of UV-induced mutability in primary CS cells have been hampered by their premature senescence. More recent studies with transformed CS cells indicate a raised mutation frequency following UV, which is elevated above normal levels, though not to the same extent as in XP[30]. It is probably the case that, whilst preferential repair has a profound effect on cell survival through the removal of lesions which inhibit transcription, for humans at least, it contributes little to suppressing mutagenesis. There are three reasons for supposing this to be so: first, mutations may still arise in active genes through lesions present in the non-transcribed strand, which is not influenced by preferential repair[71]; second, preferential repair of transcribed DNA only accelerates the removal of a subset of

DNA lesions, including pyrimidine dimers, but not the second most common UV-induced lesion, (6-4) photoproducts[72]. The removal of (6-4) photoproducts is 'fast' in both the bulk and transcribed DNA and perhaps the preferential repair pathway is targeted to lesions which are normally more difficult to repair, such as pyrimidine dimers. Third, the 'slower' overall genome repair present in CS cells will, of course, eventually remove all the lesions in both the non-transcribed and transcribed strands, averting mutagenesis over the entire genome. Far more serious, in mutagenic terms, is a defect in overall genome repair, made clear by the increased mutagenic sensitivity of XPC cells and the tumour proneness of XPC individuals. In XPC cells, there is transcription-coupled repair but overall genome repair is lacking[73].

As discussed earlier, several individuals exhibit a very rare conjunction of clinical features of both XP and CS. Three such patients comprise the XPB/CS group, while one case (two sibs) of XPD/CS has been reported together with two cases of XPG/CS[74–76]. While these patients illustrate both the neurological problems characteristic of CS and the abnormal skin pigmentation of XP, in only two cases were XP-like skin tumours found. The early deaths of the two XPG/CS individuals (at 2 and 6 years of age) would explain the absence of tumours but not in the two sibs assigned to XPB/CS who are still alive yet without XP-associated skin tumours. Of the two XPD/CS sibs, only a single tumour was reported in total though, among other members of the XPD group, the development of tumours is not inevitable[74]. The absence or low frequency of skin tumours in many of the XP/CS individuals remains an enigma, and it will require the creation and study of XP and XP/CS mouse models in order to gain further insights into the problem. Interestingly, cells from all combined XP/CS patients demonstrate a lack of both overall genome repair and of preferential repair of transcribed genes, similar to XPA cells.

The role of immune surveillance in XP

One immune surveillance mechanism thought to be critical in protecting the host against the development of neoplasia is cytotoxicity by natural killer (NK) cells. A variety of cellular immune abnormalities have been identified in XP patients[77], including reduced NK activity compared with normal controls. In contrast, a small number of patients with CS and PIBIDS showed normal immune function and normal NK activity[78]. These findings led at first to the suggestion that decreased immune function, in particular lack of NK activity, might play a role in the cancer proneness of XP compared with CS and PIBIDS[79]. Subsequent studies involving larger numbers of patients have indicated that not all cancer-prone XP patients have reduced NK activity and that four out of five patients with the non-cancer-prone disorder PIBIDS also lacked normal NK activity[80,81]. However, peripheral blood and lymphocytes from all XP patients tested showed marked reduction of interferon-γ production after stimulation with interferon inducers[81]. Whilst this latter deficiency may play a role in skin cancer susceptibility in XP, comparative studies have yet to be reported for CS and PIBIDS patients so the exact role of immune surveillance in XP remains unclear.

XERODERMA PIGMENTOSUM VARIANT

Xeroderma pigmentosum variant (XPV) patients develop similar clinical characteristics to XP patients from other complementation groups, including photosensitivity and elevated skin cancer, but differ in the absence of neurological symptoms. Unlike cells from the classical XP groups, cultured XPV cells, which all fall into a single complementation group, do not possess a defect in NER. They are only mildly UV sensitive and exhibit normal or near normal excision rates for UV photoproducts. The defect in XPV cells lies in their inability to replicate DNA containing UV-induced lesions as efficiently as normal human cells. Mammalian cells are now known to be able to replicate a genome containing large amounts of damage by simply bypassing the sites of DNA lesions. However, this operation may leave discontinuities in the newly synthesized DNA strand, which must be dealt with at a later time in a process called post-replication recovery (PRR). The defect in XPV was first observed almost twenty years ago by Lehmann and colleagues, as a slow rate of daughter strand maturation following UV irradiation[82]. In stark contrast to the dramatic progress in understanding the defects in NER underpinning the classical XP groups, little more is known today about the molecular biology of post-replication recovery in mammalian cells or of the specific defect in XPV than was known twenty years ago.

A link between the PRR deficiency of XPV cells and the cancer proneness of XPV patients is, however, provided by the hypersensitivity of skin fibroblasts from XPV patients to the mutagenic effects of UV[83]. UV-induced mutation studies involving both the endogenous HPRT locus and shuttle vectors carrying the mutagenesis market gene, SupF, have shown that the mutation spectra differ between XPV and normal cells[84,85]. XPV cells are less likely than normal cells to insert an adenine residue opposite UV photoproducts during bypass replication; under normal circumstances adenine is by far the most common base inserted opposite a non-instructional or modified base (known as the 'A' rule[56]). This suggests that a qualitatively altered DNA polymerase is involved in replication past UV photoproducts in XPV cells. It may also help to explain the elevated mutation induction since cyclobutane dimers formed between two adjacent thymine residues are the most common form of UV photoproduct, and therefore insertion of an adenine in the opposite strand will not result in a mutation. However, the insertion of non-adenine bases, in particular pyrimidines, opposite dimers will give rise to mutations. A plausible explanation for the defect in XPV is that these cells carry an alteration in a DNA polymerase or in an accessory factor which enables the replication complex to replicate past UV photoproducts in the template DNA.

DEFECT IN MISMATCH REPAIR AND COLON CANCER?

The genetic basis of cancer development is reflected in the two major premises around which investigation of the malignant phenotype is focused. First, that malignancy arises through alterations in the genetic material of the cell; and, second, that the accumulation of these mutations occurs in a multistep fashion[86].

The clinical presentation of the disease is attributed to those genetic alterations leading to perturbations in cell growth control. Progressive genetic changes in the growth-controlling genes of cells (proto-oncogenes and tumour suppressor genes) have been documented in a wide variety of human cancers. However, the molecular origins of these mutations are still poorly understood and the contribution of exogenous compared with endogenous mutagenesis is still unclear. Skin cancer in XP patients is believed to arise from defective restoration of the DNA following ultraviolet light. In contrast, the very recent discovery[87,88] of a defective gene involved in the repair of replication mismatches in the hereditary form of colon cancer (HNPCC) provides insight into the role of repair mechanisms in preventing carcinogenesis arising from endogenous mutations.

Mismatch repair in *E. coli* and man

In all cells so far studied, replication errors remaining after DNA polymerase proofreading are corrected by the mismatch repair system[13], a current model for which is depicted in Figure 8.6. In *E. coli*, the first step requires recognition of the mismatch – perhaps a T:T or A:C mispair or two or more unpaired bases looped out from the DNA – by the 97-kDa MutS protein. Binding of MutS to the mismatch recruits a homodimer of the 70-kDa MutL protein and a 25-kDa monomeric MutH protein to the location of the mismatch. MutH possesses DNA endonuclease activity and cleaves the newly synthesized DNA strand containing the mismatched base(s) at a nearby hemimethylated d(GATC) sequence. The newly replicated strand in *E. coli* is distinguishable from the old template strand due to a delay in methylation of the adenine residue in newly synthesized d(GATC) sequences by the *Dam* methylase protein. Thus, lack of methylation of d(GATC) sequences instructs the MutH protein to cleave the newly synthesized strand, hence imparting strand specificity to the reaction. The mispaired base(s) on this strand are replaced in order to preserve the original informational content of the DNA. The late steps of mismatch repair are typical of those in excision repair reactions; an oligonucleotide containing the mismatched base is unwound from the incision by the UvrD helicase and a combination of an exonuclease to degrade the displaced DNA, a polymerase (Pol III of *E. coli*) to synthesize the repair patch and DNA ligase act in concert to complete the repair reaction. The same basic model is thought to occur in mammalian cells, but, without a *Dam* methylase system, it is unclear how, if at all, strand specificity of incision is imparted.

Mismatch repair and hereditary non-polyposis colon cancer

Lynch and colleagues described two disorders characterized by an autosomal dominantly inherited predisposition to colon cancer without polyposis[89]. Together, Lynch syndromes I and II comprise hereditary non-polyposis colon cancer (HNPCC), and are among the most common cancer-predisposing syndromes, with as many as 1 affected individual in 200[90]. Both syndromes are associated with early age of diagnosis of colon cancer, particularly tumours of the

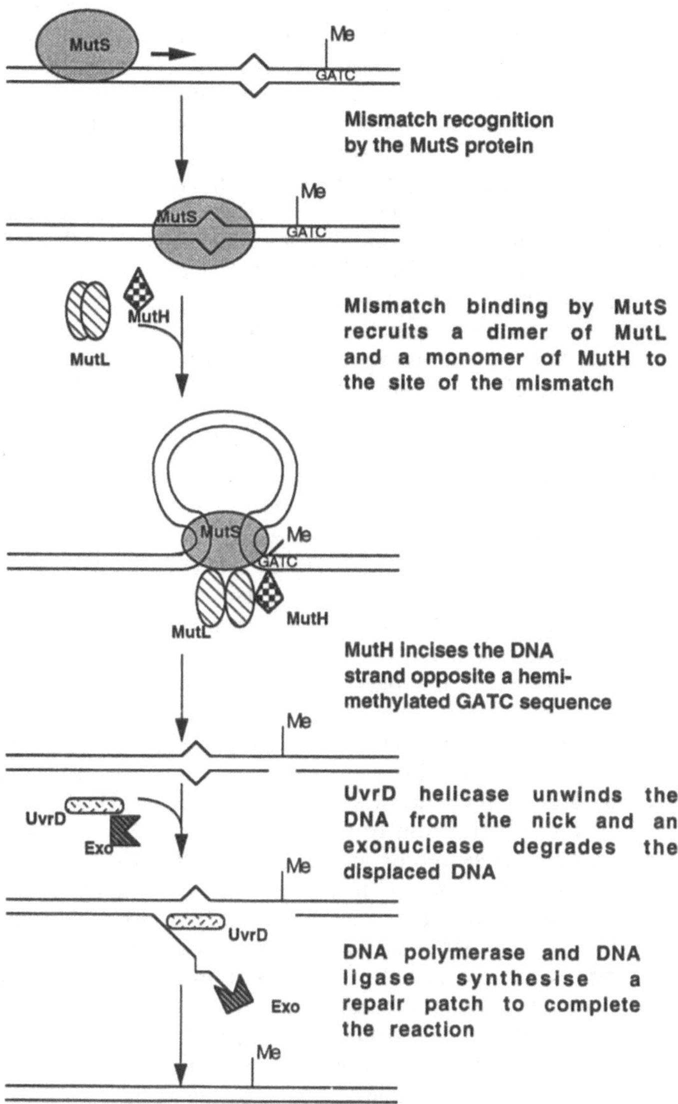

Figure 8.6 Mismatch repair in *E. coli* (see text for explanation)

right colon, and a susceptibility to multiple primary malignancies. While colonic adenomas are more common in HNPCC individuals, HNPCC is distinguished from familial adenomatous polyposis coli (FAPC) by an absence of the florid polyposis associated with the latter disease. The mean age of onset of colon cancer in the Lynch syndromes is around 44 years and the penetrance of the syndromes is thought to be 75–90%. Lynch syndrome II also predisposes to extra-colonic cancer, such as cancer of the uterus, ovary, stomach, pancreas and breast.

Physical and linkage analysis using HNPCC families was used to map the most common HNPCC gene to an 800-kb region on chromosome 2p[87,91]. The laborious task of searching this region for genes by chromosome walking seemed inevitable when a surprise discovery linking a subset of colon tumours to a defect in replication or mismatch repair was made. Using a PCR-based genomic fingerprinting technique, the laboratory of Perucho showed that 12% of colorectal carcinomas carried somatic deletions in poly(dA:dT) sequences and other simple repeats[92]. They estimated that over 100 000 such mutations were present in cells from these tumours and that all neoplasias from the same individuals contained similar levels of simple repeat instability. In addition, repeat instability correlated with a particular clinical presentation of tumours of the right colon, mainly poor differentiation and good prognosis. A number of researchers went on to establish that repeat instability was a constant characteristic of hereditary non-polyposis colorectal cancer (HNPCC) and occurred in a subset of sporadic colon cancers[93]. These tumours were designated RER$^+$, for replication error positive. Experiments in yeast had shown that while mutations in the proofreading domain of DNA polymerases had little effect on simple repeat stability, mutations in any one of three genes involved in mismatch repair (PMS1, MLH1 and MSH2) led to as much as a 700-fold increase in the rate of expansion and contraction of dinucleotide repeat sequences[94]. The similarity of DNA sequence changes between mismatch repair defective yeast cells and RER$^+$ colon cancers implicated defective mismatch repair as the likely source of DNA instability in these tumours.

The human homologue of the bacterial MutS gene (MSH2 in the yeast *Saccharomyces cerevisiae*) was cloned and mapped to human chromosome 2p22-21, the same region which contains the HNPCC gene[88]. Mutations in the human MutS homologue, hMSH2, were found in the germ-line DNA from affected individuals of HNPCC kindreds as well as in the DNA of sporadic colon tumours. A T to C transition in the splice acceptor site of an intron in front of the most highly conserved exon was found in affected members of two unrelated HNPCC kindreds[88] and a C to T transition at codon 622, resulting in substitution of leucine for proline in another highly conserved sequence of hMSH2, was found to segregate exactly with the disease in a third kindred[87]. Identical mutations were also found in some tumours from patients with no family history of colon cancer. At the same time, it was discovered that extracts from HNPCC tumour cell lines and from sporadic RER$^+$ tumours were unable to carry out mismatch recognition in a cell-free system[95]. The defect in the recognition of DNA mismatches could be complemented by the addition of protein fractions from normal cells. Purification of the complementing activity led to the isolation of the hMSH gene product[96].

Taken together, this evidence demonstrates that defects in the hMSH2 gene underlie the most common form of HNPCC and the RER$^+$ group of sporadic colon cancers. It is likely that affected individuals of HNPCC kindreds inherit a single defective hMSH2 gene and that a further somatic event is required to inactivate the second wild-type allele giving rise to a mismatch repair defective, RER$^+$ cell (the Knudsen two-hit hypothesis). To support this, most tumours from affected HNPCC individuals share similarly unstable repeats and are defective in mismatch repair *in vitro*; all non-tumour tissues from the same individuals are both RER⁻ and have normal mismatch repair capabilities, indicating a recessive phenotype for the hMSH2 gene.

The role of mismatch repair and repeat instability in colon tumorigenesis

It is widely acknowledged that the development of cancer requires multiple mutations in cellular oncogenes and tumour supressor genes. Colon cancer is no exception and the dominant oncogene, K-*ras* and the tumour suppressor genes, DCC (**D**eleted in **C**olon **C**ancer), APC (gene associated with **A**denomatous **P**olyposis **C**oli), as well as p53 have been consistently associated with colon tumours. Whilst the order in which these mutations accumulate is not critical, there is some preference for the following sequence of events: mutations inactivating APC occur at an early stage, followed by activation of K-*ras* and the inactivation of DCC and p53[97,98]. It is now known that the DNA-repeat instability characteristic of RER$^+$ tumours arises as a very early event in colon tumour development and persists after transformation[99]. The distinguishing clinical features of RER$^+$ tumours can be explained by supposing that the mode of genetic instability behind RER$^+$ tumour progression differs from that of other colon tumours. This accounts for the low correlation with p53 mutations and for the absence of gross chromosomal instability (particularly translocations and allelic loss through large deletions) in RER$^+$ tumours. Whether the RER$^+$ phenotype is generated via mutation of the remaining wild-type hMSH2 allele as the first event in colorectal cancer or whether it occurs as an early secondary event in cells already carrying a growth advantage, is not yet known. The latter hypothesis is supported by the knowledge that, in HNPCC, benign polyps in the colon undergo transformation to tumours at a higher rate than in other forms of colon cancers, whilst the frequency at which such polyps arise initially is not greater for HNPCC patients. Once the second hMSH2 allele has been inactivated, it is logical to assume that the resultant mismatch repair defect accelerates the accumulation of mutations in other critical growth-controlling genes. There are, however, a couple of unanswered questions. First, a direct link between spontaneous mutagenesis and repeat instability has yet to be firmly established. An increase in spontaneous mutation rates of around 2–4-fold has been demonstrated in two RER$^+$ tumour lines[100], but this hardly parallels the 1000-fold increase in spontaneous mutation rates in *E. coli* lacking MutS activity. A wider survey of spontaneous mutagenesis in RER$^+$ cell lines is required to ascertain the contribution of hMSH2 in suppressing mutagenesis in human cells. The predisposition of HNPCC patients to develop mainly non-polyposis colon cancer is also interesting since it is not evident why the loss of the second allele of hMSH2 should occur more or less specifically in colon tumours. We can only speculate that there may exist an as yet undefined role of hMSH2 in preventing HNPCC.

Further considerations

Mammalian cells contain at least two different homologues of the bacterial MutS gene and also two of MutL, the other bacterial gene involved in early stages of mismatch correction. Methyl-directed mismatch repair is restricted to prokaryotes and a MutH homologue is not thought to exist in mammalian cells. However, many more genes involved in mammalian mismatch correction may await discovery. In *E. coli*, genes whose products are involved in correcting specific mismatches generated by chemical modifications of DNA bases (e.g. deamination of 5-methyl-cytosine to give thymine) also have mutator phenotypes when deleted. Defects in as yet unknown genes performing similar functions in humans may underlie other cancers and cancer-prone disorders. In this respect, it is encouraging that mutations in the human mismatch repair gene homologous to MutL, hMLH1, have recently been reported to be associated with a minority of HNPCC families, where the disease locus maps to chromosome 3p21-22[101]. Finally, the tantalizing possibility also exists that some form of replication or repair abnormality underlies the sudden expansion of triplet repeats known to cause a number of human diseases, including fragile-X syndrome and Huntington chorea[102].

THE CHROMOSOME BREAKAGE DISORDERS

The breakage and reunion of chromosomes mechanistically provokes the occurrence of large-scale chromosomal alterations, such as translocations, deletions and amplifications in eukaryotic DNA. These types of genetic change, often of a non-random nature, at the level of the chromosome are often associated with specific malignancies, as well as reflecting a general genome instability common to a diverse range of tumour types. Together with tumour cells in general, a small number of human hereditary diseases are associated with spontaneously elevated levels of chromosome abnormalities and these are termed the chromosome breakage disorders[103]. Patients who suffer from three of these – ataxia telangiectasia, Bloom syndrome and Fanconi anaemia – also demonstrate high incidence of cancer. A major question remains whether elevated rates of chromosome instability are associated with DNA repair defects.

Ataxia telangiectasia

Ataxia telangiectasia (AT) is an autosomal recessive disorder (1 in approximately 300 000 live births) characterized by telangiectases, progressive cerebellar ataxia and recurrent respiratory infections. Affected children, who are generally small, usually develop telangiectases between the ages of 3 and 5 years, firstly on the bulbar conjunctiva and subsequently variably involving the ears, eyelids, cheeks and limbs. The ataxia is progressive, often first manifest as clumsiness in the second year of life, but deteriorating such that the child may be unable to walk without assistance by the age of 12. Other signs of cerebellar disease, such as nystagmus and slurred speech, occur and mental deterioration may be observed. Recurrent sinus and pulmonary infections are frequent and may be fatal. Disturbances in immunological mechanisms include thymic abnormalities, lymphocytopenia and abnormalities of the humoral and cellular immunity. A diminished or absent IgA is especially characteristic and may be detected even before other manifestations have appeared.

There is considerable evidence for an increased risk of cancer associated with the AT gene. AT homozygotes have a risk of cancer 60–184 times greater than the general US population[104] and around 1 in 10 develop a malignancy in childhood. The vast majority of tumours in AT patients are lymphoid in origin and a 70-fold and 250-fold excess of leukaemias and lymphomas, respectively, has been reported for AT patients[105]. An elevated risk of cancer of the stomach, liver, uterus and ovaries has also been observed associated with AT[106]. Studies performed on 60 AT families in the UK have led to the suggestion that AT patients with T-cell tumours can be grouped into either an older or younger category. T-cell chronic lymphocytic leukaemia (T-CLL) arises mainly in older AT patients (mean age 33 years) whilst T-cell acute leukaemia/lymphoma (T-ALL) is the predominant cancer in younger patients between 2 and 12 years of age[105]. In the heterozygous state, the AT gene has been reported to give rise to a risk of cancer 2–6 times above the average[107]. Most significantly, the heterozygous risk of breast cancer in women was found to be 6.8 times the national average. Why the AT gene in the heterozygous state should predispose to breast cancer and not to lymphoma/leukaemia, the predominant cancer in homozygotes, is not known.

Complementation studies have demonstrated the existence of at least four ataxia telangiectasia complementation groups (AT-A, AT-C, AT-D and AT-E) as well as a variant group (AT-variant). In three out of the four complementation groups, the gene locus for AT has been localized to chromosome 11q22-23 in a region associated with neurological and immune function loci[108], but, as yet, no definitive AT gene has been cloned[109]. Cultured AT cells are hypersensitive to ionizing radiation and to strand breakage agents, such as bleomycin, but are not hypersensitive to UV light or to alkylating agents [109,110]. Interestingly, AT cells also demonstrate radioresistant DNA synthesis [112] and loss of proliferative controls which normally ensure cycle arrest after damage. Normal cells respond to ionizing radiation damage by inhibiting replicative DNA synthesis, allowing for repair of the genome before replication proceeds. This is not so in AT cells which continue semiconservative replication despite a damaged DNA template. However, this is not thought to be the sole cause of hypersensitivity to ionizing radiation since delaying cell-cycle progression in AT cells does not enhance survival after irradiation[113]. One potential reason for the enhanced X-ray sensitivity of AT cells is the slow rate of repair of DNA double-strand breaks which has been demonstrated in certain AT cells[114] and which correlates with an increased frequency of residual chromosome breaks[115]. A 300-fold elevated rate of interlocus recombination has also been shown for cells from AT patients, indicating a loosening of the restrictions on inappropriate recombination[116]. Hyper-recombination activity in AT may also underlie the increased frequency of chromosome translocations characteristic of AT lymphocytes.

One important consequence of inappropriate recombination occurring in AT patients is the development of cancer. Karyotyping reveals that between 5 and 10% of the circulating T lymphocytes of AT patients carry chromosome translocations, the breakpoints typically occurring on chromosomes 7 and 14 at sites of immune gene complexes. These chromosomal rearrangements include inv(7;14)(p35,q35), t(7;7)(p13;35), t(7;14)p13q11) and t(14;14)(q11;q32).

While similar rearrangements occur in the T cells from normal individuals, the frequency in AT may be 40–50 times higher. It has been noticed that, in AT patients, cells carrying such translocations can expand to produce large clones in the circulating T-cell population. The two main types of translocation involving the immune gene clusters are rearrangements between two T-cell receptor (TCR) genes themselves or between TCR genes and unknown genes on other chromosomes[117,118]. It is only the latter type of rearrangement which produces large clonally expanded populations of translocation T cells, probably due to a growth advantage conferred on those cells by the translocation. These large clones might be considered to have taken the first step along the pathway to malignancy, and, indeed, translocation clones with t(14:14)inv14[119], t(7;14)(q35;q32)[120] and t(X;14)(q28;q11)[121] rearrangements have been reported to give rise to full malignancy. Further genetic changes are required for a complete tumour phenotype to develop from cells of these lineages, which may comprise up to 100% of peripheral T cells, and it has been observed that tumour cells from AT individuals possess a high frequency of further chromosomal abnormalities arising during progression of the disease.

Translocations also occur at high frequency in B cells at sites of V(D)J recombination, and hyper-recombination at these loci may be involved in the variable immunodeficiencies seen in AT patients. In the light of the neurodegeneration of AT patients, it is interesting to note recent evidence of somatic recombination occurring in the brains of transgenic mice[122]. In conclusion, the precise molecular defect of AT is unknown and true understanding of the disease awaits cloning of the genes corresponding to the different complementation groups.

Bloom syndrome

This rare autosomal recessive disorder is more common in males and is particularly prevalent amongst Ashkenazi Jews (carrier rate of 1 in 20). Erythema and telangiectasia affecting the face, particularly the malar area, nose and around the ears, often begin within the first weeks of life. These abnormalities are accentuated by sun exposure which may induce bullae with bleeding and crusting. Repeated sun exposure may eventually lead to reticulate pigmentation and atrophy. Whether true photosensitivity can be demonstrated by phototesting or whether abnormal light responses are restricted to the already damaged telangiectatic skin is unresolved. Bloom syndrome patients are well proportioned but small and have a long narrow head with characteristic facies consisting of a prominent nose and receding chin. Central nervous system abnormalities are uncommon and intelligence is normal.

Patients are predisposed to multiple severe infections and premature development of neoplasms. About 20% of patients develop cancers, half before the age of 20 years. There is a 150–300-fold increased frequency of development of lymphatic and non-lymphatic leukaemia, lymphosarcoma, lymphoma and carcinomas of the oral cavity and gastrointestinal tract. Immunological abnormalities include reduced immunoglobulin levels and reduced lymphocyte proliferative responses to mitogens and in the mixed dose cyte reaction.

Cells from Bloom syndrome (BS) patients fall into a single complementation group and display chromosome abnormalities characteristic of a chromosome breakage disorder. The most impressive chromosome abnormality associated with the disease is the increased level of spontaneous sister chromatid exchanges (SCEs)[123], which provides a clear diagnostic aid for the syndrome. Possibly related to the high rate of SCEs in these cells is their abnormally low rate of DNA replication[124,125]. Spontaneous chromosome aberrations, particularly interchanges between homologous chromatids, are also increased in BS cells. Bloom syndrome cell lines appear to show considerable heterogeneity of response to different DNA-damaging agents; perhaps the only report of hypersensitivity consistently observed over a wide range of BS cells is that to simple alkylating agents[126]. Chromosome aberrations and SCEs are also induced by exposure to UV and a variety of chemical agents, including the alkylating agent EMS.

Some BS cells are reported to possess low levels of DNA ligase I activity[127] but have normal levels of DNA ligase II and III activity. However, mutations have not been identified in the DNA ligase I gene in cells from Bloom syndrome patients[128]. It remains possible that an as yet unknown factor, which interacts with ligase I *in vivo* and is required for ligase activity, is lacking in these cells. No other unifying hypothesis has been put forward to explain the defect in BS cells[129] though a recent discovery has demonstrated a lack of induction of the tumour suppressor gene p53 in 2 out of 11 Bloom syndrome cells lines studied, perhaps implicating a damage-signalling defect[130]. Earlier studies[131] implicated loss of normal cycle control of DNA repair enzymes in the aetiology of Bloom syndrome. Intriguingly, a single individual whose clinical symptoms were initially reminiscent of Bloom syndrome but whose cells exhibited only slightly elevated spontaneous SCE levels has been shown to lack DNA ligase I activity and to possess mutations in both ligase I alleles[132].

The pronounced cancer proneness of Bloom syndrome patients is still a mystery, though BS cells have been shown to be spontaneously hypermutable[133,134]. Constitutively elevated c-*myc* oncogene levels, probably due to the slow repair of DNA strand breaks, have also been implicated in the cancer predisposition of BS[129]. There is also evidence for enhanced somatic recombination between homologous chromosomes in BS cells[133,134]. Somatic crossing-over, resulting in loss of heterozygosity for large regions of chromosomes, is an important mechanism in the loss of tumour supressor genes. Figure 8.7 summarizes the factors which may contribute to cancer proneness in Bloom syndrome. None of the chromosomal abnormalities associated with BS are present in cells from BS heterozygotes and there is no evidence for an increase in malignancy in these individuals.

Fanconi anaemia

The age of onset of this autosomal recessive disorder, which is more common in boys, is usually between 4 and 10 years. Patients with Fanconi anaemia (FA) are characteristically small, hyperpigmented especially around the lower trunk and neck, and possess skeletal abnormalities, notably of the thumb and radius. Microcephaly, mental retardation and hypergonadism are also common. A

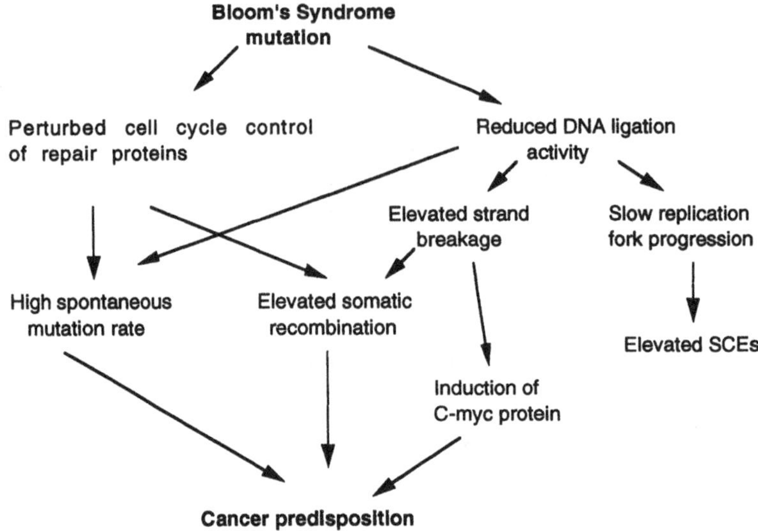

Figure 8.7 Cancer predisposition in Bloom syndrome (see text for further details)

constant feature is progressive hypoplastic anaemia with neutropenia and thrombocytopenia, usually presenting as an increased bleeding tendency. Complete bone marrow failure (pancytopenia) usually causes death within 2–5 years. In addition, FA patients are particularly at risk from myelodysplasia (MDS) and/or acute myelogenous leukaemia (AML) compared with the normal population. Of 371 FA patients analysed in one study, 84% possessed haematological abnormalities and 14% developed MDS or AML; interestingly, risk of cancer was greater in those patients without prior haematological abnormalities[135].

Cutured cells from FA patients show spontaneous chromosome instability in the form of elevated chromatid-type chromosome aberrations; these cells are also hypersensitive to bifunctional DNA crosslinking agents, such as mitomycin C, diepoxybutane, photoreactivated psoralen derivatives and cisplatin. The measurement of chromosome breakage and cellular sensitivity to diepoxybutane (DEB) is used as a diagnostic aid for FA as well as in prenatal screening for the disease[103]. FA cells have been shown to fall into at least four complementation groups[136] and one of the genes (FA group C) has been cloned. This gene encodes a 63-kDa protein, which shares no homology with known proteins and whose function in the cell is still a mystery[137]. Sensitivity to crosslinking agents suggests a defect in the repair of these DNA adducts, and an altered DNA endonuclease complex which recognizes intrastrand crosslinks produced by 8-methoxypsoralen and UVA irradiation has been identified in FA group A cells[135,138]. In addition, FA cells have been reported to be unusually sensitive to high oxygen tensions, to have increased rates of spontaneous intrachromosomal mitotic recombination[135] and to lose the ability to repair DNA interstrand crosslinks during prolonged culture *in vitro*[139], all factors which could contribute to the cancer proneness of the disease. Further attempts at cloning FA genes are likely, though it will probably prove necessary to create mouse models of FA in order to understand the complex mixture of developmental and DNA repair abnormalities associated with this disease.

CONCLUDING REMARKS

We began this chapter with an overview of DNA repair mechanisms and have presented evidence that these processes are a vital resource in protecting human cells against malignant transformation. Extrapolating from *in-vitro* studies[140], the antimutagenic properties of the nucleotide-excision repair process protect against the shorter wavelengths of sunlight, while the mismatch correction system compensates for the limited fidelity of DNA replication. Deficiencies in NER or mismatch repair result in cancer proneness through the accumulating load of mutations; defects in NER may also be associated with complex disease phenotypes. We have also discussed the role of DNA strand breakage in mutation and human cancer. Increased chromosomal instability promotes the progression of many tumours through the amplification, rearrangement and deletion of oncogenes and tumour suppressor genes. Such large-scale mutations may arise from the aberrant rejoining of broken chromosomes through ill-defined mechanisms, and further investigation into the basic processes of DNA breakage and repair will be required to understand fully the reasons behind such forms of genetic instability. In the next few years, we may anticipate good progress in understanding mechanisms of double-strand break repair and the relationship of these operations to recombination. Defects in such processes are likely to cause chromosome instability. A further mechanism of DNA surveillance and damage correction is the base-excision repair (BER) of DNA following oxidation, hydrolysis or non-enzymatic methylation[7]. As yet, no human syndromes have been assigned as defective in BER, probably reflecting the essential nature of this form of repair. On the other hand, it has been suggested that, since a variety of DNA glycosylases act to initiate BER at particular lesions, the loss of one may not affect cell survival but might allow the more rapid accumulation of mutations associated with such lesions. Indeed, defects in *E. coli* glycosylases confer strong mutator phenotypes. Thus, subtle defects in the gene products involved in BER may be associated with specific forms of human cancer, while germ-line mutations in genes encoding BER proteins may be found in any of the 50 or so as-yet unexplained human cancer-prone syndromes[141].

References

1. Friedberg EC. DNA repair. Oxford, UK: W.H. Freeman; 1985.
2. Cleaver JE. Defective repair replication of DNA in xeroderma pigmentosum. Nature. 1968;218:652–656.
3. Fishel R, Lescoe MK, Rao MRS *et al.* The human mutator gene homolog MSH2 and its association with hereditary nonpolyposis colon cancer. Cell. 1993;75:1027–1036.
4. Sancar A. Structure and function of DNA photolyase. Biochemistry. 1994;33:2–9.
5. Margison GP, Brennand J, Ockey CH, O'Connor PJ. Complementation of mammalian DNA repair defects by a prokaryotic gene. BioEssays. 1989;11:58–63.

6. Hoejmakers JHJ. Nucleotide excision repair I: from *E.coli* to yeast. Trends Genet. 1993;9:173–177.
7. Lindahl T. Instability and decay of the primary structure of DNA. Nature. 1993;362:709–715.
8. Obe G, Johannes C, Schulke-Frohlinde D. DNA double strand breaks induced by sparsely ionizing radiation and endonucleases as critical lesions for cell death, chromosome aberrations, mutations and oncogenic transformations. Mutagenesis. 1992;7:3–12.
9. Haber JE. Exploring the pathways of homologous recombination. Curr Opin Cell Biol. 1992;4:401–412.
10. Roth DB, Wilson J. Illegitimate recombination in mammalian cells. In: Kucherlapati R, Smith GR, ed. Genetic recombination. Washington DC: American Society of Microbiology;1988.
11. Kaufmann WK. Pathways of human post-replication repair. Carcinogenesis. 1989;10:1–11.
12. Kornberg A, Baker T. DNA replication. 2nd edn. Oxford, UK:W.H. Freeman; 1992.
13. Modrich P. Mechanisms and biological effects of mismatch repair. Ann Rev Genet. 1991;25:229–253.
14. Kreamer KH, Lee MM, Scotto J. Xeroderma pigmentosum. Cutaneous, ocular and neurologic abnormalities in 830 published cases. Arch Dermatol. 1987;123:241–250.
15. Kreamer KH, Lee MM, Scotto J. DNA repair protects against cutaneous and internal neoplasia: Evidence from xeroderma pigmentosum. Carcinogenesis. 1982;5:511–514.
16. Hakamada S, Watanabe K, Soboe G, *et al.* Xeroderma pigmentosum: Neurological, neurophysiological and morphological studies. Eur Neurol. 1982;21:69–76.
17. Roytta M, Anttinan A. Xeroderma pigmentosum with neurological abnormalities. A clinical and neuropathological study. Acta Neurol Scand. 1986; 73:191–199.
18. Reed WB, May SB, Nickel WB. Xeroderma pigmentosum with neurological complications: the de Sanctis–Cacchione syndrome. Arch Dermatol. 1965;91:224–226.
19. Tanaka K, Wood RD. Xeroderma pigmentosum and nucleotide excision repair of DNA. Trends Biochem Sci. 1994;19:83–86.
20. Cleaver JE, Kraemer KH. In: Scriver CR, Beaudet AL, Sly WS, Valle D, eds. The metabolic basis of inherited disease, Vol II. Maidenhead: McGraw Hill; 1989.
21. Ramsey CA, Cotart TM, Blunt S, Pawsey SA, Giannelli F. Prenatal diagnosis of xeroderma pigmentosum. Report of the first successful case. Lancet. 1975;2:1109–1112.
22. Hoeijmakers JHJ. Nucleotide excision repair I: from E.coli to yeast. Trends Gene. 1993;9:173–177.
23. Shivji MKK, Kenny MK, Wood RD. PCNA is required for DNA excision repair. Cell. 1992;69:367–374.
24. Coverley D, Kenny MK, Munn M, Rupp WD, Lane DP, Wood RD. Requirement for the replication protein SSB in human DNA excision repair. Nature. 1991;349:538–541.
25. Downes CS, Ryan AJ, Johnson RT. Fine tuning of DNA repair in transcribed genes: mechanisms, prevalence and consequences. BioEssays. 1993;15:209–216.
26. Selby CP, Sancar A. Molecular mechanism of transcription-repair coupling. Science. 1993;260:53–58.
27. Hanawalt PC, Cooper PK, Ganesan AK, Smith CA. DNA repair in bacteria and mammalian cells. Annu Rev Biochem. 1979;48:783–836.
28. Nance MA, Berry SA. Cockayne syndrome: review of 140 cases. Am J Med Genet. 1992;42:68–84.
29. Venema J, Mullenders LHF, Natarajan AT, Van Zeelan AA, Mayne LV. The genetic defect in Cockayne syndrome is associated with a defect in repair of UV-induced DNA damage in transcriptionally active DNA. Proc Natl Acad Sci USA. 1990;87:4707–4711.
30. Arlett CF, Harcourt SA. Variations in response to mutagens amongst normal and repair defective human cells. In: Lawrence CW, ed. Induced mutagenesis. Molecular mechanisms and their implications for environmental protection. New York: Plenum Press; 1983:249–266.
31. Rebora A, Crovato F. Trichothiodystrophy, xeroderma pigmentosum and PIBI(D)S syndrome. Hum Genet. 1988;78:106–108.
32. Tanaka K, Satokato I, Ogito Z, Uchida T, Okado Y. Molecular cloning of a mouse DNA repair gene that complements the defect of group-A xeroderma pigmentosum. Proc Natl Acad Sci USA. 1989;86:5512–5516.
33. Tanaka K, Miura N, Satokata I, *et al.* Analysis of a human excision repair gene involved in group A xeroderma pigmentosum and containing a zinc finger domain. Nature. 1990;348:73–76.

34. Robins P, Jones CJ, Biggerstaff M, Lindahl T, Wood RD. Complementation of the DNA repair defect in a xeroderma pigmentosum group A cell extract by a protein with affinity for damaged DNA. EMBO J. 1991;10:3913–3921.
35. Nishigori C, Moriwaki S, Takebe H, Tanaka T, Imamura S. Gene alterations and clinical characteristics of xeroderma pigmentosum group A patients in Japan. Arch Dermatol. 1994;130:191–197.
36. Hwang BJ, Chu G. Purification and characterisation of a human protein that binds to damaged DNA. Biochemistry. 1993;32:1657–1666.
37. Weeda G, van Ham RCA, Vermeulen W, Bootsma D, van der Eb AJ, Hoeijmakers JHJ. A presumed DNA helicase encoded by ERCC-3 is involved in the human repair disorders xeroderma pigmentosum and Cockayne's syndrome. Cell. 1990;62:777–791.
38. Flejter WL, McDaniel ID, Johns D, Friedberg EC, Schultz RA. Correction of xeroderma pigmentosum complementation group D mutant cell phenotypes by chromosome and gene transfer: involvement of the human ERCC2 DNA repair gene. Proc Natl Acad Sci USA. 1992;89:261–265.
39. Sung P, Bally V, Weber C, Thompson LH, Prakash L, Prakash S. Human xeroderma pigmentosum group D gene encodes a DNA helicase. Nature. 1993;365:852–855.
40. Schaeffer L, Roy R, Humbert S, *et al.* DNA repair helicase: A component of BTF2 (TFIIH) basic transcription factor. Science. 1993;260:58–63.
41. Drapkin R, Reardon JT, Ansari A, *et al.* Dual role of TFIIH in DNA excision repair and in transcription by RNA polymerase II. Nature. 1994;368:769–772.
42. Matson SW, Bean DW, George JW. DNA helicases: enzymes with essential roles in all aspects of DNA metabolism. Bio Essays. 1994;16:13–22.
43. Li L, Bales ES, Peterson CA, Legerski RJ. Characterisation of molecular defects in xeroderma pigmentosum group C. Nature Genet. 1993;54:413–417.
44. Prakash S, Sung P, Prakash L. DNA repair genes and proteins of *Saccharomyces cerevisiae*. Annu Rev Genet. 1993;27:33–70.
45. Chikahide M, Sugasawa K, Yanagisawa J, *et al.* Purification and cloning of a nucleotide excision repair complex involving the xeroderma pigmentosum group C protein and a human homologue of yeast RAD23. EMBO J. 1994;13:1831–1843.
46. Bootsma D, Hoeijmakers JHJ. Engagement with transcription. Nature. 1993;363:114–115.
47. Scherly D, Nouspikel T, Corlet J, Ucla C, Bairoc A, Clarkson SG. Complementation of the DNA repair defect in xeroderma pigmentosum group G cells by a human cDNA related to yeast RAD2. Nature. 1993;363:182–188.
48. van Duin M, Vredeveldt G, Mayne LV, *et al.* The cloned human DNA excision repair gene ERCC-1 fails to correct xeroderma pigmentosum complementation groups A through I. Mutat Res. 1989;83–89.
49. Biggerstaff M, Szymkowski D, Wood RD. Co-correction of the ERCC1, ERCC4 and xeroderma pigmentosum group F repair defects in vitro. EMBO J. 1993;12:3685–3692.
50. Van Vuuren AJ, Appledoorn E, Odijk H, *et al.* Evidence for a repair enzyme complex involving ERCC1 and complementing activities of ERCC4, ERCC11 and xeroderma pigmentosum group F. EMBO J. 1993;12:3693–3701.
51. Tomkinson AE, Bardwell AJ, Bardwell L, Tappe NJ, Friedberg EC. Yeast DNA repair and recombination proteins Rad1 and Rad10 constitute a single stranded-DNA endonuclease. Nature. 1993;360:860–862.
52. Troelstra C, van Gool A, de Wit J, Vermeulen W, Bootsma D, Hoeijmakers JHJ. ERCC6 a member of a subfamily of putative helicases, is involved in Cockayne's syndrome and preferential repair of active genes. Cell. 1992;71:939–953.
53. Mitchell DL, Nairn RS. The biology of the (6-4) photoproduct. Photochem Photobiol. 1989;49:805–819.
54. Mitchell DL. The relative cytotoxicity of (6-4) photoproducts and cyclobutane dimers in mammalian cells. Photochem Photobiol. 1988;48:51–57.
55. Hart RW, Setlow RB, Woodhead AD. Evidence that pyrimidine dimers in DNA can give rise to tumours. Proc Natl Acad Sci USA. 1977;74:5574–5578.
56. Strauss BS. The 'A rule' of mutagen specificity: a consequence of DNA polymerase bypass of non-instructional lesions? BioEssays. 1991;13:79–84.
57. Cole J, Arlett CF, Norris PG, *et al.* Elevated hprt mutant frequency in circulating T-lymphocytes of xeroderma pigmentosum patients. Mutat Res. 1992;273:171–178.

58. Bredberg A, Kraemer KH, Seidman NM. Restricted ultraviolet mutational spectrum in a shuttle vector propagated in xeroderma pigmentosum cells. Proc Natl Acad Sci USA. 1986;83:8273–8277.
59. Seetheram S, Protic-Sablijc M, Seidman M, Kraemer KH. Abnormal ultraviolet mutagenic spectrum in plasmid DNA replicated in cultured fibroblasts from a patient with skin cancer-prone disease, xeroderma pigmentosum. J Clin Invest. 1987;80:1613–1617.
60. Dumaz N, Drolgard C, Sarasin A, Daya-Grosjean L. Specific UV-induced mutation spectrum in the p53 gene of skin tumours from DNA repair deficient xeroderma pigmentosum patients. Proc Natl Acad Sci USA. 1993;90:10529–10533.
61. Tyrrel RM, Pidoux M. Action spectra for human skin cells: estimates of the relative cytotoxicity of the middle ultraviolet and violet regions of sunlight on epidermal karatinocytes. Cancer Res. 1987;47:1825–1829.
62. Setlow RB, Grist E, Thompson K, Woodhead AD. Wavelengths effective in induction of malignant melanoma. Proc Natl Acad Sci USA. 1993;90:6666–6670.
63. Peall MJ, Peall DG, Carves BA. Induction of direct and indirect single strand breaks in human cell DNA by far- and near-ultraviolet radiation: action spectrum and mechanisms. Photochem Photobiol. 1987;45:381–387.
64. Tyrell RM, Pidoux M. Correlation between endogenous glutathione content and sensitivity of cultured human skin cells to radiation at defined wavelengths in the solar ultraviolet range. Photochem Photobiol. 1988;47:405–412.
65. Vuillaume M, Calvayrac R, Beit-Belpomme M, *et al.* Deficiency in catalase activity of xeroderma pigmentosum cell and simian virus 40-transformed human cell extracts. Cancer Res. 1986;46:538–544.
66. Swift M, Chase C. Cancer in families with xeroderma pigmentosum. J Natl Cancer Inst. 1978;62:1415–1421.
67. Pippard EC, Hall AJ, Barker JP, Bridges BA. Cancer in homozygotes and heterozygotes of ataxia-telangiectasia and xeroderma pigmentosum in Britain. Cancer Res. 1988;48:2929–2932.
68. Pawsey SA, Magnus IA, Ramsey CA, Benson PF, Giannelli F. Clinical, genetic and DNA repair studies on a consecutive series of patients with xeroderma pigmentosum. Clin J Med. 1979;48:179–210.
69. Rainbow AJ. Reduced capacity to repair irradiated adenovirus in fibroblasts from xeroderma pigmentosum heterozygotes. Cancer Res. 1980;40:3945–3949.
70. Squires S, Johnson RT. Kinetic analysis of UV-induced incision discriminates between fibroblasts from different xeroderma pigmentosum complementation groups/xeroderma pigmentosum heterozygotes and normal individuals. Mutat Res. 1988;193:181–192.
71. Mellon I, Spivak G, Hanawalt PC. Selective removal of transcription-blocking DNA damage from the transcribed strand of the mammalian DHFR gene. Cell. 1987;51:241–249.
72. Link Jr CJ, Mitchell DL, Nairn RS, Bohr VA. Preferential and strand specific DNA repair of (6-4) photoproducts detected by a photochemical method in the hamster DHFR gene. Carcinogenesis. 1992;13:1975–1980.
73. Venema J, van Hoffen A, Karcagi V, Natarajan AT, van Zeeland AA, Mullenders LHF. Xeroderma pigmentosum complementation group C cells remove pyrimidine dimers selectively from the transcribed strand of active genes. Mol Cell Biol. 1991;11:4128–4134.
74. Johnson RT, Squires S. The XPD complementation group. Insights into xeroderma pigmentosum, Cockayne's syndrome and trichothiodystrophy. Mutat Res. 1992;273:97–118.
75. Lehmann AR. Three complementation groups in Cockaynes syndrome. Mutat Res L. 1982;106:347–356.
76. Vermeulen W, Jacken J, Jaspers NGJ, Bootsma D. Xeroderma pigmentosum complementation group G associated with Cockayne's syndrome. Am J Hum Genet. 1993;53:185–192.
77. Wysenbek AJ, Weiss H. Immunologic alterations in xeroderma pigmentosum patients. Cancer. 1986;5:219–221.
78. Norris PG, Limb GA, Hamblin AS, *et al.* Immune function, mutant frequency and cancer risk in the DNA repair defective genodermatoses xeroderma pigmentosum, Cockaynes syndrome and trichothiodystrophy. J Invest Dermatol. 1990;94:94–100.
79. Lehmann AR, Norris PG. DNA repair and cancer. Speculations based on studies with xeroderma pigmentosum, Cockayne's syndrome and trichothiodystrophy. Carcinogenesis. 1989:10:1353–1356.

80. Mariani E, Facchini A, Honorati A, *et al.* Immune defects in families and patients with xeroderma pigmentosum and trichothiodystrophy. Clin Exp Immunol. 1992:88:376–382.
81. Gaspari A, Fleisher T, Kraemer K. Impaired interferon production and natural killer cell activation in patients with the skin cancer prone disorder, xeroderma pigmentosum. J Clin Invest. 1993;92:1135–1142.
82. Lehmann AR, Kirk-Bell S, Arlett CF, *et al.* Xeroderma pigmentosum cells with normal levels of excision repair have a defect in DNA synthesis after UV irradiation. Proc Natl Acad Sci USA. 1975;72:219–233.
83. Maher VM, Ouellette LM, Curren RD McCormick JJ. Frequency of ultraviolet light-induced mutations is higher in xeroderma pigmentosum variant cells than in normal human fibroblasts. Nature. 1976;261:593–595.
84. Wang YC, Maher VM, McCormick JJ. Xeroderma pigmentosum variant cells are less likely than normal cells to incorporate dAMP opposite photoproducts during replication of UV-irradiated plasmids. Proc Natl Acad Sci USA. 1991;88:7810–7814.
85. Wang YC, Maher VM, Mitchell DL, McCormick JJ. Evidence from mutation spectra that UV hypermutability of xeroderma pigmentosum variant cells reflects abnormal, error-prone replication on a template containing photoproducts. Mol Cell Biol. 1993;13:4276–4283.
86. Goddard AD, Solomon E. Genetic aspects of cancer. In: Harris H, Hirschen K, eds. Advances in human genetics, Vol 21. New York: Plenum Press; 1993:321–376.
87. Leach FS, Nicolaides NC, Papadopoulos N, *et al.* Mutations of a mutS homolog in hereditary nonpolyposis colorectal cancer. Cell. 1993;75:1215–1225.
88. Fishel R, Lescoe MK, Rao MRS, *et al.* The human mutator gene homolog MSH2 and its association with hereditary nonpolyposis colon cancer. Cell. 1993;75:1027–1038.
89. Lynch HT, Albano WA, Lynch JF, *et al.* Recognition of the cancer family syndrome. Gastroenterology. 1983;84:672–673.
90. Lynch HT, Smyrk Tc, Watson P, *et al.* Genetics, natural history, tumour spectrum and pathology of hereditary non-polyposis colorectal cancer: an updated review. Gastroenterology. 1993;104:1535–1549.
91. Aaltonen LA, Peltomaki P, Leach FS, *et al.* Clues to the pathogenesis of familial colorectal cancer. Science. 1993;260:812–816.
92. Ionov Y, Peinado MA, Malkhosyan S, Shibata D, Perucho M. Ubiquitous somatic mutations in simple repeated sequences reveal a new mechanism for colon carcinogenesis. Nature. 1993; 363:558–561.
93. Thibodeau SN, Bren G, Schaid D. Microsatellite instability in cancer of the proximal colon. Science. 1993;260:816–819.
94. Strand M, Prolla TA, Liska, RM, Petes TD. Destabilisation of tracts of simple repetitive DNA in yeast by mutations affecting DNA mismatch repair. Nature. 1993;365:274–6.
95. Parsons R, Guo-Min L, Longley MJ, *et al.* Hypermutability and mismatch repair deficiency in RER$^+$ tumour cells. Cell. 1993;75:1227–1236.
96. Palambo F, Hughes M, Jiricny J, Truong O, Hsuan J. Mismatch repair and cancer. Nature. 1993;367:417–419.
97. Fearon E, Vogelstein B. A genetic model for colorectal tumouregenesis. Cell. 1990;61:759–761.
98. Fearon E, Jones PA. Progressing towards a molecular model of colorectal cancer development. FASEB J. 1992;6:2783–2790.
99. Shibata O, Peinado MA, Ionov Y, Malkhhosyan S, Perucho M. Genomic instability in repeated sequences is an early somatic event in colorectal tumourigenesis that persists after transformation. Nature Genet. 1994;6:273–281.
100. Branch P, Aquilina G, Bignami M, Karren P. Defective mismatch binding and a mutator phenotype in cells tolerant to DNA damage. Nature. 1993;362:652–654.
101. Bronner CE, Baker SM, Morrison PT, *et al.* Mutation in the DNA mismatch repair gene homologue hMLH1 is associated with hereditary non-polyposis colon cancer. Nature. 1994;368:258–261.
102. Bates G, Lehrach H. Trinucleotide repeat expansions and human genetic disease. Bioessays. 1994;16:277–284.
103. Taylor AMR, McConville CM. Chromosome breakage disorders. In: Brock CJH, Rodeck C, Fergusson-Smith M, eds. Prenatal diagnosis and screening. Edinburgh: Churchill-Livingstone; 1992:405–421.

104. Morrel D, Cromartie E, Swift M. Mortality and cancer incidence in 263 patients with ataxia telangiectasia. J Natl Cancer Inst. 1986;77:89–92.
105. Taylor AMR. Ataxia telangiectasia genes and predisposition to leukaemia, lymphoma and breast cancer. Br J Cancer. 1992;66: 5–9.
106. Spector BD, Filipovich AH, Perr GS, Kersey KH. Epidemiology of cancer in ataxia telangiectasia. In: Bridges BA, Harnden G, eds. Ataxia telangiectasia – a cellular and molecular link between cancer, neuropathology and immune deficiency. Chichester: John Wiley and Sons; 1982:103–138.
107. Swift M, Morrell D, Massey RB, Chase CL. Incidence of cancer in 161 families affected by ataxia telangiectasia. N Engl J Med. 1991;325:1831–1836.
108. Gatti RA, Berkal I, Boder E, *et al.* Localisation of an ataxia telangiectasia gene to chromosome 11q222-23. Nature. 1988;336:577–580.
109. Taylor AMR, Jaspers NGJ, Gatti RA. Fifth international workshop on ataxia–telangiectasia. Cancer Res. 1993;53:438–441.
110. Cox R. A cellular description of the repair defect in ataxia telangiectasia. In: Bridges BA, Harnden DG, eds. Ataxia Telangiectasia. New York: Wiley;1982:141–153.
111. McKinnon PJ. Ataxia telangiectasia: an inherited disorder of ionising radiation sensitivity in man. Hum Genet. 1987;75:197–208.
112. Young BR, Painter RB. Radioresistant DNA synthesis and human genetic diseases. Hum Genet. 1989;82:113–117.
113. Cox R, Masson WK, Weichselbaum RR, Nove J, Little JB. Repair of potentially lethal damage in X-irradiated cultures of normal and ataxia telangiectasia fibroblasts. Int J Radiat Biol. 1981;39:357–365.
114. Blocher D, Sigut D, Hannan MA. Fibroblasts from ataxia telangiectasia (AT) and AT heterozygotes show an enhanced level of residual DNA double strand breaks after low dose-rate gamma irradiation as assayed by pulse field gel electrophoresis. Int J Radiat Biol. 1991;60:791–802.
115. Cornforth MN, Bedford JS. On the nature of the defect in cells from individuals with ataxia telangiectasia. Science. 1985;227:1589–1591.
116. Meyn SM. High spontaneous intrachromosomal recombination rates in ataxia telangiectasia. Science. 1993;260:1327–1330.
117. Baer R, Heppell A, Taylor AMR, Rabbitts PH, Boullier B, Rabbitts TH. The breakpoint of an inversion chromosome 14 in a T cell leukaemia; sequences downstream of the immunoglobulin heavy chain locus implicated in tumourigenesis. Proc Natl Acad Sci USA. 1987;84:9066–9073.
118. Heppel A, Butterworth SV, Hollis RJ, Kennaugh AA, Beatty DW, Taylor AMR. Breakage of the T-cell receptor alpha chain locus in non malignant clone from patients with ataxia telangiectasia. Hum Genet. 1988;79:360–364.
119. Taylor AMR, Butterworth SV. Clonal evolution of T cell chronic lymphocytic leukemia in a patient with ataxia telangiectasia. Int J Cancer. 1986;37:511–516.
120. Russo G, Isobe M, Pegoraro L, Finan J, Nowell PC, Croce CM. Molecular analysis of a t(7;14)(q35;q32) chromosome translocation in a T cell leukemia of a patient with ataxia telangiectasia. Cell. 1988;53:137–144.
121. Thick J, Sherrington PD, Fisch P, Taylor AMR, Rabbitts TH. Molecular analysis of a new translocation, t(x;14)(q28;q11), in premalignancy and in leukemia associated with ataxia telangiectasia. Genes Chrom Cancer. 1992;5:321–325.
122. Matsuoka M, Nagawa F, Okazaki K, *et al.* Detection of somatic recombination in the transgenic mouse brain. Science. 1991;254:81–86.
123. Chaganti RSF, Shonberg S, German J. A many fold increase in sister chromatid exchanges in Bloom's syndrome lymphocytes. Proc Natl Acad Sci USA. 1974;71:4508–4572.
124. Giannelli F, Benson F, Pawsey SA, Polani PD. Ultraviolet light sensitivity and delayed DNA chain maturation in Bloom's syndrome fibroblasts. Nature. 1977;265:466–469.
125. Ockey CH, Saffhill R. Delayed DNA maturation, a possible cause of the elevated sister chromatid exchange in Bloom's syndrome. Carcinogenesis. 1986;7:53–57.
126. Willis AE, Spurr NF, Lindahl T. Concomitant reversion of the characteristic phenotypic properties of a cell line of Bloom's syndrome origin. Carcinogenesis. 1989;10:217–219.
127. Willis AE, Lindahl T. DNA ligase I deficiency in Bloom's syndrome. Nature. 1987;325:355–357.

128. Petrini JHJ, Huwiler KG, Weaver DT. A wild type ligase I gene is expressed in Bloom's syndrome. Proc Natl Acad Sci USA. 1988;88:7615–7619.
129. Sullivan NF, Willis AE. Cancer predisposition in Bloom's syndrome. BioEssays. 1992;14:333–336.
130. Lu X, Lane DP. Differential induction of transcriptionally active p53 following UV or ionising radiation: defects in chromosome instability syndromes? Cell. 1993;75:765–778.
131. Gupta PK, Sirover MA. Altered temporal expression of DNA repair in hypermutable Bloom's syndrome cells. Proc Natl Acad Sci USA. 1984;81:757–761.
132. Barnes DE, Tomkinson AE, Lehman AR, Webster DB, Lindahl T. Mutations in the DNA ligase I gene of an individual with immunodeficiencies and cellular hypersensitivity to DNA damaging agents. Cell. 1992;69:495–503.
133. Bubley GJ, Schnipper LE. Effects of Bloom's syndrome fibroblasts on genetic recombination and mutagenesis of Herpes Simplex Virus type I. Som Cell Mol Gen. 1987;13:111–117.
134. Langlois RG, Bigbee WL, Jenson RH, German J. Evidence for increased in vivo mutation and somatic recombination in Bloom's syndrome. Proc Natl Acad Sci USA. 1989;86:670–674.
135. Levine AS. Workshop on molecular, cellular and clinical aspects of Fanconi anaemia. Exp Hematol. 1993;21:703–726.
136. Strathdee CA, Duncan AMV, Buchwald M. Evidence for at least four Fanconi anaemia genes including FACC on chromosome 9. Nature Genet. 1992;1:196–198.
137. Strathdee CA, Gavish H, Shannon WR, Buchwald M. Cloning of cDNAs for Fanconi anaemia by functional complementation. Nature. 1992;356:763–767.
138. Sakaguchi SA, Harris PV, Ryan C, Buchwald M, Boyd JB. Alteration of a nuclease in Fanconi anaemia. Mutat Res. 1991;255:31–38.
139. Sognier MA, Hittelman WN. Loss of repairability of DNA interstrand crosslinks in Fanconi's anaemia cells culture age. Mutat Res. 1983;108:383–393.
140. Maher VM, Dorney DJ, Mendrake AL, Kanze-Thomas B, McCormick JJ. DNA excision repair processes in human cells can eliminate the cytotoxic and mutagenic consequences of ultraviolet radiation. Mutation Res. 1979;62:311–323.
141. Lindahl T. DNA surveillance defect in cancer cells. Curr Biol. 1994;4:249–251.

9
Implications of studies of inherited predisposition for prevention and treatment

C.M Steel

ALL OR NOTHING?

At one extreme, the reaction to identification of constitutional genetic factors increasing cancer susceptibility is to advocate 'gene therapy', meaning replacement of the mutant gene with a normal copy. While this would have obvious attractions, everything that is known about the practicalities of gene therapy suggests that hereditary cancer will be one of the last areas where it will find a place. Even assuming that removal of the inherited mutation is unnecessary (and this would probably be a false assumption in certain instances, such as MEN 2 or Li-Fraumeni syndrome), introduction of any new gene construct is limited by the efficiency of the transfection step. Under the most favourable conditions, using a retroviral vector and being prepared to accept insertion of multiple copies of the construct into some cells, the efficiency of *in-vivo* transfection never reaches 100%[1,2]. In the case of a cancer, escape of even a tiny number of cells from genetic 'correction' would defeat the purpose of the therapy.

In any event, since, in familial cancer, the mutation is a constitutional one, completely successful transfection of tumour cells would still leave the individual susceptible to further episodes of malignant change. If this route is to be followed, therefore, we shall have to contemplate germ-line therapy which, at present, is regarded by the regulatory bodies of most countries as being ethically unacceptable[3,4]. Furthermore, as 50% of the offspring of an affected family member will not carry the mutation, some form of zygote selection is likely to be a much more straightforward option than germ-line manipulation of the genome.

At the other extreme, it is sometimes argued that publicizing the hereditary element of certain cancers, in the absence of any guarantee of protection for those found to be at high risk, merely generates anxiety and places burdens on health care organizations to no good purpose. It would follow from this view that nothing should be done for most cancer families and that much of cancer genetics should be treated as a theoretical and experimental concept with no clinical dimension. In practice, it is far too late to implement such a policy, even if it were logically sound. Many – if not most – members of affected families are already well aware of their inherited predisposition to cancer. Indeed, they have often been ahead of the medical profession in this respect and, in the past, may have been offered false reassurance that the clusters of cases in close relatives have been chance events with no prognostic significance. It has, in fact, been known for several years that members of these families have increased levels of anxiety and need appropriate counselling which includes estimation and explanation of risks, together with whatever type of screening seems to offer the best prospect of detecting early (preferably premalignant) tumours[5,6]. There are inevitably some individuals whose response to their perception of a genetic predisposition to disease is denial or avoidance, and *ipso facto* their opinions are under-represented in any survey of cancer family members[6,7]. Nevertheless, the message that has emerged from several substantial clinic-based studies is that most people with a strong family history of cancer wish to discuss the position with interested health care professionals, that they often overestimate the level of their own risk (some are convinced that they will inevitably develop cancer themselves) and that, even where the counselling process confirms the existence of a substantial risk, measures of anxiety tend to show improvement rather than the reverse[5–9].

The establishment and running of a 'cancer family' clinic is a very substantial undertaking, demanding a commitment of time and resources from individuals with expertise in a range of different areas (see Table 9.1). Many such clinics now operate throughout the UK and, without exception, they have been inundated with 'clients' whose needs had not been met previously. The fact that they

Table 9.1 Some practical issues in setting-up and running a 'cancer family' clinic

1. Publicizing the clinic	Letters to local primary care physicians Participation in medical education seminars Leaflets/posters, e.g. in 'well-woman' centres Articles in local press or on radio, etc.
2. Clinic facilities on-site	A contact person for each client (nurse/counsellor or 'genetics associate') plus written material for information Specialist services: Medical geneticist Surgeon, gynaecologist or medical oncologist Psychology support Radiology (may be off-site as backup)
3. Backup facilities	Biochemical screening Molecular genetics laboratory Long-term at-risk genetics register Epidemiological data collection Verification of medical histories (contact with GPs, hospital pathology records) Genealogy services for verification and extension of family trees Expertise in data handling and analysis

See also References 26 and 50

fulfil both research and service functions creates difficulties in identifying an appropriate mechanism for funding them and this is currently one of the major unresolved problems in cancer genetics.

In all dealings with members of cancer families, it is important to remember that their personal experience of the disease is often extensive and harrowing. They may have nursed several close relatives dying from cancer at an early age and the entire course of their lives may well have been altered by the presence in the family of a 'cancer gene'. Their perspective on the issue is therefore quite distinct from that of an average member of the public, or even of a cancer researcher, and it is no less valid. It is remarkable how few such individuals come to cancer family clinics with the expressed intention of seeking protection for themselves and how many are motivated by what may be achieved for the next generation. Given the formidable obstacles to be overcome before we can anticipate substantial clinical benefits, it is reassuring to find that the expectations of those most closely concerned are realistic.

APPROACHES TO PREVENTION

Genetic registers and DNA banks

On the basis that, in a condition such as cancer, prevention would be the preferred option, the first issue to be addressed is how to ascertain the population at risk. In most circumstances, the only practical approach is to extend the family tree, where the history points to a genetic predisposition and, applying the likeliest segregation model (usually autosomal dominant with limited penetrance), to identify every member whose chance of having inherited the trait approaches 50%[10]. Where a specific gene has already been implicated in a familial cancer and there is a manageable technique for identifying relevant mutations (a situation that will become increasingly common), there is, at least in theory, the option of applying total population screening for the presence of these mutations. However, except where the prevalence of cancer-associated mutations is high, it is likely that some form of selection, based on family history and structure, will still be applied.

The entire population of Iceland is already documented on a register that defines family structure and health records over several generations so that identification of those at risk from genetic disorders becomes a straightforward excercise[11]. That, of course, is an exceptional situation. Most communities have some form of public records but not organized in a format that assists the medical geneticist to quite the same degree. We are therefore dependent on the willing participation of family members and their doctors. This creates ethical dilemmas[12]. In taking an initial history from a client who has sought referral to a 'cancer family' clinic, it may be immediately apparent that several other family members are at substantial risk. Extension of the pedigree may be highly desirable in order to increase the accuracy of risk estimates and may well reveal still more individuals at risk. Who, if anyone, is entitled to approach these people – who may be blissfully unaware of the position and who may not wish to have this state of happy ignorance disturbed? If they are relatives already known to the original client, then the position is best resolved within the family and, indeed, relevant discussions have often taken place before the first clinic visit. Nevertheless, the situation commonly arises where different branches of an extended family do not know each other personally. In the UK, the general practitioner ('primary care physician' or 'family doctor') with whom a given individual is registered, is an invaluable source of guidance as to whether, and how, he/she might be approached.

Similarly, verification of medical records (an essential part of the excercise since word-of-mouth histories of cancer are notoriously unreliable) commonly requires confidential enquiries of individual doctors and of hospitals where treatments were undertaken. Ideally, permission should be sought from the patient concerned, if he/she is alive, but, once again, sensitivity is needed, particularly if the patient may have been unaware of the diagnosis (or even suspicion) of cancer. Hence, prior consultation with the general practitioner is wise.

When dealing with conditions such as familial polyposis coli or MEN 2, where there is unequivocal evidence of the benefits of screening, little serious debate arises over the practice of family tracing. The ethical position is less clear in the case of breast or ovarian cancer families which comprise a large proportion of the clientele of most cancer genetics clinics. Authoritative legal and philosophical opinion offers the assurance that where, in the course of investigating any family with a genetic disorder, an individual who has no personal contact with the members being counselled is found to be at risk, then it is the duty of the doctors undertaking the clinical study to inform that individual of his/her risk status. To withold the information might well be treated as a misdemeanour, whereas to impart it, while possibly earning hostility, is entirely defensible[12,13]. It is fair to say that not all geneticists – or indeed doctors from other disciplines – feel totally comfortable with this position but there is no simple formula that will be right for all situations.

In view of the long-term nature of most studies on familial cancer, it is highly desirable to ensure that registers of affected families are maintained in such a way that they can be updated continuously over several decades. Obviously, the risk status of individual family members will change over such a time span as they grow older and as new cases of cancer arise. Few research programmes are funded for more than five years so it is important to establish close links with a department that enjoys a greater degree of permanence – often the regional genetics service – which can accept responsibility for the next generation. Family members who come to a genetics clinic will almost always agree to have information about themselves entered on such a register. Data concerning family structure is in the public domain so that recording of pedigrees *per se* does not require the express permission of every member. However, medical information is in a different category and great care must be taken to obtain consent for its inclusion in a genetics register, wherever practicable, and to protect its confidentiality at all times[12].

The taking and storing of blood specimens (or even buccal scrapes or mouthwashings) as sources of DNA for linkage studies and mutation analyses is almost a reflex action on the part of modern geneticists. There is a powerful temptation to take samples from all available family members 'while they are around' and most subjects are willing or at least acquiescent. Few, unfortunately, fully appreciate the implications (current or future) of donating to a DNA bank and it is doubtful whether valid consent can be given for investigations that may become feasible at some later date but which cannot be envisaged at the time the specimens were taken. Similarly, the prospect of a definitive test for a cancer-predisposing mutation may look attractive from a safe distance but when it becomes an immediate reality some family members will wish to think long and hard before submitting themselves to it. As a general rule, therefore, even when a sample has been stored, fresh permission should be sought for any new test that may have a bearing on the individual's risk status before such a test is carried out[13].

Primary prevention by lifestyle changes

Where exogenous factors can be implicated in causation of a particular type of cancer, it is logical to recommend that anyone at increased risk (because of their family history) should make special efforts to avoid exposure to these factors. Thus, for example, individuals whose genetic constitution determines that nitrosamines and polycyclic aromatic hydrocarbons in tobacco smoke are metabolized to produce particularly high or persistent levels of carcinogens, definitely should not smoke[14], while members of melanoma families should protect themselves from strong sunlight[15]. There is, however, no clear epidemiological evidence to show that such measures, applied selectively to high-risk groups, are effective in reducing the incidence of cancers. Antismoking and sun-avoidance campaigns, where prosecuted with vigour, have undoubtedly influenced cancer statistics in whole populations but the question of whether the same environmental considerations apply to the genetically susceptible subpopulation remains open[14–16].

In some rare hereditary conditions, such as ataxia telangiectasia, xeroderma pigmentosum, Gorlin syndrome, Bloom syndrome and Fanconi anaemia, increased sensitivity to ultraviolet light, ionizing radiation, crosslinking agents or alkylating agents is very obvious[17,18]. On the other hand, when we consider the common cancers, with the exception of lung and melanoma, there is much less certainty about the identity of environmental contributions to aetiology and less still about the advice that might be appropriate for those at increased familial risk. There are correlations, for example between high animal fat/low-fibre diets and the incidence of large bowel cancer but only very limited data to suggest that dietary modification might protect members of colon cancer families[19]. The incidence of breast cancer has risen dramatically over the past fifty years in most advanced western countries and the change has been associated with several secular trends, among which are increasing birth weight, earlier age of menarche, reduced parity and later age at first pregnancy, decline in breast feeding, reduced consumption of fresh fruit and vegetables (anti-oxidants), use of oral contraceptives or postmenopausal hormone replacement therapy and increased consumption of alcohol[20–22]. Some studies indicate that the penetrance of the familial breast cancer trait has increased and the mean age of presentation of familial cases has declined over a similar period, implying an interaction between genetic and environmental factors[23,24]. At least one report[25] disagrees, however, and, given the evidence for genetic heterogeneity in familial breast cancer, we should not be surprised if it is eventually found that only some families show enhanced sensitivity to hormonal and other exogenous carcinogenic influences[26–28]. General risk factors for ovarian cancer include low parity and late age at first birth but these do not seem to apply to women with a strong family history[23].

One conclusion must be that, until much stronger evidence is forthcoming, members of breast, ovarian or colorectal cancer families cannot be offered advice on diet, reproductive behaviour or any other aspect of their lifestyle that carries with it any guarantee of even a modest degree of protection from cancer. The general health benefits of reducing dietary fats and increasing fresh fruit and vegetables and of avoiding smoking are, of course, sufficient in themselves to justify encouragement of anyone who wishes to follow that route.

A second conclusion is that we require much more comprehensive epidemiological data on the social circumstances, dietary and reproductive practices of people at increased genetic risk of common cancers[29]. Ideally, such studies should be population based, to avoid biases introduced by concentrating upon families that include particularly large numbers of affected members. The latter, though very useful for genetic linkage analyses, may be atypical with respect to penetrance of the trait and hence with respect to gene/environment interactions.

Primary prevention by drugs

The observation that both calcium supplements and low-dose aspirin can reduce the proliferation rate of epithelial cells in the intestinal crypts has led to the suggestion that they may be of value in protecting at-risk individuals from colorectal cancer[19,30,31]. There is indeed some evidence for their efficacy, both in the general population and in those who have inherited the *apc* (polyposis coli) mutation but large-scale trials have yet to be reported. Both have the merit of being relatively innocuous and therefore acceptable as potential preventive agents.

Much more controversial is the proposed trial of tamoxifen in women at increased genetic risk of breast cancer[32–34]. This oral anti-oestrogen has a proven track record in established breast cancer and, in particular, has been shown to reduce the incidence of second primaries in women who have already had curative resection of a first tumour. However, it can be associated with symptoms of premature menopause and recent data have raised anxieties, particularly about increased risks of endometrial cancer. Furthermore, the prophylactic effect demonstrated so far applies only to the five-year maximum duration of drug administration in any published trial, and although, in some studies, benefit persisted for at least ten years after tamoxifen was stopped[34], we cannot predict whether it is likely to afford the lifelong protection required by someone with a genetic predisposition to breast cancer. All these issues have to be discussed fully with any woman invited to enter the tamoxifen trial.

Other forms of hormonal manipulation proposed (and indeed in use) for people at increased genetic risk of cancer include gonadotrophin releasing hormone (GnRH) agonists for breast cancer and finasteride (a 5-α reductase inhibitor), which blocks conversion of testosterone to the more potent androgen dihydrotestosterone, for prostate cancer[35]. These interventions are best described as experimental at present and results are awaited with interest. The combined oral contraceptive pill, which, by inhibiting ovulation, reduces the incidence of ovarian cancer, might be regarded as a prophylactic measure against that tumour in women with a positive family history. Unfortunately, most ovarian cancer families also show an excess of breast cancers, usually linked to the BRCA 1 locus. There are accounts of large multigeneration breast/ovarian cancer families in whom the relative incidence of breast cancer has increased markedly among the present generation[36–38]. Whether these can be attributed to the effects of oral contraceptive use is unknown but it seems prudent to advise against reliance on the 'pill' as a long-term measure to reduce genetically determined ovarian cancer risk.

Prophylactic surgery

In someone with a family history suggestive of predisposition to melanoma, few would argue against a policy of excising any melanotic skin lesions, especially if they are raised or show any recent change in appearance and provided they are not present in such profusion as to preclude effective surgery. Similarly, the removal of any intestinal polyps detected at endoscopy in members of colorectal cancer families is clearly beneficial. For other types of familial cancer, prophylactic surgery is more controversial. In the case of breast cancer, some surgeons advocate bilateral mastectomy at the time of initial surgery in younger women presenting with a first tumour, if they also have a family history of the disease, arguing that the lifetime risk of a second primary in carriers of a breast-cancer gene mutation is 80% or more. There is even a case to be made for bilateral prophylactic mastectomy before any tumour has developed if the family history is sufficiently striking[26,39,40]. A few women who have thought through the issues with great care request this procedure for themselves even when they realise that there is a 50% chance that they do not actually carry the predisposing mutation. In that situation, the condition being treated is perhaps anxiety rather than precancer. Nevertheless, if the anxiety is sufficiently disabling, the treatment may well be justified and, in the author's experience, women who have followed this course after adequate counselling do not regret their decision.

It should be borne in mind that prophylactic mastectomy is a procedure for the highly skilled surgical specialist. Incomplete removal of breast epithelium, perhaps as a 'trade-off' for what is expected to be a better cosmetic result, may be associated with a substantial residual risk of breast cancer[40].

Oophorectomy, as a prophylaxis against familial ovarian cancer, is obviously a simpler operation for both surgeon and patient[36]. It may also carry the benefit, if undertaken at a relatively early age (before age 40) of offering some protection against breast cancer in those at increased risk of both diseases, though this is as yet unproven. Reports of 'primary peritoneal' cancer following prophylactic oophorectomy in genetically predisposed women rightly cause concern[23]. A frequency of under 3% is quoted in one large series[41] but it is not known how many of the women who underwent oophorectomy were actually at risk. It would certainly have been less than half so that the true incidence of subsequent peritoneal cancer in susceptible individuals probably approaches 10%. It is possible that, at least in some instances, apparently primary multifocal peritoneal cancer in these women is actually due to spread from an occult ovarian primary, present at the time of oophorectomy but too small to be detected even on careful pathological examination of the excised tissue. If this is so, it argues for early oophorectomy and against reliance on ultrasound screening which can only detect macroscopically evident tumours.

Total or subtotal colectomy is the standard management for familial adenomatous polyposis once the condition has become clinically evident. This policy, which has served polyposis families well, is unlikely to change in the near future. A slightly more contentious issue is whether some members of hereditary non-polyposis colorectal cancer (HNPCC) families may also require prophylactic colectomy. Clearly, the preferred option for those at risk will be regular flexible colonoscopy at intervals determined by the findings on each occasion (numbers, size and site of polyps) but there may well be patients whose disease is not controlled by repeated polypectomy or in whom carcinomas arise without an evident preceding adenoma. Even the most effective screening protocol is therefore unlikely to obviate the need for more radical surgery in a proportion of those with an inherited predisposition to colon cancer[31,42].

In terms of strict cost–benefit analysis, a very strong case can be made in favour of prophylactic surgery (i.e. polypectomy or colectomy, as appropriate) for those at high risk of colorectal cancer but, as regards familial breast or ovarian cancer, the jury is still out[43]. There are at least two reasons for the difference. First, individuals genetically predisposed to bowel cancer can be identified, both phenotypically and by molecular techniques, with a high degree of accuracy[31] whereas, at present, most members of breast or ovarian cancer families have at least a 50% chance of being unaffected. Second, existing evidence for a protective effect of surgery is compelling in the case of familial colorectal cancer but merely persuasive for breast or ovary cancer. The position is likely to change, on both counts, within a few years but, until that happens, women who are concerned about their family histories of breast or ovarian cancer face difficult choices and the most that their medical advisers can do to resolve the uncertainties is to ensure that relevant data are collected and analysed systematically, preferably through multicentre collaborative studies, since this must be the quickest route to the urgently needed answers.

SECONDARY PREVENTION (SCREENING WITH TREATMENT OF 'EARLY' LESIONS)

The rationale behind screening for cancer is that tumours detected at an early stage of development are likely to be amenable to curative treatment. As already discussed, this reasoning is sound in the case of colorectal cancer but rather less is known about the biology of some other cancers that also occur in familial forms, notably breast, ovarian or prostate[23,44–46]. It is likely that these are heterogeneous and that some cases carry a poor prognosis even if detected at an apparently early stage. Conversely, some screen-detected tumours might never progress to frank malignancy. For instance, three out of six ovarian tumours detected on ultrasound screening of a population of young women with a positive family history were of borderline histology[47]. Not only do these have low malignant potential, they do not appear, in other studies, to be associated with genetic predisposition[23]. In the case of prostate cancer, use of the prostate-specific antigen (PSA) screening test or postmortem histological examination of 'normal' glands both detect 'early cancers' at rates that far exceed the incidence of clinically evident disease and there is no evidence as yet that PSA measurement will have particular value for men at increased genetic risk[46,48,49]. These examples illustrate some of the difficulties in assessing the success or otherwise of screening campaigns.

Nevertheless, it makes sense to target screening at the highest-risk groups which, for virtually all common cancers, includes those with a family history of the disease. Various criteria have been proposed for inclusion in screening programmes, based on numbers of affected relatives, closeness of the relationship and age at diagnosis. These have to be interpreted with a degree of flexibility, not least because family histories often prove to be inaccurate. For this reason, simple guidelines are to be preferred[50]. It would, however, defeat the purpose of the exercise if screening were universally available since the sensitivity and specificity of almost any protocol will decline as the frequency of positives drops. All screening procedures carry a cost and some are also associated with measurable risk. Thus, even in skilled hands, colonoscopy is associated with a perforation rate of about 0.2%, some 7% of these proving fatal[51]. The radiation exposure involved in mammography carries a minute, but calculable, risk of inducing breast cancer and this is cumulative so that the earlier a woman enters a mammographic screening programme the greater her chance, over a lifetime, of acquiring a significant radiation dose[52].

Meta-analysis of many large-scale mammographic screening programmes shows convincing evidence of a reduction in subsequent mortality in those aged fifty or over at entry[53]. Studies of women in younger age groups have produced less conclusive data[54]. This is really to be expected, partly because interpretation of images from the younger breast can be difficult and partly because the age–incidence curve predicts a much lower pick-up rate. One widely-quoted Canadian trial suggested that screening younger women was counterproductive since, on follow-up, mortality was significantly higher in the screened group[55]. That study has been heavily criticized on several grounds[56] and its findings appear to be refuted by a number of carefully conducted trials in 40–49-year-olds that show trends towards significant benefits for the screened group (about 15% better survival) on prolonged follow-up[57,58]. This is an important issue because current estimates suggest that 70% of breast cancers arising in genetically predisposed women present before age fifty[59]. A very large study from California recorded similar mammographic detection rates (9 per 1000) for cancer in women aged 40–49 with a family history of breast cancer (defined as at least one first-degree relative affected at any age) and for unselected women aged 50 or over[60]. Most centres seeing women with a family history of breast cancer will arrange regular mammography for those at substantial risk (>2× population level), starting at age 35 or 5 years younger than the youngest age at diagnosis in a close relative (whichever is the earlier). Screening may be recommended at two-year intervals up to age 40 and annually thereafter to age 50, when, in the UK, they join the national screening programme. The results of such a policy may not emerge for more than a decade but, in our present state of knowledge, this approach appears sensible[26].

Despite the wide publicity given to mammographic screening and its limitations, there is still a popular misconception that it should be infallible and this applies equally to women with a positive family history of breast cancer. Some cautionary words are therefore in order when mammography is offered. It also seems wise to teach women attending a breast cancer family clinic how to carry out breast self-examination. The value of this procedure in the general population has been questioned but, among the highly-motivated 'breast-aware' group, it may well be a useful supplement to mammography.

Screening for early ovarian cancer is advocated because the prognosis in this disease is closely related to its stage at diagnosis. Transabdominal ultrasound scans are of rather low sensitivity. A transvaginal probe will usually give a clearer image of the ovaries and, where there is any doubt about the significance of a small irregularity or enlargement, colour Doppler analysis can be helpful in defining the pattern of blood flow to distinguish, for example, between a simple cyst and a tumour[47]. Women with a strong family history of ovarian cancer ought to be prime candidates for screening programmes of this type. In order to generate sufficient data to test the effectiveness of the approach, however, we probably require a number of specialist centres, working together on an agreed protocol and applying uniform criteria for proceeding to more invasive investigations. Findings from the Kings College Hospital (London) pilot studies[47] have been sufficiently encouraging to warrant further development but a large-scale programme of the type described will be logistically demanding and is not yet under way.

Many centres make use of serum 'markers' for ovarian cancer screening. The most popular of these is CA 125, assayed immunochemically, which is certainly of value in following the response of established tumours to surgery and chemotherapy[61]. Whether it will prove sufficiently sensitive to identify very early lesions is doubtful since the serum level tends to reflect extent of disease. However, other monoclonal antibodies defining ovarian tumour markers are under trial, singly or in combination and may have a place in screening protocols[62,63].

One of the most successful applications of a phenotypic marker for early diagnosis of a familial cancer syndrome has been the use of plasma calcitonin level to detect carriers of the MEN 2 trait among relatives of patients with the full-blown disorder[10,64] but this form of screening has been superseded by direct molecular diagnosis now that the gene responsible for MEN 2 has been identified as *ret*[65]. Similarly, phenotypic prediction of the development of adenomatous polyposis coli (APC), based on the presence of patches of retinal pigmentation (CHRPEs) and/or osteomas of jaw or skull, while still of clinical interest, has given way in practice to gene sequencing, which is applicable to all APC families and carries a greater degree of certainty[66]. Recent identification of the human mutator–suppressor gene family holds out the prospect of screening relatives of young colon cancer patients, or members of HNPCC and multi-cancer (Lynch Type 2) kindreds, directly for lesions in these genes or using constitutional microsatellite instability as a surrogate molecular marker for the trait[31]. This general trend towards molecular rather than phenotypic screening of populations at increased risk of cancer is bound to continue as more and more cancer genes are isolated. It has enormous practical, financial and psychological implications, as discussed below.

THE CONSEQUENCES OF DEFINITIVE MOLECULAR DIAGNOSIS

As mentioned earlier, the majority of current referrals to cancer genetics clinics are women with a family history of breast and/or ovarian cancer. Empirical assessment of individual risk usually requires a computation based on three elements, set out in Table 9.2. The concept of risk is thus a difficult one to communicate and to grasp, whether it is expressed in terms of 'lifetime', over the next decade, by age 60, or in any other form[71]. The essential distinction between this approach and one based on molecular identification of a specific relevant mutation is that the former retains a substantial chance that the individual being counselled is not in fact at any greater risk than the general population. Identification of carrier status through linkage analysis, for example in BRCA 1-linked breast/ovarian cancer families, is a 'half-way-house' where the degree of certainty depends on the informativeness of the family (itself determined by numbers of affected individuals, accessibility of DNA samples and distribution of alleles at close flanking markers). It is a serious option for only a small minority of those attending the clinic[26].

Table 9.2 Empirical risk assessment in a member of a breast cancer family

Component of risk level	*Factors determining risk*
Chance that there *is* a gene segregating in this family predisposing to breast cancer	Numbers of affected family members; pattern of cancers in the family; ages of onset; affected members with bilateral disease; affected members with multiple relevant primary tumours
Chance that this individual family member has inherited that gene	Predicted mode of inheritance (usually autosomal dominant); position within the family, in relation to affected members; current age, in relation to age of onset in affected members
Chance that the disease will be expressed in a gene carrier	Published estimates of penetrance for breast cancer genes; apparent penetrance level within this family; ? exposure to environmental risk factors

Notes:
The ways in which these components of risk and factors that determine risk levels are used to compute an individual risk estimate are discussed more fully in References 26 and 67–70. It should be noted that, in many breast-cancer families, there is an excess of other cancer also[11]. Female members of breast/ovarian families (usually BRCA 1-linked) should be assessed for ovarian cancer risk, with a view to ultrasound screening or prophylactic oophorectomy. According to data collected by the Breast Cancer Linkage Consortium, the lifetime risks of prostate or colorectal cancer in BRCA 1 carriers are probably less than 10%, which might not be considered high enough to justify intensive screening but should certainly be borne in mind if symptoms referable to either organ should develop

Commonly, women coming for counselling have an empirical lifetime risk of cancer in the range 20–40% and, as far as psychological measurements can tell us, they generally cope well with that information[6–9]. Few press for active prophylactic measures though the great majority are glad of the opportunity to participate in screening programmes. There is, however, a feeling, sometimes openly admitted, that both the family members and their medical advisers are conducting a 'holding operation' against the day when definitive molecular diagnosis will be possible, and that decisions, particularly about prophylactic surgery, are being put off until then. The belief that discovery of BRCA 1 was imminent has probably contributed to this frame of mind. Perhaps some reappraisal will be undertaken in view of the four-year gap between mapping and cloning of that gene and as estimates of its contribution to the totality of familial breast cancer appear to be diminishing (Reference 23 and unpublished data from the international breast cancer linkage consortium). Not surprisingly, attitudes to screening or intervention are affected by recent events within the family, such as the death of a close relative from cancer, new diagnosis of the disease in another or deterioration in the condition of someone already known to be affected[72]. There are few quantitative data on this phenomenon but it is a universal experience in the practice of cancer genetics and needs to be recognized to avoid the implementation of decisions, taken under stress, which may be regretted later.

The big question is, 'What will happen as BRCA 1 and other breast cancer genes are identified?' Women who are clearly members of cancer families face the option of converting their current empirical risk estimate into a definitive one that will be either much higher or much lower. If, as seems likely, some of the relevant mutations have a population frequency that would justify large-scale screening[70], then many women who had no previous inkling of their increased risk status may make the discovery in the context of an impersonal survey, with little in the way of preparatory counselling. In both situations, the reactions are bound to be closely related to the effectiveness or otherwise of measures to protect those found to be at high risk.

The worst case is probably exemplified by the Li Fraumeni syndrome associated with constitutional mutations of the p53 gene. At present, there is no known mechanism for preventing the development of cancers in carriers of the mutation. The best that can be done is to alert general practitioners and other medical personnel involved with these families to investigate any possible early signs of malignancy with great vigour. Molecular testing should not be offered, even to members of families in whom the precise mutation is known, without most careful discussion of the implications. Any attempt to introduce constitutional p53 sequencing as merely a 'routine diagnostic test', for example in young patients with a sarcoma, should be resisted and there is certainly no justification for embarking on wholesale population screening[73].

At the other extreme, molecular diagnosis of *apc* mutation status spares half the potentially affected family members the discomfort of annual sigmoidoscopy while ensuring that all who require regular follow-up are identified correctly. Surgery is protective in the great majority of cases so there are benefits all round.

The situation in respect of familial breast/ovarian cancer is less clearcut. It seems likely that many of those proved to be at high risk of ovarian cancer will opt for prophylactic oophorectomy as soon as they have completed their families. Where breast cancer is the major hazard, the forseeable options, as already discussed, will include oophorectomy, prophylactic mastectomy, long-term tamoxifen or surveillance by mammography and regular physical examination. It will be of interest to discover whether a randomized trial (for example of tamoxifen) will be possible once risk status has been defined more precisely. Women who have inherited a breast cancer gene mutation, given their personal experience of the disease, may have strong views on which route they personally wish to take. Breast surgeons too are likely to adopt a more interventionist stance when faced with patients who do not simply have a 50/50 chance of being at high risk but are *known* to be so.

The foregoing assumes that most women potentially at risk will wish to undergo definitive testing. This seems likely to be the case but only time will tell. One potential disincentive may be the attitude of life assurance companies (and of health insurance companies in countries where this is relevant). From the insurer's point of view, any information that has a bearing on the insured risk must be sought and disclosed. Most of us probably harbour genes that will have an adverse influence on our future health and it is perhaps unfair that those whose deleterious genes happen to be among the first to be identified should effectively suffer discrimination. When the entire genome has been sequenced, the position may revert to the original concept of insurance, i.e. that risks are randomly distributed and cover should be shared out by roughly equal contributions from everybody[12,13]. With this in mind, certain communities (the Netherlands and some American states) have reached agreements with insurance companies or have enacted legislation that precludes the use of genetic information in quoting for life assurance policies up to a certain value. It remains to be seen how long such arrangements will hold. In any event, while insurance companies might base their loading on family history rather than a molecular test, they seem to find the latter much easier to understand and tend to adapt their strategies in response to discoveries of new genes[12]. This means that members of cancer families currently undergoing counselling and investigation can be advised to buy all the insurance they are likely to need before the gene responsible for their familial disorder has been discovered. Again, the situation may change and there is a real danger that participation of cancer family members in research programmes could be inhibited by concerns over the effect that attendance at a genetic clinic may have on insurability.

Surprisingly, perhaps, the subject of prenatal diagnosis of cancer susceptibility is seldom raised in the cancer family clinic though women often cite 'decisions about whether to have children' when asked why they would wish to have a definitive genetic diagnosis. For familial tumours with exclusively adult onset – and particularly for those where prophylactic measures are already effective – selective abortion is unlikely to be contemplated, while, in many of the rarer syndromes, where infants may be severely handicapped as well as being at increased risk of cancer, variability in the phenotype makes prediction of severity uncertain even if the genetic status is clear[17]. In these circumstances, the personal experience of the prospective parents is bound to be the over-riding factor in the decision-making process.

A related issue is the question of genetic testing of children. Parents, adoption agencies and others may, for various reasons, wish to know whether a child is likely to be affected, at some future date, with a familial cancer. Unless there is an advantage to the child himself (e.g. the opportunity for screening or prophylaxis that ought to be instituted at a young age), such requests should be turned down and testing deferred until the individual is old enough to take the decision on his own behalf[11,12,73].

DISTANT PROSPECTS

Discovery of breast/ovarian cancer genes will eventually answer questions about the prevalence of mutations that confer a modest, but clinically and epidemiologically important, increase in risk, as has been suggested, for example, in the case of ataxia telangiectasia heterozygotes[70]. It seems quite conceivable that mammographic screening will ultimately be directed towards the most susceptible group defined, not by age alone, but by a population-based molecular screen. This could coincide with technical developments in breast imaging (e.g. MRI scanning coupled with automated computer analysis) that will improve the sensitivity of detection of early lesions, particularly in younger women[26,74]. The scale of the breast cancer problem in most developed countries and the cost of treatment of advanced disease justifies the massive investment that will be required to develop and implement such programmes.

Studies of women shown to carry breast cancer gene mutations will be of paramount importance both for our understanding of the basic biology of the disease and for working out effective strategies to counter the risks that these mutations confer. At present, analysis of the relative importance of various environmental risk factors is hampered by the facts that most 'high-risk' populations are genetically heterogeneous and that, as a rule, only a subgroup is genuinely at increased risk. Molecular identification of that subgroup – and particularly of those members from families where penetrance of the trait has been relatively low[70] – should make it much easier to determine whether, for example, certain mutations confer a risk that is clearly influenced by reproductive history while others do not.

In the longer term – in time perhaps for the generation now being born – the purpose of tracking down the genes responsible for inherited predisposition to cancer must be to work out precisely what functions these genes perform at the cellular level and how those functions are disturbed by the observed mutations. Once that has been achieved, we can have confidence in the skill and ingenuity of pharmacologists whose task it will be to design drugs to compensate for the defined biochemical defects[75]. This will lead to true primary prevention of the disease, rendering obsolete our current obsessions with screening or prophylactic surgery.

References

1. Friedman T. A brief history of gene therapy. Nature Genet. 1992;2:93–98.
2. Marrouche Y, Favrot MC. Meeting report: retroviral gene therapy and its application in onco-haematology. Hum Gene Ther. 1992;3:285–291.

3. HMSO. Report of the committee on ethics of gene therapy. (The Clothier Report). January 1992.
4. Wivel NA, Walters L. Germ-line gene modification and disease prevention: some medical and ethical perspectives. Science. 1993;262:533–537.
5. Kelly PT. Counselling needs of women with a maternal history of breast cancer. Patient Counselling Health Educ. 1980;3:118–124.
6. Kash KM, Holland JC, Halper MS, Miller DG. Psychological distress and surveillance behaviors of women with a family history of breast cancer. J Natl Cancer Inst. 1992;84:24–30.
7. Lerman C, Daly M, Sands C, *et al.* Mammography adherence and psychological distress among women at risk for breast cancer. J Natl Cancer Inst. 1993;85:1074–1080.
8. Evans DGR, Burnell LD, Hopwood P, Howell A. Perception of risk in women with a family history of breast cancer. Br J Cancer. 1993;67:612–614.
9. Anderson EDC, Steel CM, Smyth E, Cull A. Knowledge, attitudes, health-related behaviour and emotional status of women with a family history of breast cancer. Paper presented at 3rd Nottingham International Breast Cancer Conference, 1993.
10. Ponder BAJ. Inherited predisposition to cancer. Trends Genet. 1990;6:213–218.
11. Tulinius H, Egilsson V, Olafsdottir GH, Sigvaldson H. Risk of prostate, ovarian and endometrial cancer among relatives of women with breast cancer. Br Med J. 1992:305:855–857.
12. Nuffield Council on Bioethics. Genetic screening: ethical issues. London: Nuffield Council on Bioethics; 1993.
13. Steel CM, Ed and UK Cancer Family Study Group. Seminar on ethical issues arising from molecular studies in human genetic disease. Dis Markers. 1992;10:185–228.
14. Wolf RC, Smith AD, Forman D. Metabolic polymorphisms in carcinogen metabolising enzymes and cancer susceptibility. Br Med Bull. 1994;50:718–731.
15. Newton JA. Genetics of melanoma. Br Med Bull. 1994;50:677–687.
16. Marks R. Primary prevention of skin cancer. Br Med J. 1994;309:285–286.
17. Birch JM. Familial cancer syndromes and clusters. Br Med Bull. 1994;50:624–639.
18. Taylor AMR, McConville CM, Byrd PJ. Cancer and DNA processing disorders. Br Med Bull. 1994;50:708–717.
19. Wynder EL. Primary prevention of cancer: planning and policy considerations. J Natl Cancer Inst. 1991;83:475–479.
20. Adami H-O, Adams G, Boyle P, *et al.* Breast cancer etiology. Int J Cancer Suppl. 1990;5:22–39.
21. Harris JR, Lippman ME, Veronesi U, Willett W. Breast cancer (Part 1). N Engl J Med. 1992;327:319–328.
22. Ewertz M, Duffy SW. Incidence of female breast cancer in relation to prevalence and risk factors in Denmark. Int J Cancer. 1994;56:783–787.
23. Narod SA. Genetics of breast and ovarian cancer. Br Med Bull. 1994;50:656–676.
24. Clayton JA. Segregation analysis of familial breast cancer ascertained from a consecutive series of Scottish probands. [Paper in preparation].
25. Brinton LA, Hoover R, Fraumeni JF. Interaction of familial and hormonal risk factors for breast cancer. J Natl Cancer Inst. 1982;69:817–822.
26. Evans DGR, Fentiman IS, McPherson K, *et al.* Familial breast cancer. Br Med J. 1994;308: 183–187.
27. Steinberg KK, Thacker SB, Smith SJ, *et al.* A meta-analysis of the effect of oestrogen replacement therapy on the risk of breast cancer. JAMA. 1991;265:1985–1990.
28. La Vecchia C. Oral contraceptives and breast cancer. Breast. 1992;2:76–81.
29. Eckhardt S, Badellino F, Murphy GP. UICC meeting on breast cancer screening in premenopausal women in developed countries. Int J Cancer. 1994;56:1–5.
30. Rosenberg L, Palmer JR, Zauber AG, *et al.* A hypothesis: nonsteroidal anti-inflammatory drugs reduce the incidence of large-bowel cancer. J Natl Cancer Inst. 1992;83:355–358.
31. Cunningham C, Dunlop MG. Genetics of colorectal cancer. Br Med Bull. 1994;50:640–655.
32. Nayfield SG, Karp JE, Ford LG, Dorr A, Kramer BS. Potential role of tamoxifen in prevention of breast cancer. J Natl Cancer Inst. 1991;83:1450–1459.
33. Fugh-Berman A, Epstein S. Tamoxifen: disease prevention or disease substitution? Lancet. 1992;340:1143–1144.
34. Morrow M, Jordan VC. Risk factors and the prevention of breast cancer with tamoxifen. Cancer Surveys. 1993;18:211–229.

35. Henderson BE, Ross RK, Pike MC. Hormonal chemoprevention of cancer in women. Science. 1993;259:633–638.
36. Evans DGR, Donnai D, Ribiero G, Warrell D. Ovarian cancer family and prophylactic choices. J Med Genet. 1992;29:416–418.
37. Milner B, Allan L, Kelly K, *et al.* Linkage studies with 17q and 18q markers in a breast/ovarian cancer family. Am J Hum Genet. 1993;52:761–766.
38. Narod SA, Lynch HT, Conway T, *et al.* The incidence of cancer is increasing in a large family with hereditary breast–ovarian cancer. Lancet. 1993;341:1101–1102.
39. Lynch HT, Watson P, Conway TA, *et al.* Pilot study of DNA screening for breast/ovarian cancer susceptibility based on linked markers. Arch Int Med. 1993;153:1979–1987.
40. Harris JR, Lippman ME, Veronesi U, Willett W. Breast cancer (Part 3). N Engl J Med. 1992;327:473–480.
41. Piver MS, Jishi MF, Tsukada Y, Nava G. Primary peritoneal carcinoma after prophylactic oophorectomy in women with a family history of ovarian cancer. Cancer. 1993;71:2751–2755.
42. Selby JV. Disease prevention: screening sigmoidoscopy for colorectal cancer. Lancet. 1993;341:728–729.
43. Rees GJG. Cancer treatment: deciding what we can afford. Br Med J. 1991;302:797–800.
44. Anderson TJ. Genesis and source of breast cancer. Br Med Bull. 1991;47:305–318.
45. Piver MS, Baker TR, Jishi MF, *et al.* Familial ovarian cancer. A report of 658 families from the Gilda Radner Familial Ovarian Cancer Registry 1981–1991. Cancer. 1993;71:582–588.
46. Carter BS, Steinberg GD, Beaty TH, Childs B, Walsh PC. Familial risk factors for prostate cancer. Cancer Surveys. 1991;11:5–13.
47. Bourne TH, Campbell S, Reynolds KM, *et al.* Screening for early familial ovarian cancer with transvaginal ultrasonography and colour flow imaging. Br Med J. 1993;306:1025–1029.
48. Catalona WJ, Smith DS, Ratliff TL, *et al.* Measurement of prostate-specific antigen as a screening test for prostate cancer. N Engl J Med. 1991:324:1156–1161.
49. Siddall R. Time to screen for prostate cancer? New Scientist. 1993;137:27–30.
50. Ponder BAJ. Setting up and running a familial cancer clinic. Br Med Bull. 1994;50:732–745.
51. Ransohoff DF, Lang CA, Kuo HS. Colonoscopic surveillance after polypectomy: considerations of cost-effectiveness. Ann Intern Med. 1991;114:177–182.
52. Law J. Variations in individual radiation dose in a breast screening programme and consequences for the balance between associated risk and benefit. Br J Radiol. 1993;66:691–698.
53. Day NE. Screening for breast cancer. Br Med Bull. 1991;47:400–415.
54. Ellwood JM, Cox B, Richardson AK. The effectiveness of breast screening by mammography in younger women. Online J Curr Clin Trials. (Serial online). 1993;2: Doc NR 32.
55. Miller AB, Baines CJ, To T, Wall C. Canadian National Breast Screening Study: breast cancer detection and death rates among women aged 40 to 49 years. Can Med Assoc J. 1992;147:1459–1476.
56. Stacey-Clear A, McCarthy HA, Hall DA, *et al.* Breast cancer survival among women under age 50: is mammography detrimental? Lancet. 1992;340:991–994.
57. Nystrom L, Rutqvist LE, Wall S, *et al.* Breast cancer screening with mammography: overview of Swedish randomised trials. Lancet. 1993;341:973–978.
58. Fletcher SW, Black W, Harris R, *et al.* Report of the International Workshop on Screening for Breast Cancer. J Natl Cancer Inst. 1993;85:1644–1656.
59. Easton DF, Bishop DT, Ford D, Crockford GP, and the Breast Cancer Linkage Cosortium. Genetic linkage analysis in familial breast and ovarian cancer: results from 214 families. Am J Hum Genet. 1993;52:678–701.
60. Kerilkowske K, Grady D, Barclay J, *et al.* Positive value of screening mammography by age and family history of breast cancer. JAMA. 1993;270:2444–2450.
61. Rustin GJS. Impact of tumour marker measurements upon management of patients with carcinoma of the ovary. Dis Markers. 1991;9:153–158.
62. Scott IV. Advantages and disadvantages of randomised controlled trials of ovarian cancer screening. In: Sharp F, Mason P, Creasman G eds. Ovarian Cancer 2. London: Chapman & Hall; 1992:277–287.
63. Bast R Jr, Xu S, Woolas R, *et al.* Complementary and co-ordinate markers for detection of epithelial ovarian cancer. In: Sharp F, Mason P, Blackett A, Berek J eds. Ovarian cancer 3. London: Chapman & Hall; 1994:189–192.
64. Gagel RF, Tashijan AH Jr, Cummings T, *et al.* The clinical outcome of prospective screening for multiple endocrine neoplasia type 2a. N Engl J Med. 1988;318:478–484.

65. Mulligan LM, Kwok JBJ, Healey CS, *et al.* Germ-line mutations of the RET proto-oncogene in multiple endocrine neoplasia type 2A. Nature. 1993;363:458–460.
66. Olschwang S, Tiret A, Laurent-Puig P, *et al.* Restriction of ocular fundus lesions to a specific subgroup of FAP mutations in adenomatous polyposis coli. Cell. 1993;75:959–968.
67. Claus EB, Risch N, Thompson WD. Age of onset as an indicator of familial risk of breast cancer. Am J Epidemiol. 1990;131:961–972.
68. Houlston RS, McCarter E, Parbhoo S, Scurr JH, Slack J. Family history and risk of breast cancer. J Med Genet. 1992;29:154–157.
69. Bishop DT. The importance of inherited predisposition to cancer. Cancer Topics. 1991;8:66–68.
70. Easton D, Ford D, Peto J. Inherited susceptibility to breast cancer. Cancer Surveys. 1993;18:95–113.
71. Swanson GM. Breast cancer risk estimation: a translational statistic for communication to the public. J Natl Cancer Inst. 1993;85:848–897.
72. de Wit ACD, Meijers-Heijboer EJ, Tibben A, *et al.* Effect on a Dutch family of predictive DNA testing for hereditary breast and ovarian cancer. Lancet. 1994;344:197.
73. Li FP, Garber J, Friend SH, *et al.* Recommendations on predictive testing for germ line p53 mutations among cancer-prone individuals. J Natl Cancer Inst. 1992;84:1156–1160.
74. Wu Y, Giger ML, Doi K, *et. al.* Artificial neural networks in mammography. Radiology. 1993;187:81–87.
75. Workman P, Harris A. Translating advances in molecular oncology into improved therapy: new targets for drug discovery. Cancer Topics. 1993;9:97–99.

10
Mutagenic properties of anticancer drugs

L.R. Ferguson

INTRODUCTION

Anticancer drugs are among the earliest recognized and strongest mutagens. They have been extensively studied. For example, mustard gas is a sulphur mustard that was widely used as a poison gas in the first world war. It became apparent that the systemic effects of this compound were related to inhibition of cell division, and this in turn was used as a rationale for testing it as an antitumour agent, with some limited degree of success[1]. In 1946, studies on mustard gas in *Drosophila melanogaster* provided the first ever report of mutagenesis induced by a chemical[2]. In this same year, the first use of the related nitrogen mustards as antitumour drugs was reported[3]. These mustards were the prototype of a variety of compounds tested as anticancer drugs, with very different chemical structures (Figure 10.1), but having in common that they functioned as DNA alkylating agents under physiological conditions and possessed mutagenic potential[4].

Since that time, a wider range of anticancer drugs has been developed, examples of which target not only DNA but also DNA-associated species, including the mitotic spindle and topoisomerase enzymes. For example, a breakdown of the anticancer drugs used in a single year (1993) at a typical New Zealand hospital is given in Table 10.1. Of 23 drugs routinely used, 8 are alkylating agents (a total of 1564 doses annually), 8 are topoisomerase II poisons (2432 doses annually), 4 are antimetabolites (7300 doses annually), 2 are mitotic spindle inhibitors (1376 doses annually) and 1 is a DNA-strand cutting agent (bleomycin; 284 doses annually).

It became apparent at an early stage that clinically used alkylating agents were carcinogenic and probably had other long-term consequences relating to their mutagenic potential. One of the justifications for developing other types of therapy was to reduce these risks. However, it is becoming increasingly apparent that most of these other types of chemicals also have long-term effects, and these are probably related to their mutagenic potential.

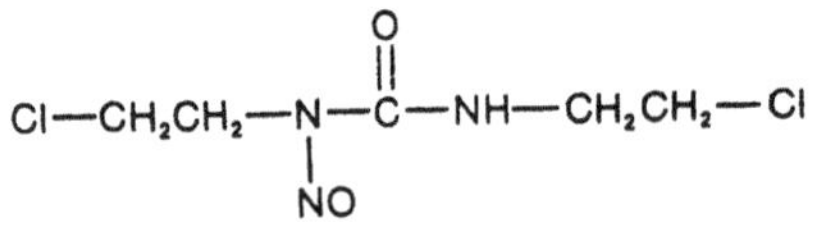

Cl—CH_2CH_2—N(NO)—C(=O)—NH—CH_2CH_2—Cl

Carmustine
(BCNU)

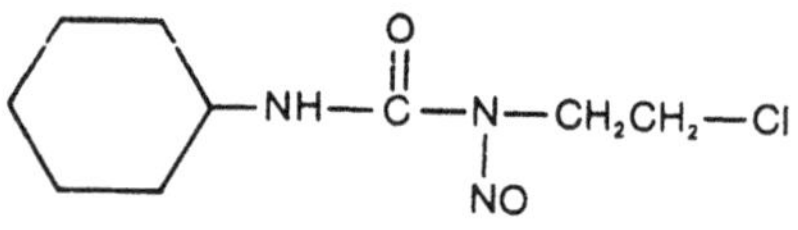

Cyclohexyl—NH—C(=O)—N(NO)—CH_2CH_2—Cl

Lomustine
(CCNU)

CH_2OH, OH, OH, HO, NO, NH—C(=O)—N—CH_3

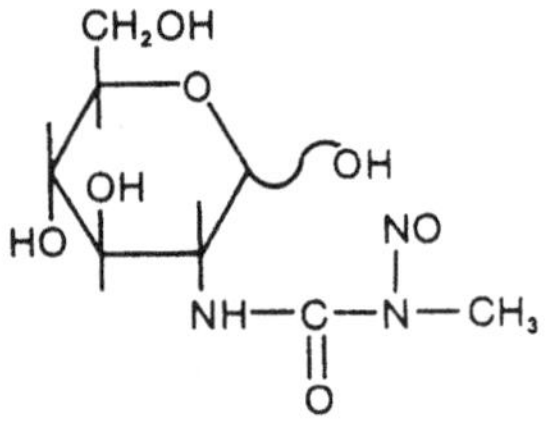

Streptozotocin

Figure 10.1 Structures of some alkylating agents. (a) nitrosoureas

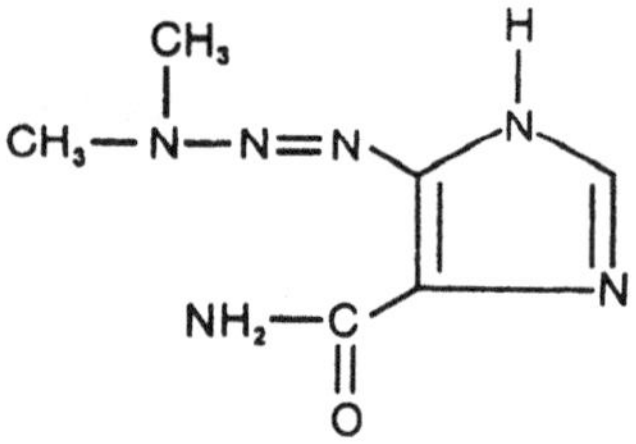

CH_3—N(CH_3)—N=N—, H, N, N, NH_2—C(=O)

DTIC
(Dacarbazine)

CH_3—NH—NH—CH_2—C6H4—C(=O)—NH—CH(CH_3)—CH_3

• HCl

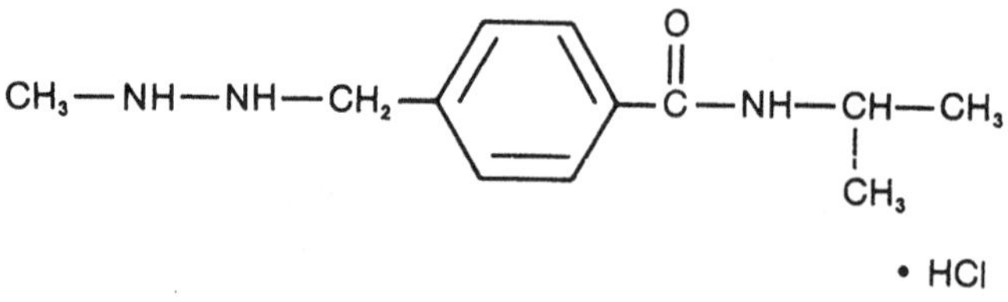

Procarbazine

(b) Dacarbazine and procarbazine

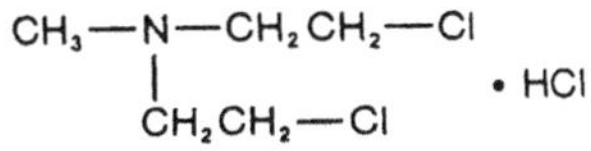

$CH_3-N(CH_2CH_2-Cl)-CH_2CH_2-Cl \cdot HCl$

Nitrogen mustard

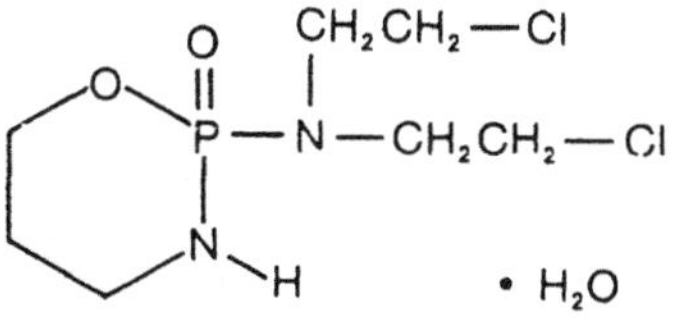

Cyclophosphamide $\cdot H_2O$

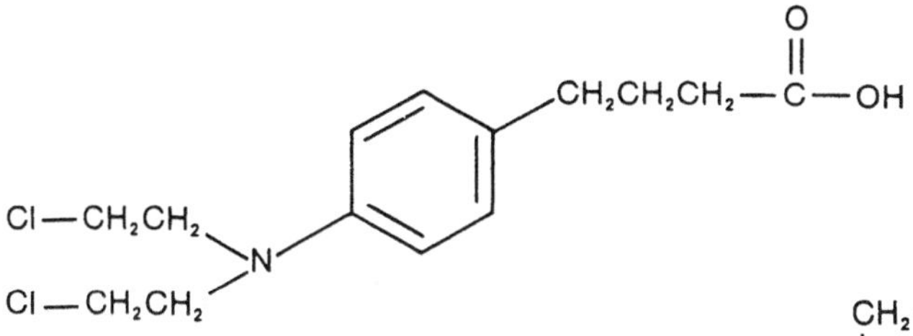

Chlorambucil

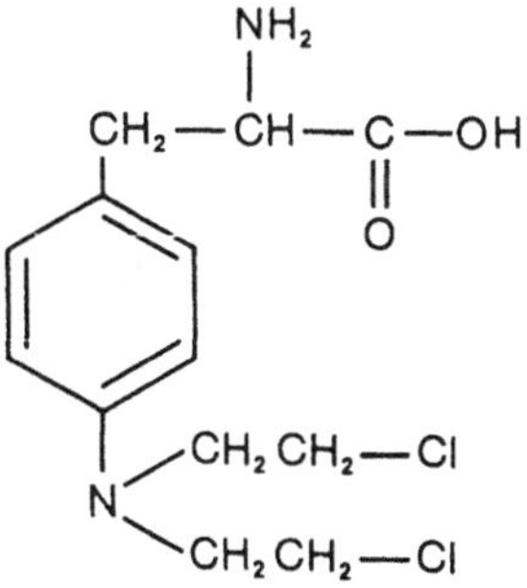

Melphalan

Figure 10.1 *cont.* (c) Nitrogen mustards

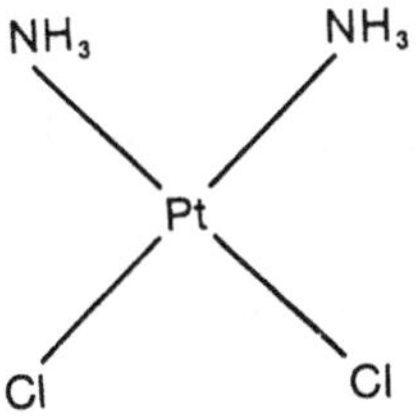

cis-Platin

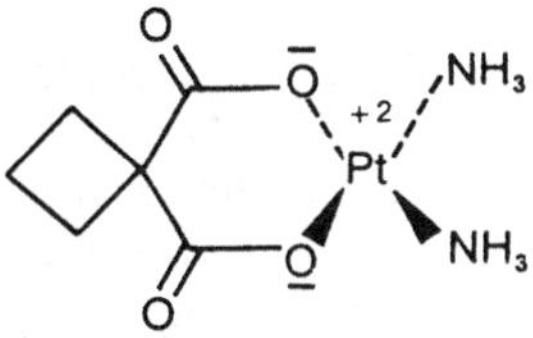

Carboplatin

(d) Platinum co-ordination complexes

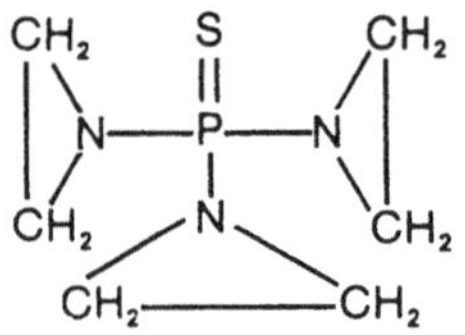

Thio-TEPA

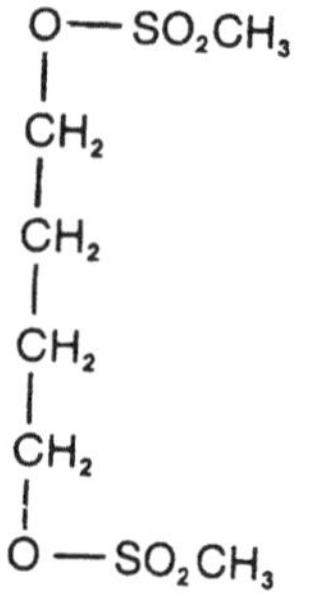

Busulfan
(Myleran)

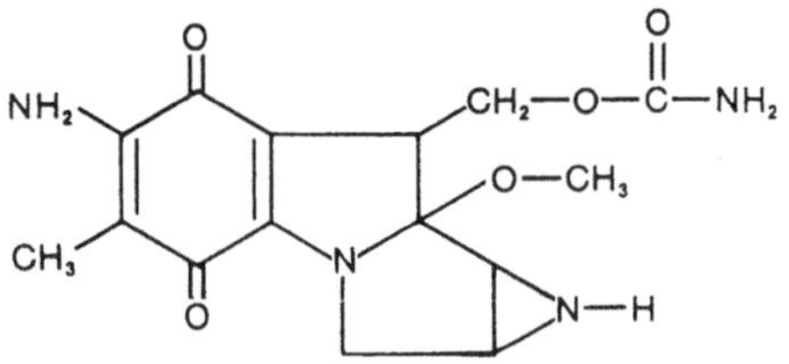

Mitomycin C

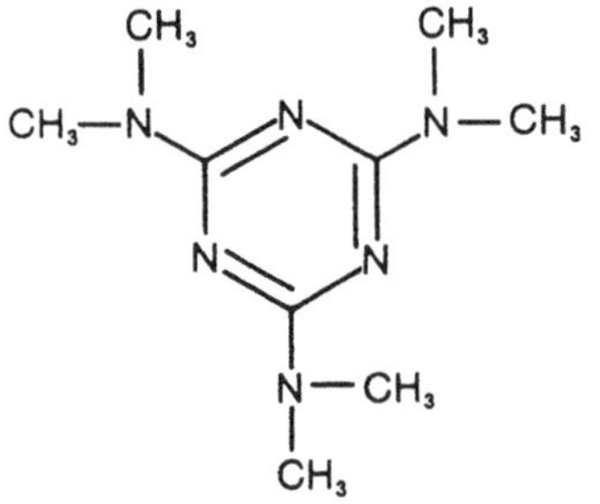

Hexamethyl melamine

Figure 10.1 *cont.* (e) Other drugs

MAJOR CLASSES OF ANTITUMOUR DRUGS AND THEIR MODES OF ACTION

Alkylating agents

Monofunctional alkylating agents which are used clinically include the nitrosoureas (BCNU, CCNU and streptozotocin), as well as dacarbazine and procarbazine. This latter chemical is metabolized into a methylating agent via a rather complex pathway. The most effective clinical alkylating agents are bifunctional, and their anticancer effects are largely due to their ability to form crosslinks in cellular DNA[5]. These crosslinks involving DNA may be within a single strand, between two complementary strands, or between DNA and other molecules[6–8]. The nitrogen mustards include nitrogen mustard (mustine), cyclophosphamide (and its geometric isomer, ifosfamide), melphalan and chlorambucil. These drugs form interstrand crosslinks at the N-7 of guanines, preferentially at 5′-GNC sites[9]. Other known clinical bis-alkylating agents include thiotepa, busulphan (Myleran), mitomycin C, and hexamethylmelamine. There was originally some dispute as to whether the latter acted as an alkylating agent but it is now known to be metabolized to a hydroxymethyl

Table 10.1 Annual consumption of anticancer drugs at Auckland Hospital

Drug	*Mode of action*	*Number of doses*	*Total used (mg)*
Amsacrine	Topo II poison	80	1300
Bleomycin	DNA cutting agent	284	6852
Carboplatin	Alkylating agent	420	214360
Carmustine	Alkylating agent	4	1980
Cisplatin	Alkylating agent	192	26960
Cyclophosphamide	Alkylating agent	764	830996
Cytarabine	Antimetabolite	1496	526076
Dacarbazine	Alkylating agent	36	18252
Daunorubicin	Topo II poison	184	9596
Doxorubicin	Topo II poison	632	32246
Epirubicin	Topo II poison	64	4508
Etoposide	Topo II poison	1056	178952
Floxuridine	Antimetabolite	16	4000
5-Fluorouracil	Antimetabolite	3860	2730140
Fludarabine	Antimetabolite	144	6300
Idarubicin	Topo II poison	24	322
Ifosfamide	Alkylating agent	96	126800
Melphalan	Alkylating agent	4	400
Methotrexate	Antimetabolite	1784	742632
Mitoxantrone	Topo II poison	88	1460
Nitrogen mustard	Alkylating agent	48	544
Teniposide	Topo II poison	304	49184
Vinblastine	Mitotic spindle inhibitor	256	2116
Vincristine	Mitotic spindle inhibitor	1120	1589

derivative which can release formaldehyde, known to have DNA alkylation activity[10].

The platinum co-ordination complexes, *cis*-platin and carboplatin, are converted to alkylating agents within the cell. *cis*-Platin makes intrastrand links in DNA by binding to N-7 of adjacent guanosine residues. However, it has been suggested that the cytotoxic event in the cell may occur rather differently than for many of the other alkylators. A structure-specific recognition protein, SSRP1, binds to DNA modified with *cis*-platin[11], possibly at recombination signal sequences.

Crosslinks are more difficult to repair and more cytotoxic than a single adduct[12–14]. Crosslinking is a two-step process, with the first step (monofunctional adduct formation) being more rapid than the second (crosslinking). Thus, most bifunctional alkylators produce about 20-fold more mono-adducts than bis-adducts[15].

Although the main target for biological activity of alkylating agents is DNA, such chemicals can also alkylate other cell components[16]. Additionally, the site of reaction within the DNA varies with the nature of the drug and different sites of alkylation have different significance for various types of biological activity. For example, it has been suggested that the O-6 position of guanine is a major target for mutagenesis[17], while the N-7 position may be important for chemotherapy[16]. However, this may no longer hold true for some of the newer types of experimental anticancer drugs[18,19].

Topoisomerase inhibitors

Topoisomerases are enzymes which relieve the torsional stress generated in double-stranded DNA during both transcription and replication. Topoisomerase II (topo II) enzymes are an important part of the mitotic chromosome scaffold and are thought to be essential for mitotic chromosome assembly and condensation[20–22]. They act by transiently breaking two DNA strands and attaching themselves to the free ends of the broken DNA via the amino acid tyrosine[23]. A second DNA helix is then able to pass between the two enzyme protein subunits, allowing both swivelling and also untangling of DNA[24]. The cleavage process is normally spontaneously reversible, restoring DNA to its original form.

Although there are a number of ways in which topo II enzymes can be inhibited, the clinically used topo II inhibitors (Figure 10.2) are all thought to act through the formation of a ternary complex of DNA–drug–topo II, which prevents the DNA breaks from rejoining. They are sometimes described as 'topo II poisons' in order to distinguish them from other types of topo II inhibitor[25]. The 'cleavable complex' initially formed can be irreversibly converted to topoisomerase-linked DNA breaks upon addition of a strong protein denaturant. This type of lesion differs from the covalent lesions associated with alkylating agents in its reversibility, as it disappears upon removal of the inhibitor. In the absence

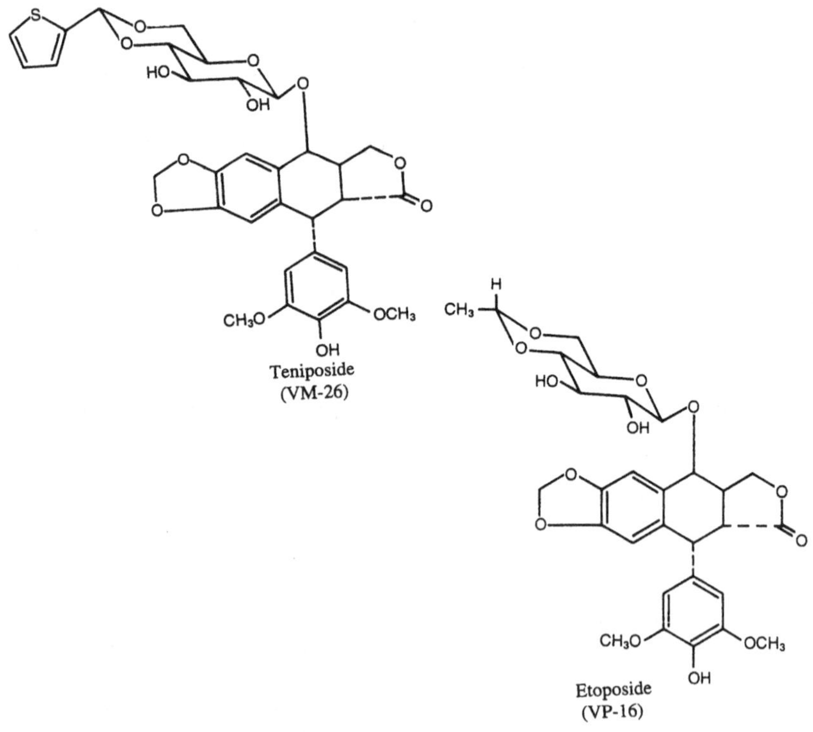

Teniposide (VM-26)

Etoposide (VP-16)

Figure 10.2 Structures of some topo II poisons

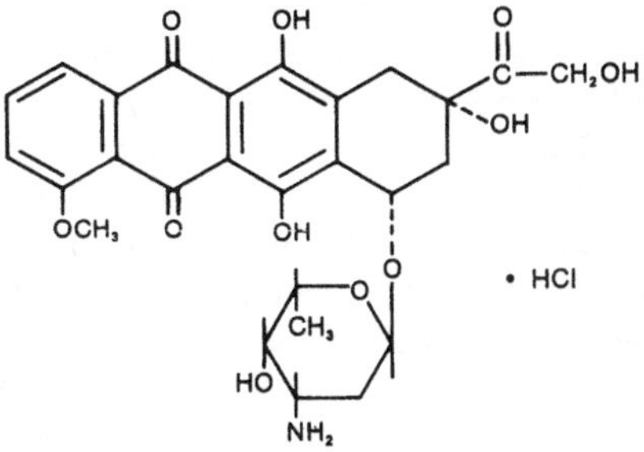

Doxorubicin
(Adriamycin)

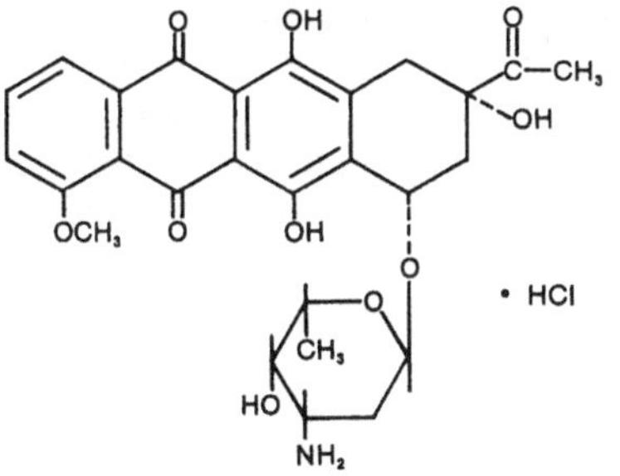

Daunorubicin
(Daunomycin)

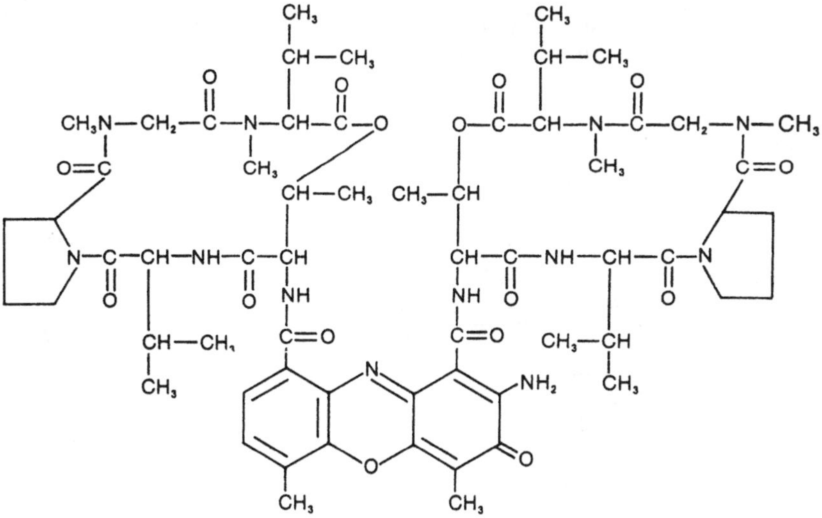

Dactinomycin
(Actinomycin D)

Figure 10.2 *cont.*

of DNA replication, the drug would eventually dissociate by itself, permitting the normal repair processes. However, when topo II enzymes are inhibited during progression of DNA polymerase along the DNA, the DNA damage and/or cell death may occur. The recent review by Ralph and co-workers[26] provides substantially more detail on the molecular action of topo II inhibitors.

The epipodophyllotoxins, etoposide (VP-16) and teniposide (VM-26), target the topo II enzyme without DNA intercalation. However, all the other important clinical topo II poisons (illustrated in Figure 10.2) intercalate into DNA. Those commonly used are the anthracyclines including doxorubicin (Adriamycin) and daunorubicin (daunomycin); the acridine which is variously known as amsacrine, m-AMSA or Cain's acridine; and dactinomycin (actinomycin D). There are also a number of new drugs currently in clinical trial and many experimental agents which target topo II or even topo I enzymes (e.g. camptothecin). The actions of these newer types of chemicals were reviewed recently[26].

The sensitivity of cells to topo II poisons changes in relation to cell cycle progression, at least partly because levels of topo II change with time[27]. Cells exposed to topoisomerase poisons before or during the S (DNA synthetic) phase of the cell cycle undergo abnormal DNA replication and become irreversibly blocked in the G2 (premitosis) phase. Treatment of G2-phase cells, at least with etoposide or teniposide, prevents the condensation of chromosomes and entry into mitosis[20,28,29].

Bleomycin and other free radical generating agents

Bleomycin is a radiomimetic anticancer antibiotic. The clinical formulation, blenoxane, is a mixture of polypeptides, primarily bleomycins A2 and B2[30] (Figure 10.3). The drug interacts with DNA in the presence of certain redox

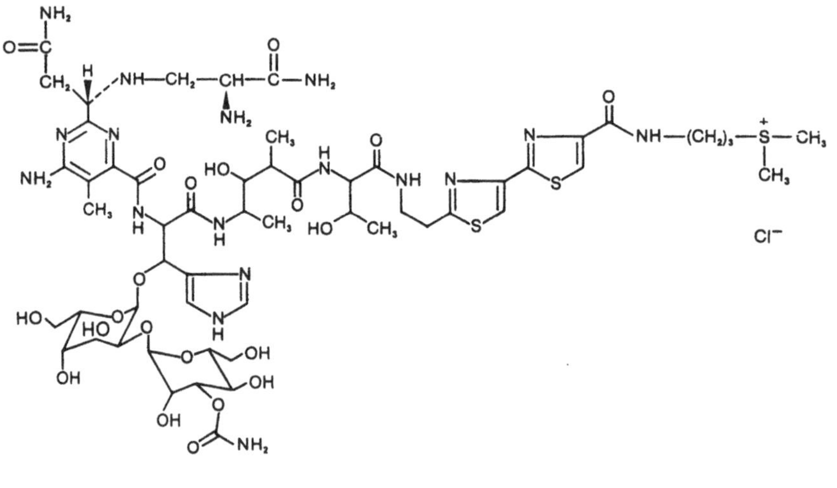

Bleomycin A2

Figure 10.3 Structure of bleomycin A2

active metals such as iron and an oxygen source, generating radicals primarily at the C-4′ position of the deoxyribose. Oxidation of these radicals then leads to a sequence of events resulting in single- and double-strand DNA breaks and also in apurinic sites with closely opposed strand breaks[30]. DNA cleavage by bleomycin occurs preferentially at 5′-GC and 5′-GT sequences[31]. More details on the molecular events associated with bleomycin can be found in the recent review by Natrajan and Hecht[30].

Although the production of the free radicals is not thought to be the primary mode of action of clinical anticancer drugs other than bleomycin, it may well be a side-effect of a number of drugs and may also cause some of their observed mutagenic effects. For example, within the group of topo II poisons, phenolic or anilino groups are commonly present and are easily and reversibly oxidizable. Such groups are found in amsacrine and an analogue currently undergoing clinical trial (CI-921)[32], the anthracyclines, epipodophyllotoxins, ellipticines and anthracenediones.

Mitotic spindle inhibitors

Vinblastine and vincristine are closely related chemicals (Figure 10.4) which do not react with DNA but instead bind to tubulin, a key component of microtubules. They both produce metaphase arrest during the cell cycle leading to an increase in the number of cells in mitosis. Wendell and co-workers[33] studied vinblastine-treated cells using electron microscopy. They showed that vinblastine did not affect the structure of the microtubules or of the kinetochores, although the number of microtubules attached to the kinetochores was significantly decreased. Both the centrosomes and the association between mother and daughter centrioles were altered, with many of the centrioles having abnormal ultrastructure. These data support the suggestion that vinblastine (and probably also vincristine) acts through inhibition of the polymerization dynamics of the mitotic spindle microtubules and possibly also the centriole microtubules, rather than through microtubule depolymerization[33,34].

Antimetabolites

Most antimetabolites bear strong structural similarities to endogenous nucleic acid precursors. Those commonly used include the pyrimidine analogues 5-fluorouracil (5-FU), 5-fluorodeoxyuridine (floxuridine; FUdR) and cytarabine (ara-C); and the purine analogues, fludarabine (F-ara-A), 6-mercaptopurine and 6-thioguanine. Hydroxyurea and methotrexate are also antimetabolites, although structurally rather different from others in the group. All these examples are illustrated in Figure 10.5.

Although the cytotoxicity of antimetabolites is generally cell cycle phase-specific, the individual mechanisms of action of these agents differ. Methotrexate acts as a potent inhibitor of dihydrofolate reductase, blocking the conversion of 2-deoxyuridylate (dUMP) to thymidylate (dTMP), an essential component of DNA. The fluorinated pyrimidines also play a key role in nucleic

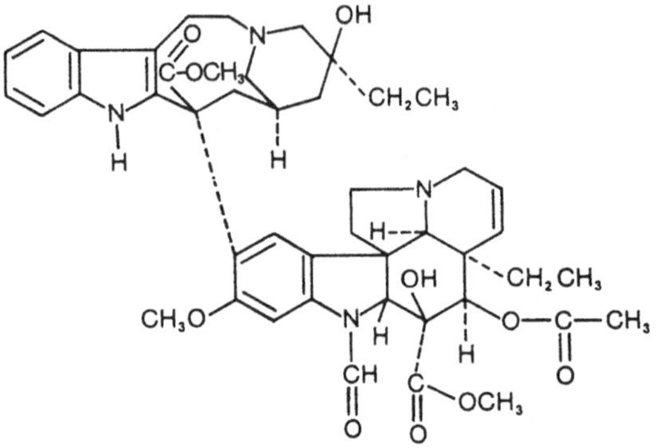

Vincristine

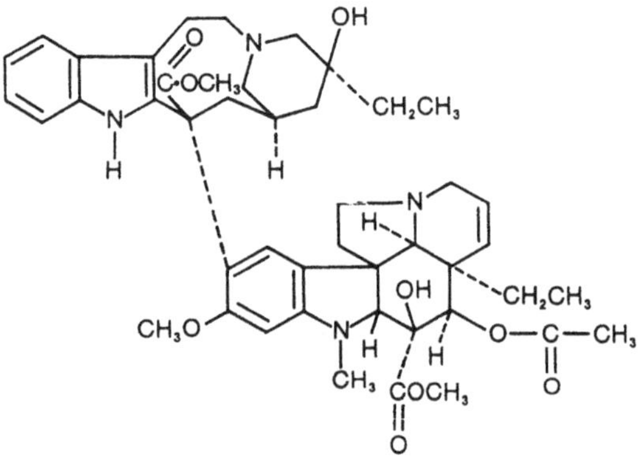

Vinblastine

Figure 10.4 Structures of two mitotic spindle inhibitors

acid metabolism[35]. FUdR is converted by thymidine kinase to FdUMP, a thymidylate synthase inhibitor. 5-FU similarly blocks the thymidylate synthase enzyme, again preventing the conversion of dUMP to dTMP. Hydroxyurea is an inhibitor of ribonucleotide reductase. Each of these four chemicals leads to thymidylate stress, which has direct implications for mutagenesis[36].

Cytarabine and fludarabine are cytosine and adenine nucleoside analogues respectively. Fludarabine is thought to inhibit DNA replication by blocking the synthesis of nuclear matrix-associated primer RNA and RNA-primed Okazaki fragments[37]. Both cytarabine and fludarabine are transported into cells and converted to the 5′-triphosphate. 6-Mercaptopurine and 6-thioguanine are both substrates for the enzyme hypoxanthine-guanine phosphoribosyltransferase, which acts to convert various purines (including guanine but not adenine) to their corresponding 5′-ribonucleotides. Effectively, each of the

(a)

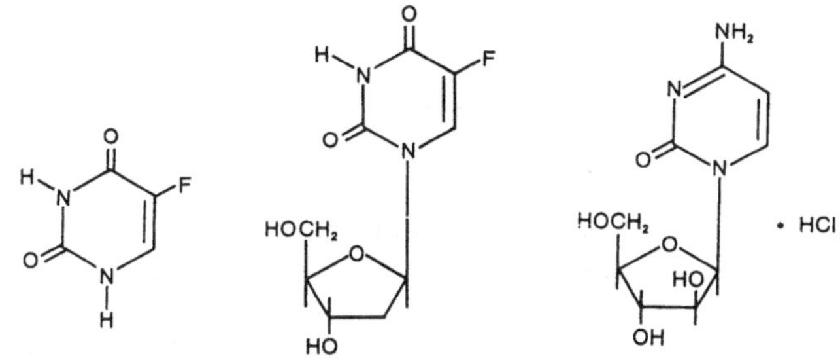

5-Fluorouracil (5-FU)

5-Fluorodeoxyuridine (FUdR)

Cytarabine (Cytosine arabinoside, Ara-C)

(b)

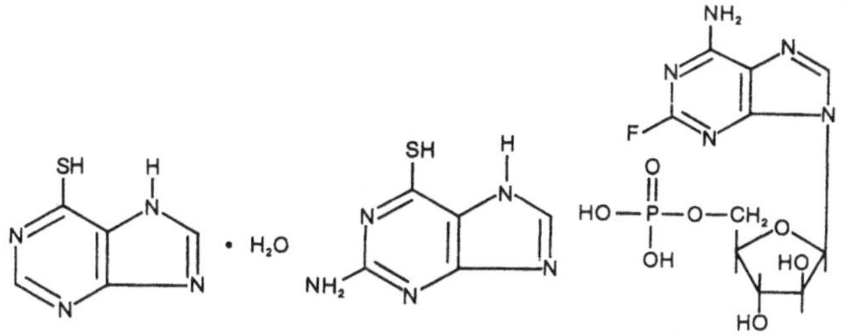

6-Mercaptopurine

6-Thioguanine

Fludarabine (F-ara-A)

(c)

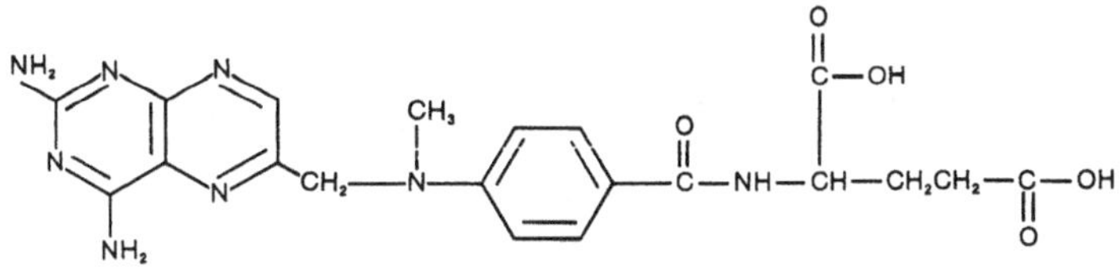

Methotrexate

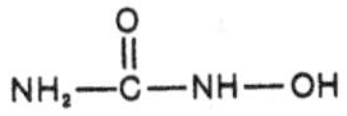

Hydroxyurea

Figure 10.5 Structures of some antimetabolites. (a) Pyrimidine analogues. (b) Purine analogues. (c) Others

antimetabolites inhibits DNA synthesis and may lead to changes in nucleotide pools in the cell.

POSSIBLE CONSEQUENCES OF THE MUTAGENIC EFFECTS OF ANTICANCER DRUGS

As will be discussed later, anticancer drugs can potentially cause various types of mutations, dependent upon their chemical nature and mode of action. The alterations may involve a single gene (gene mutation), blocks of genes (chromosome mutation) or the gain or loss of a whole chromosome (genome mutation or aneuploidy). Effects involving single genes may be a consequence of effects on a single DNA base (point mutations) or of larger changes, such as deletions, within the gene. Gene amplification may also be affected, i.e. the process by which the number of copies of a specific gene within the cell can be increased. The effect of a gene may also be modified through recombination. The ability of an anticancer drug to cause these various effects may have implications for the successful conclusion of treatment, may affect reproduction, or may be involved in the subsequent development of a second treatment-related cancer as follows.

Development of anticancer drug resistance

A major limitation to successful cancer chemotherapy is the development of resistance to drugs being used to treat it. There are often drug-resistant cells originally present in the tumour and these will increase in proportion as the sensitive cells are killed. Additionally, many of the anticancer drugs are able to create mutations in surviving cells, thereby potentially enhancing the development of resistance to other agents during subsequent cycles of chemotherapy.

There are a number of mechanisms by which drug resistance occurs. Possibly the best characterized general mechanism is development of the multiple drug resistance (mdr) phenotype, which leads to simultaneous resistance to a range of different anticancer drugs. Mdr commonly occurs through gene amplification, which can be demonstrated cytogenetically as either homogeneously staining regions or as double minute chromosomes[38,39].

For any given drug, there may be multiple mechanisms by which resistance arises, involving different types of mutations. For example, resistance to the antimetabolite 6-thioguanine can be caused by mutation at the level of the gene or the chromosome[40]. Resistance to another antimetabolite, methotrexate, commonly occurs through gene amplification[41] or through specific types of gene mutation[42].

Infertility and spontaneous abortion

It has been estimated that a minimum of 15% of all known pregnancies are lost before term, and that up to 50% of those lost have detectable chromosome anomalies[43]. Additionally, approximately 30–50% of conceptuses are thought to be lost before pregnancy is recognized, and these are also likely to involve a high proportion of chromosome anomalies, including both chromosomal aberrations and aneuploidy[44]. These figures are likely to increase with the use of mutagenic drugs.

Birth defects

Many genetic diseases in man are known to be caused by chromosome anomalies, including both stuctural and numeric alterations. The most common numeric chromosome alteration is trisomy 21 (Down syndrome), while structural mutations may occur in one third of all defective live births[45]. Other defects are due to single genes of large effect, including autosomal dominant diseases such as Huntington disease, or autosomal recessive disorders, such as phenylketonuria. These may be due to point mutations involving single DNA base changes or larger changes, such as deletions within the gene, which again could be related to the use of mutagenic drugs.

Carcinogenesis

Proto-oncogenes are a highly conserved group of normal cellular genes, the majority of which are probably involved in normal cell growth and differentiation. They can, however, be activated to forms which play a role in carcinogenesis. Mechanisms of activation include point mutations, chromosome translocation or gene amplification. A range of human cancers commonly shows increased dosage of cellular oncogenes resulting from gene amplification, although it is not clear at which stage this occurs[46].

Tumour suppressor genes act to prevent cells from becoming malignant and both copies of the gene must be inactivated before this happens. Once the first copy of the gene is inactivated in some manner, then loss of heterozygosity can occur through various mechanisms, including point mutations, chromosome loss, chromosomal deletions, gene conversion or mitotic recombination. A variety of specific mutations in the p53 tumour suppressor gene has been identified in a range of human cancers[47].

Au[48] studied the sequence of events leading to the development of malignant characteristics in cultured cells from irradiated male mice. He found that aneuploidy and extensive chromosome breakage occurred early, followed by inactivation of the retinoblastoma tumour suppressor gene. Amplification of the *myc* oncogene preceded expression of the tumour phenotype. Similarly, a sequence of different events (including both mutation and gene expression) has been associated with the development of colorectal cancer in humans[49].

TESTING SYSTEMS FOR MUTAGENICITY, AS RECOMMENDED FOR REGULATORY PURPOSES

A battery of mutagenicity tests is usually considered necessary for assessing the genotoxic potential of any given chemical, including anticancer drugs. The exact nature of the test battery varies according to the specific requirements of each country[45,50].

The current UK regulations suggest two stages in testing[50]. An initial *in-vitro* screen would involve testing gene mutation in the *Salmonella* mutagenicity assay developed by Ames and co-workers[51]. A second *in-vitro* assay should estimate chromosomal aberrations in mammalian cells. It is recognized that this combination of assays may not detect a small proportion of agents with the potential for *in-vitro* mutagenicity, and it may be appropriate to supplement these assays with a mammalian mutation assay and/or data on gene recombination events.

The mutation endpoint which is not adequately considered in current regulations is at the level of the genome. Neither *in-vivo* nor *in-vitro* recommended testing methods provide information on interaction with the mitotic spindle or on the induction of aneuploidy.

A second stage in mutagenicity testing requires an *in-vivo* assay for chromosome damage (using metaphase analysis or the micronucleus test) in the bone marrow of a rodent. In some cases, other assays, such as measurement of unscheduled DNA synthesis in rat liver, may also be desirable.

Not all somatic cell mutagens are germ-cell mutagens. For chemicals such as anticancer drugs, it is desirable to proceed to a third stage of testing and assess germ-cell effects. It is important to distinguish assays that look at genetic damage in germ cells from those which provide evidence for the heritable component of induced damage[50]. It is also important to recognize that the various stages of spermatogenesis in the male as well as the different stages in maturation of the female oocyte can each show differing sensitivities, even towards potent mutagens[52]. Two of the recommended assays directly estimate chromosomal events, including reciprocal translocations (cytogenetics in spermatogonia and cytogenetics in spermatocytes for reciprocal translocations[50]). The recommended *in-vivo* mammalian germ-cell assay is the dominant lethal assay[53], and it may also be appropriate to progress to the heritable translocation assay[54] and the morphological specific locus test[55].

The performance of anticancer drugs in these recommended test systems (as summarized in Tables 10.2–4) is largely related to their chemical type. Over the last 10 years, reviews have been published on the mutagenicity of busulphan[56], procarbazine[57], cyclophosphamide[58], bleomycin[59] and 6-mercaptopurine[60]. We recently reviewed the more general topic of mutagenicity and topo II enzymes[25] while other general reviews are available on the genetic consequences of nucleotide pool imbalances[36] and the genetic toxicology of fluorinated pyrimidines[35].

GENE MUTATIONS IN *SALMONELLA TYPHIMURIUM*

A considerable amount of mutagenicity data on anticancer drugs derives from the *Salmonella* assay developed by Ames and co-workers and sometimes known as the Ames test[51]. There are considerable advantages in using this assay. Firstly, there is an enormous body of data on a wide range of chemical types, so that the work on anticancer drugs can be placed in perspective. Secondly, information as to which strain preferentially shows mutation can be used to understand the likely

Table 10.2 Mutagenic activity of anticancer drugs in *Salmonella typhimurium*

	Bacterial strain								
	TA1537		*TA98*		*TA100*		*TA102*		*References*
Drug	*– S9*	*+ S9*	*– S9*	*+ S9*	*– S9*	*+ S9*	*– S9*	*+ S9*	
Alkylating agents									
Busulphan	+	–	–	–	++	++			153, 154
Carboplatin			–	–	+	+	+	+	155
Carmustine	–	–	–	–	+	+			156, 157
Chlorambucil	–	–	–	–	–	+	+	+	153, 158
Cisplatin	–	–	+	+	+	+	+	+	155, 159, 160
Cyclophosphamide	–	–	–	–	–	+			161, 162
Dacarbazine			+	+	+	+			163
Hexamethylmelamine	–	–	–	–	–	–			153
Lomustine			–	–	+	+			156
Melphalan	–	–	–	–	+	+			160, 164
Mitomycin C	–	–	–	–	–	–	+		64, 154, 160
Nitrogen mustard			–	–	+	+			164
Procarbazine	–	–	–	–	–	–			160, 162
Streptozotocin			–	–	+++	+++			156, 160
Thiotepa	–		–		+				160
Topo II inhibitors									
Amsacrine	+++	++	–	–	–	–	+		165
Dactinomycin	–	–	–	–	–	–	–		154, 160, 166
Daunorubicin	–+		++	++	–+	–+	+		160, 167
Doxorubicin	–+	+	++	++	–+	–+	+		160, 168
Etoposide			–	–	–	–	–	–	169
Teniposide							–	–	169
Bleomycin	–	–	–	–	–	–	+		160, 166
Mitotic spindle inhibitors									
Vinblastine	–		–	–	–	–			154, 160
Vincristine	–		–	–	–	–			154, 160
Antimetabolites									
Cytarabine	–	–	–	–	–	–	–	–	154, 160
Hydroxyurea	–	–	–	–	–	–	–		160, 161
Floxuridine	–	–	–	–	–	–			170
Fludarabine									
5-Fluorouracil	–	–	–	–	–	–	–	–	160, 171
6-Mercaptopurine	–	–	–	–	+	–	–		154, 160, 172
Methotrexate	–	–	–	–	–	–	–		154, 160
6-Thioguanine	–	–	–	–	–	–			170

Notes:
Results from the assays are recorded in the table as follows: –, maximum reversion frequency less than 2× that in the negative control; +, maximum reversion frequency 2– <10 × that in the negative control; ++ maximum reversion frequency 10– <100x that in the negative control; +++, maximum reversion frequency 100 or more times that in the negative control. Data have only been taken from studies using the standard methodology, with or without supplementation with S9 mix, the microsomal activating preparation.

Table 10.3 Mutagenic activity of anticancer drugs in mammalian *in–vitro* assays

	SCE[a]				*Gene mutation*[b]				*Chromosomal aberrations*[b]				*Reference*
	Chinese hamster		*Human*		*Chinese hamster 6tg resistance*		*L5187Y TK +/–*		*Chinese hamster*		*Human*		
Exogenous metabolic activation:	–	+	–	+	–	+	–	+	–	+	–	+	
Alkylating agents													
Busulphan	++				+/++	++	++	++	++		++		112, 173–175
Carboplatin	++				++								176
Carmustine			++		++								177, 178
Chlorambucil	++/++ +		++		++						++		112, 174, 179
Cisplatin	+++		++		++						++		112, 174, 179
Cyclophosphamide	–	++			–	++	–	++	–	+++			112, 175, 180–182
Dacarbazine	+				–/+	++	+	++					174, 183, 184
Hexamethylmelamine													
Lomustine	+				+		++	++	+++		+		174, 178, 183
Melphalan	+++		++				++	++	+++		+		112, 179, 183, 185, 186
Mitomycin C	+++		+++		+		+	+	++		++		112, 175, 187–189
Nitrogen mustard	+++		++		+				–/+		++		12, 181, 188, 190–192
Procarbazine	++				+		+	++			+	+	193–196
Streptozotocin					+								178
Thiotepa	++		+		+				++		+		112, 185, 188, 197

Table 10.3 *Continued*

	SCE[a]				*Gene mutation*[b]				*Chromosomal aberrations*[b]				*Reference*
	Chinese hamster		*Human*		*Chinese hamster 6tg resistance*		*L5187Y TK +/–*		*Chinese hamster*		*Human*		
Exogenous metabolic activation:	–	+	–	+	–	+	–	+	–	+	–	+	
Topo II inhibitors													
Amsacrine	++		+		++		+++		+++		+++		40, 79, 198–200
Dactinomycin	++		–		+	–	++		+++		+++		40, 112, 174, 186, 191
Daunorubicin	++		++		+	–	++	++			++		40, 112, 167, 174, 183, 191
Doxorubicin	+/++	+	++		+/++/	+	++/++	++	++/++	++	++		168, 174, 181, 183,
					+++		+		+				189, 191, 201, 202
Etoposide	+++				+		++		++				169, 174, 198, 202
Teniposide	+++				+/++		++/++						80, 169, 174, 202
							+						
DNA cutting agent													174, 181, 185, 186
Bleomycin	–/+		+		+		++		+/+++		++		189, 197, 202
Mitotic spindle inhibitors													
Vinblastine					–				+				190, 203
Vincristine	–		+		–	–	+	+	–		++		180, 183, 185, 190, 204

Table 10.3 *Continued*

	SCE[a]				*Gene mutation*[b]				*Chromosomal aberrations*[b]				*Reference*
	Chinese hamster		*Human*		*Chinese hamster 6tg resistance*		*L5187Y TK +/–*		*Chinese hamster*		*Human*		
Exogenous metabolic activation:	–	+	–	+	–	+	–	+	–	+	–	+	
Antimetabolites													112, 180, 187, 189
Cytarabine	+		–/+		++	–	++		+++		+++		205, 206
Hydroxyurea			++				+						206, 207
Floxuridine					++				+++				187, 208
Fludarabine					++								209
5-Fluorouracil									+++				187, 210
6-Mercaptopurine	–/+				+	+			++/++		++		60, 112, 180, 185, 187
									+				
Methotrexate			–		+	+	+	+	++/++		+		112, 175, 180,
									+				183, 186, 210
6-Thioguanine	+								+++				185, 187

Notes:

[a] Results from sister chromatid exchange (SCE) assays are recorded in the tables as follows: –, maximum reversion frequency less than 1.5× that in the negative control; + maximum reversion frequency 1.5– <2× that in the negative control; ++, maximum reversion frequency 2– <10x that in the negative control.

[b] Results from mutagenicity and chromosomal assays are recorded in the tables as follows: –, maximum reversion frequency less than 2× that in the negative control: + maximum reversion frequency 2– <10× that in the negative control; ++, maximum reversion frequency 10– <100× that in the negative control: +++, maximum reversion frequency 100 or more times that in the negative control. Data have only been taken from studies using the standard methodology

Table 10.4 Mutagenic activity of anticancer drugs in *in-vivo* assays

	Chromosomal effects[a, b]			*Germ cell effects*[c]			
Drug	*SCE*	*MN*	*CA*	*DLA*	*CA in S*	*CA in O*	*References*
Alkylating agents							
Busulphan		+–++	+++	+	+	+	53, 173, 211–213
Carboplatin							
Carmustine	+++	++			+		214, 215
Chlorambucil					+		116, 214
Cisplatin	++		+		+		214, 216
Cyclophosphamide	+++	+++	+++	+	+	+	211, 212, 217–221
Dacarbazine							
Hexamethylmelamine							
Lomustine				+			53
Melphalan					+		118
Mitomycin C		+++	+++	+	+	+	53, 212, 214, 217, 218, 220, 221
Nitrogen mustard				–/+			212, 222
Procarbazine	++	+/++		–/+			212, 218, 219, 223
Streptozotocin	++			–			212, 224
Thiotepa		+++		+	+		210, 212, 214
Topo II poisons							
Amsacrine	++	++	++				225, 226
Dactinomycin				+			212
Daunorubicin				+			212
Doxorubicin		++/+++	+++	+	+		210, 227–229
Etoposide		++				+	82, 230, 231
Teniposide			+				231
DNA cutting agent							
Bleomycin		–			+		210, 232
Mitotic spindle inhibitors							
Vinblastine		++	++	–		+	212, 217, 218, 233
Vincristine	–	++	+			–	210, 231, 234, 235
Antimetabolites							
Cytarabine	++	+/++	++		+		88, 210, 236
Hydroxyurea				–			212
Floxuridine							
Fludarabine							
5-Fluorouracil		+/++	+++	–/+		–	210, 236–238
6-Mercaptopurine		+/++	++	–/+	+		212, 236, 239–241
Methotrexate		+/++	+++			+	210, 221, 236, 238, 242
6-Thioguanine							

[a] Results from SCE assays are recorded in the table as follows: –, maximum reversion frequency less than 1.5× that in the negative control; +, maximum reversion frequency 1.5– <2× that in the negative control; ++, maximum reversion frequency 2– <10× that in the negative control; +++, maximum reversion frequency 10 or more times that in the negative control.

[b] Results from MN and chromosomal assays are recorded in the table as follows: –, maximum reversion frequency less than 2× that in the negative control; +, maximum reversion frequency 2– <10× that in the negative control; ++, maximum reversion frequency 10– <100× that in the negative control; +++, maximum reversion frequency 100 or more times that in the negative control.

[c] Results from dominant lethal assays or estimates of chromosomal aberrations in various stages of spermatogenesis and oogenesis or in early embryos have been scored as positive if positive results were seen in any study. It should be noted that there are differences between susceptibility to chromosome damage between various stages of spermatogenesis and oogenesis.

Abbreviations used are: SCE: sister chromatid exchange; MN: micronuclei; CA: chromosomal aberrations; DLA: dominant lethal assay; CA in S: chromosomal aberrations in any stage of spermatogenesis; CA in O: chromosomal aberrations in any stage of oogenesis or in early embryos

nature of the mutagenic event. A mutagenic response in *Salmonella typhimurium* strains TA98 and/or TA1537 is usually considered to indicate that a chemical is a frameshift mutagen. More specifically, strain TA1537 detects frameshift mutations in a CCCC-rich region of the DNA, an event which has been considered largely characteristic of acridines[61] and other DNA intercalators[62,63]. Response in TA100 may indicate base-pair substitution mutagenesis[51]. Strain TA102 is generally thought to detect mutation through oxygen radicals[64].

Comparative data are given in Table 10.2 for anticancer drugs in their respective classes, when tested in strains TA1537, TA98, TA100 and TA102.

The alkylating agents

For the most part, the alkylating agents failed to provide evidence for frameshift mutagenesis in strains TA1537, TA1538 or TA98. The exceptions to this were busulphan, which caused frameshift mutations in TA1537, and *cis*-platin, which gave strongly positive results in TA98. More of the alkylators were weakly positive in TA100, suggesting that these had a modest ability to cause base-pair substitution mutations in bacteria. Streptozotocin gave strongly positive and busulphan moderately positive results in this strain. There were only sporadic data available for these chemicals in strain TA102, but those which were tested yielded positive results.

Among those drugs for which positive responses were reported, two (chlorambucil and cyclophosphamide) required exogenous metabolic activation. Although procarbazine appeared negative in these assays, this is because it is metabolized to a methylating agent by an unusual pathway, and that reaction does not occur using standard Ames test (or most other mutagenicity) protocols[65]. This problem has caused considerable confusion in interpreting much of the literature on procarbazine[57]. Both procarbazine and hexamethylmelamine could be demonstrated to be positive with appropriately modified protocols[10,66].

Topo II poisons

When bacterial mutagenicity tests were first applied in comparative studies of antitumour drugs such as topo II poisons, it was hoped that they could be used in order to identify non-mutagenic (and possibly non-carcinogenic) chemicals[67–69]. Unfortunately, however, while it proved relatively easy to develop drugs that were non-mutagenic in the Ames test, it seems increasingly likely that these Ames-negative drugs are still hazardous and that point mutations are a relatively minor contributor to the overall mutagenicity of topo II poisons.

As summarized in Table 10.2, topo II poisons give no consistent pattern in bacterial mutagenicity tests. Bacterial gyrases are relatively insensitive to inhibitors of mammalian topoisomerases, and therefore bacterial mutagenicity tests may be only poor indicators of mutagenicity through interactions with topo II. However, many of the clinical topo II poisons have other activities, including intercalation, production of active oxygen species and possibly DNA alkylation[25,70]. The latter authors suggested that bacterial assays on topo II poisons may indicate mutagenic activity mediated through these alternative mechanisms.

Dactinomycin appeared to be non-mutagenic, while amsacrine caused mutagenesis only in strain TA1537. Doxorubicin and daunorubicin caused weak and variable mutagenesis in strain TA1537 but showed up as much more effective frameshift mutagens in strain TA98. Several of the drugs evoked a weak mutagenic response in strain TA102, probably through oxygen radical-induced damage[64].

Bleomycin

This drug gave very strong effects in TA102, again consistent with mutagenesis through oxygen radical production[64].

Mitotic spindle inhibitors

There were no suggestions of positive results in any of the Ames test strains for these drugs.

Antimetabolites

With the exception of a positive response to 6-mercaptopurine in TA100, the antimetabolites generally give negative responses in *Salmonella*. However, it seems that many of the antimetabolites *can* cause point mutations[36,71]. It has been suggested[36] that this negative response in *Salmonella* may be caused, not by intrinsic lack of mutagenesis, but by secondary effects that interfere with the detection of induced mutations. For example, methotrexate has repeatedly given negative results in these assays (Table 10.2). The assays are generally performed using minimal media with specific supplements which may override the consequences of thymidylate stress[36]. When the test procedure was varied by modifying the nutrients in the media, methotrexate appeared mutagenic[72].

GENE AND CHROMOSOMAL MUTATIONS IN MAMMALIAN CELLS

There are several well-established mammalian mutagenesis assays which have been used in comparative studies on anticancer drugs. Those for which the most data are available are the mouse lymphoma L5178Y $TK^{+/-}$ assay[73] (which estimates resistance to trifluorothymidine through mutations at the thymidine kinase (TK) locus) and the HPRT system (which estimates resistance to the antimetabolite, 6-thioguanine, through mutations at the hypoxanthine-guanine phosphoribosyl transferase (HGPRT) locus) in either CHO or V79 Chinese hamster cells[40]. Although assays such as these are generally described as 'gene mutation' assays, this may not be strictly true. In some cases, they may be revealing chromosomal mutations or even recombinogenic events. For example, preferential formation of small colony mutants in the mouse lymphoma assays is thought to indicate chromosomal mutations[73].

Estimates of ability to cause events at the chromosomal level may often be made in parallel with mammalian mutagenesis assays. Although chromosomes may be studied directly, it may be more convenient to measure micronuclei (MN) as an index of clastogenesis. Micronuclei are commonly formed from acentric fragments induced by clastogens although they may also derive from entire lagging chromosomes induced by aneugens[74]. Sister chromatid exchange (SCE) is often used as a very sensitive indicator of effects on the chromosome, although SCE has no genotoxic consequences in its own right.

Data for anticancer drugs in these common mutagenesis assays, i.e. estimates of sister chromatid exchange and of clastogenic activity in selected mammalian cells, are summarized in Table 10.3. Some *in-vivo* data are shown in Table 10.4.

Alkylating agents

Alkylating agents have generally proved positive in mutagenicity assays but differ significantly in the magnitude of mutagenic response. For example, Sanderson and co-workers[75] compared the effects of eight alkylating agents in human lymphoblastoid cells. At equitoxic doses (killing 50% of the cells), the frequency of induction of 6-thioguanine-resistant mutants ranged from approximately 3×10^{-6} for BCNU to 2×10^{-5} for busulphan and *cis*-platin.

Where molecular analyses have been performed, these generally showed that the clinically used drugs cause mutations at the level of the chromosome rather than the gene[76]. For example, mitomycin C caused mostly small colony thymidine kinase-deficient mutants in L5178Y ($TK^{+/-}$) mouse lymphoma cells which resulted from large deletions[76]. This was in contrast to the monoalkylating agent ethyl methane sulphonate, tested in parallel, which caused mostly point mutations[76]. deBoer and Glickman[77] showed that *cis*-platin caused a range of transversions, transitions, frameshifts and short deletions and duplications of DNA in the *aprt* gene of CHO cells.

It has often been assumed that, whereas DNA monoadducts lead to mutations, DNA crosslinks lead to cytotoxicity through inhibition of DNA replication and gross chromosomal damage including unbalanced structural chromosomal aberrations[6–8]. Both bacterial and mammalian assays confirm that bis-alkylating anticancer drugs are less likely to cause point mutations than do related monoalkylating chemicals. However, despite cytotoxicity, there are a considerable number of cells with heavily damaged chromosomes that survive treatment by these crosslinking drugs. It may be spurious to conclude that they have lower mutagenic potential than the monoalkylators. Instead, they appear to cause a different spectrum of mutagenic events that may not have been as well recognized as point mutations in the past.

Topo II poisons

In Chinese hamster V79 cells, amsacrine and analogues showed weak but significant activity at the HGPRT locus. All drugs were potent clastogens as indicated by micronucleus assays. There was a highly significant relationship between mutation frequency (measured as resistance to 6-thioguanine) and either cytotoxicity or clastogenicity, suggesting that chromosomal events may be both killing and mutating the cells[78]. DeMarini and co-workers compared various topo II poisons in L5178Y/TK$^{+/-}$3.7.2C mouse lymphoma cells[79–81]. Each of the topo II inhibitors produced large numbers of small colony TK mutants but relatively few large colony mutants, again suggesting that chromosome mutations were a primary event. There was also a very large excess of chromosomal compared with gene mutation events for etoposide[82]. From these data, as well as results presented in Table 10.3 and 10.4, it would appear to be generally true that topo II poisons cause chromosomal aberrations in cultured cell lines and also *in vivo*, and that these are probably responsible for most of the mutations recovered in the common mammalian 'gene mutation' assays. All the clinical topo II poisons which have been tested also induced moderately high levels of sister chromatid exchanges (SCE) both *in vitro* and *in vivo*.

Two studies on the molecular nature of topo II poison-induced[83,84] gene alterations showed predominantly small deletion and insertion mutations, which were thought to result from recombinatorial events. These effects of topo II poisons are cell cycle specific. For example, Deaven and co-workers[85] suggested that amsacrine was particularly effective at times when chromatin was undergoing structural modifications (G1-S and S-G2 boundaries).

Bleomycin

This antibiotic is an effective clastogen and mammalian mutagen, almost certainly through the generation of oxygen radicals[86]. It is not effective in production of SCEs.

Mitotic spindle inhibitors

Although primarily aneugens, both vincristine and vinblastine caused a small amount of chromosome damage at high doses *in vitro*, but were not generally mutagenic in the commonly used test systems.

Antimetabolites

Interpretation of mutagenicity data pertaining to chemicals which interfere with metabolism is complicated by the fact that the intracellular activities of certain enzymes, and their contributions to particular pathways, vary greatly among different organisms and different cell types, or even within the same cell in different parts of the cell cycle[36].

Methotrexate, 5-FU, FUdR and hydroxyurea cause nucleotide pool imbalances which affect the fidelity of DNA replication and thereby induce point mutations[36]. In mammalian cells, however, it seems that this group of chemicals predominantly induces chromosomal mutations. For example, methotrexate induced high frequencies of large colony mutants at the thymidine kinase (TK) locus, although it was weakly or non-mutagenic at the hemizygous HGPRT locus in these same cells[87]. Similarly, cytosine arabinoside appeared to be predominantly a chromosomal mutagen, possibly through inhibiting DNA repair[88]. It appears that the nucleotide pool imbalances caused by these drugs can lead to a range of genetic effects, including mutation, recombination, chromosome rearrangement, breakage and loss. Gross forms of damage appear to be more common than point mutations[36].

RECOMBINATION AND GENE AMPLIFICATION

Interchromosomal recombination includes both reciprocal (crossing-over) and non-reciprocal (gene conversion) events occurring between two homologous regions of DNA located on homologous chromosomes. Intrachromosomal recombination can occur between repeated genes on the same chromosome or chromatid or between sister chromatids. Although these types of homologous recombination will not create new genetic material, they could lead to the expression of a recessive gene which was previously masked in a heterozygote. In relation to cancer, mitotic recombination has been particularly associated with activation of tumour suppressor genes, often associated with hereditary cancers.

Illegitimate recombination has been defined as a DNA rearrangement between non-homologous and non-specific sequences[89,90]. It is thought to lead to deletions, duplications, insertions, substitutions and inversions of DNA, as well as gene amplification. These types of events may have substantially more drastic long-term consequences than homologous recombination.

There have been few systematic studies of the relative abilities of anticancer drugs to promote recombination. The ideal system would involve mammalian cells, but such assays are still technically cumbersome, and there have only been sporadic studies of anticancer drugs in these. For example, a polymerase chain reaction-based method has been used for classifying mutations at the HLA-A locus in human T lymphocytes[91].

Alkylating agents

As many as 82% of the mutations induced by mitomycin C at the HLA-A locus in human T lymphocytes were found to be caused by mitotic recombination and a further 8% by deletions[92].

Much of the evidence for homologous recombination by alkylating agents has come from assays with the yeasts *Saccharomyces cerevisiae* or *Candida albicans*. We compared a range of anticancer drugs for their ability to cause mitotic recombination, using the *S. cerevisiae* strain D5[93]. The nitrosoureas, especially BCNU and nitrogen mustard, were particularly effective, as was *cis*-platin. *cis*-Platin also induced high levels of both reciprocal and non-reciprocal mitotic recombination in *C. albicans*[94] and in other strains of *S. cerevisiae*[95]. Chlorambucil, dacarbazine, mitomycin C and thiotepa caused substantial amounts of mitotic crossing over in our studies, while hexamethylmelamine was inactive[93].

Topo II poisons

Providing the yeast was growing during treatment, amsacrine, daunorubicin and doxorubicin, but not etoposide, caused moderate levels of homologous recombination in *S. cerevisiae* strain D5[93]. In addition to homologous recombination, there is now strong evidence that illegitimate recombination events are a common consequence of treatment of mammalian cells by topo II poisons[83,84].

Bleomycin

At the HLA-A locus, bleomycin induced a lower frequency of mutants compared with the alkylating agent mitomycin C[92]. However, mitotic recombination was again the major mechanism, accounting for 77% of all mutants recovered, while 14% were due to deletions[92]. In our yeast assays, bleomycin was one of the strongest recombinogens tested, showing comparable activity to the alkylating agents[93].

Mitotic spindle inhibitors

Neither vinblastine nor vincristine caused recombination in the yeast D5 assay[93].

Antimetabolites

Some of these are highly recombinogenic in either yeast or mammalian assays, often without point mutation activity[36]. Thymidylate stress leads to the formation of DNA strand breaks, which are themselves known to stimulate genetic exchange[36]. When thymidylate stress was induced in mammalian cells with floxuridine, this significantly enhanced homologous recombination activity[96]. Using *S. cerevisiae*, we found that 5-FU, methotrexate and hydroxyurea (but not 6-thioguanine) were effective recombinogens, providing the yeast was growing during treatment[93]. Similar results were obtained with hydroxyurea in the yeast, *C. albicans*[97].

Gene amplification

Gene amplification may arise through recombinatorial events. This has only rarely been studied as an endpoint in its own right except after treatment with mitomycin C[98], hydroxyurea[99] or some of the topo II poisons[100].

ANEUPLOIDY

The long-term consequences of aneuploidy which have been best recognized are infertility and birth defects. The mitotic spindle inhibitors, vincristine and vinblastine, have been unambiguously shown to cause aneuploidy[101] but the situation for other anticancer drugs is less clear. Several of the alkylators, including cyclophosphamide and mitomycin C, as well as the topo II poison amsacrine, can damage the synaptonemal complex[102]. For example, mitomycin C binds to heterochromatin and causes the trilamellar plates to become detached from the chromosome[103]. These chemicals may also be aneugens.

The most direct method of estimating aneuploidy simply involves looking at chromosomes. For example, vincristine causes changes in chromosome numbers in primary Chinese hamster embryonic cells[101]. Looking directly for changed numbers of chromosomes is relatively easy when dealing with an agent that specifically affects the mitotic spindle. However, this approach is almost impossible for cells treated with chemicals that cause massive amounts of chromosomal fragmentation, in addition to being potential aneugens. More modern assays involve the use of antibodies to detect whether micronuclei contain centromeres, or the use of fluorescent *in-situ* hybridization. Such approaches have confirmed that busulphan[104], mitomycin C[105] and also the topo II poisons, etoposide and amsacrine[106], can induce aneuploidy as well as chromosomal aberrations.

Other authors have avoided these technical problems by using fungal systems to investigate the induction of aneuploidy by various anticancer drugs. Cyclophosphamide failed to induce mitotic or meiotic chromosome gain in the diploid *S. cerevisiae* strain BR1669[107]. Similarly, mitomycin C caused no chromosome loss in the yeast strain D61.M[108]. However, hydroxyurea induced aneuploidy in yeast[109], as did bleomycin in *Aspergillus*[110].

REPRODUCTION AND BIRTH DEFECTS

Anticancer drugs have been commonly used to treat patients of reproductive age. Since these chemicals are most active against rapidly dividing cells, male germ cells might be considered a particularly vulnerable target. A large number of reports has appeared in the literature claiming adverse effects of various chemotherapeutic agents and regimens on human reproduction[111,112]. Unfortunately, however, most of these are case reports or studies on small numbers of patients, where the data fail to reach statistical significance. It becomes important to rely on animal germ-cell assays in order to predict these effects.

A combination of genetic, cytogenetic and molecular analyses have shown the nature of events in the most commonly used animal assays[113,114]. The dominant lethal assay primarily detects chromosomal mutations or aneuploidy[115], while the mouse translocation assay more specifically detects reciprocal chromosome exchanges that are transmitted to the F1 generation[54]. The morphological specific locus test detects mutations due to damage as small as a few base changes (e.g. A-T transversion or deletion of a few bases) or as large as multigenic deletions and rearrangements[116].

Alkylating agents

Those alkylating anticancer drugs which have been adequately tested (according to the criteria of Green *et al.*[53]) have all shown some germ-cell effects including dominant lethal mutations. The data suggest a significant role for crosslinks, not only in cytotoxicity but also in the formation of hereditary genetic damage[117]. Russell and co-workers found chlorambucil and melphalan to be two of the most highly mutagenic chemicals known for male mouse germ cells, and significantly more effective than radiation[116]. They were also the only two chemicals they found for which specific-locus mutation induction in the mouse reaches a maximum in early spermatids[118]. Chlorambucil exerted strong effects on postmeiotic germ cells and early spermatids, and mutant cells showed predominantly chromosomal rearrangements (deletions and translocations)[116]. Melphalan induced high frequencies of specific-locus mutations in postspermatogonial germ cells of the mouse, and was also mutagenic in spermatogonial stem cells. At least 12 of 15 melphalan-induced mutations recovered from postspermatogonial stages (but only 1 of 7 mutations recovered from stem-cell or differentiating spermatogonia) gave evidence of being deletions or other rearrangements[113].

Mitomycin C induced heritable mutations and translocations in male germ cells, and high numbers of abnormal spermatogonia in male mice[119,120]. In the germ cells of *Drosophila*, all 37 mutations induced by hexamethyl melamine were either intra- or inter-locus deletions, with no point mutations yet identified[117].

Topo II poisons

These have highly significant effects on human reproduction[70] but there have been no comprehensive comparative studies on topo II poisons in germ cells using animal models. All three topo II poisons tested showed dominant lethal effects in rodents. Etoposide inhibited premitotic DNA synthesis at specific stages during rat spermatogenesis, but premeiotic DNA synthesis was less effectively inhibited[121]. Etoposide induced micronuclei in meiotic cells in an *in-vitro* system and predicted similar effects on male germ cells[122]. Teniposide had a range of effects on nuclear events during oocyte maturation, fertilization, and early embryonic development of fertilized *Spisula solidissima* oocytes[123].

In view of the absolute requirement for cell division to show topo II inhibitor effects, it is surprising that dominant lethal effects of doxorubicin were seen when the female was the exposed partner but not the male[124].

Bleomycin

This agent also caused female-specific dominant lethal effects in mice[125].

Mitotic spindle inhibitors

These also affect germ cells, although vinblastine gave negative results in a dominant lethal assay. It has been suggested that vincristine affects the fertilization capability of all germ-cell stages in male mice[126]. Hyperploidy was demonstrated in germ cells of male Chinese hamsters treated with vincristine[127]. In the germ cells of female mice, vinblastine induced a significant increase in the frequency of ovulated MI oocytes and of hyperploid MII oocytes compared with controls[128].

Antimetabolites

Clinically, these drugs are known to have effects on human fertility and reproductive outcome[36,112]. Where they have been tested in animal models, they also have a range of effects on germ cells[112].

CANCER

Alkylating agents

Chemicals which can crosslink DNA are among the most potent carcinogens in rodents[129] and humans[130,131]. There is a problem in scrutinizing patient data to identify anticancer drugs as human carcinogens because most of these chemicals are used as part of combination chemotherapy. Nevertheless, of 24 substances or groups of substances that are known to be human carcinogens, 6 are alkylating antitumour drugs (busulphan, chlorambucil, methylCCNU, cyclophosphamide, melphalan and nitrogen mustard)[132]. There are a further 156 substances or groups of substances which the Department of Health and Human Sciences[132] considers may reasonably be expected to be human carcinogens, of which a further 8 are antitumour drugs. These include the alkylating agents, BCNU, CCNU, *cis*-platin, dacarbazine, procarbazine, streptozotocin and thiotepa. Compared with other types of alkylating agents which form monoadducts, bis-alkylators have a relatively high 'carcinogenic potency', as indicated by a low threshold dose in rodents[133]. Acute myeloid leukaemia (AML) occurs commonly following therapy by alkylating agents, after a lag period of 4–5 years. These leukaemias are often associated with chromosomal deletions, especially in chromosomes 5 and 7[134,135].

Topo II poisons

These have been only rarely studied in animal systems, and the only one listed in the 'could reasonably be expected to be a carcinogen' class is doxorubicin[132]. However, there is increasing evidence from second malignancies in survivors of initial chemotherapy that a range of topo II poisons do themselves induce cancer[136–139]. The epipodophyllotoxins, etoposide and teniposide, appear to induce secondary AML, with a shorter (2–3 years) latency of onset than alkylator-induced leukaemia, and with a number of different characteristics[134,135,138,139]. The cells also have a characteristic morphology and balanced chromosomal translocations involving bands 11q23 or 21q22[137,139–141]. Secondary AML following treatment with intercalating agents, such as doxorubicin, often appears to involve the same chromosomal translocations that are involved in *de-novo* AML (t(9;11), t(8;21), t(15;17))[139]. The topoisomerase inhibitors, doxorubicin, mitoxantrone and (less commonly) etoposide, also induce secondary acute promyelocytic leukaemia (APL) with an abnormality at the t(15;17) chromosomal location[142].

Bleomycin

Bleomycin caused a variety of tumours in rats, and also enhanced the formation of tumours by some alkylating agents, although it is not considered as a proven human carcinogen[132,143,144].

Mitotic spindle inhibitors

At least in the traditionally-used animal systems, vincristine and vinblastine are not themselves carcinogenic[145]. However, it seems that they may either reduce or enhance the effects of other chemicals, depending partly upon the timing of administration[146]. Vincristine caused morphological transformation in Syrian hamster embryo cells, despite failing to cause unscheduled DNA synthesis or gene mutations at two loci[147].

Antimetabolites

Methotrexate tested alone showed no oncogenic potential in Sprague–Dawley rats[148]. However, the clinical use of methotrexate has been linked with the subsequent development of lymphomas, leukaemias and carcinomas[112,149]. In animal systems, some of the antimetabolites have been shown to enhance the carcinogenicity of alkylating chemicals such as procarbazine[150]. Again, these effects may depend upon the relative timing of exposure to the two chemicals. For example, Iverson found that hydroxyurea enhanced alkylator-induced skin carcinogenesis when given shortly before the carcinogen, but not after[151].

CONCLUSIONS

Much of the previous research on mutagenicity and carcinogenicity has centred around monoalkylating chemicals which are not often used as anticancer drugs. This review has covered the most widely-used anticancer drugs with a range of different modes of action. Not only do these compounds affect a wide spectrum of tumours, but they also induce a whole spectrum of mutagenic events. Between them, they are capable of causing all the various types of mutational and recombinational events that have been implicated in human disease. Their mutagenic potential may have been underestimated because they have been primarily tested in assays that were developed and optimized using monoalkylating chemicals. With the exception of the alkylating agents, none of these chemicals would trigger the structural alerts to carcinogenicity and other hazards associated with electrophilic species[152]. Different testing strategies may well be needed if we are to understand the long-term implications of prolonged use of these other classes of mutagenic chemicals.

Acknowledgements

I wish to thank Professor W.A. Denny for helpful discussions and Amira Pearson for helping to produce the Tables. I also thank the Auckland Division, Cancer Society of New Zealand for their financial support.

References

1. Adair FE, Bogg HJ. Experimental and clinical studies on the treatment of cancer by dichloroethylsulphide (mustard gas). Ann Surg. 1931;93:190–9.
2. Auerbach C, Robson JM. Chemical production of mutations. Nature. 1946;157:302.
3. Gilman A, Phillips FS. The biological actions and therapeutic applications of b-chloroethylamines and sulphides. Science. 1946;103:409–13.
4. Goldin A, Wood HBJ. Preclinical investigation of alkylating agents in cancer chemotherapy. Ann NY Acad Sci. 1969;163:954–95.
5. Sharma M, He QY, Tomasz M. Effects of glutathione on alkylation and cross-linking of DNA by mitomycin C. Isolation of a ternary glutathione–mitomycin–DNA adduct. Chem Res Toxicol. 1994;7:401–7.
6. Brookes P, Lawley PD. The reaction of mono- and di-functional alkylating agents with nucleic acids. Biochem J. 1961;80:496–503.
7. Hemminki K, Kallama S. Reactions of nitrogen mustards with DNA. In: Schmahl D, Kaldor JM, eds. Carcinogenicity of alkylating cytostatic drugs. Lyon: International Agency for Research on Cancer; 1986:55–70. (IARC Scientific Publications; No 78).
8. Singer B, Grunberger D. Molecular biology of mutagens and carcinogens. 1st edn. New York: Plenum Press; 1983.
9. Millard JT, Raucher S, Hopkins PB. Mechlorethamine crosslinks deoxyguanosine residues at 5′-GNC sequences in duplex DNA fragments. J Am Chem Soc. 1990;112:2459–60.
10. Ashby J, Callander RD, Rose FL. Weak mutagenicity to Salmonella of the formaldehyde-releasing anti-tumour agent hexamethylmelamine. Mutat Res. 1985;142:121–5.
11. Bruhn SL, Pil PM, Essigmann JM, Housman DE, Lippard SJ. Isolation and characterization of human cDNA clones encoding a high mobility group box protein that recognizes structural distortions to DNA caused by binding of the anticancer agent cisplatin. Proc Natl Acad Sci USA. 1992;89:2307–11.
12. Lawley PD, Brookes P. Molecular mechanism of the cytotoxic action of difunctional alkylating agents and of resistance to this action. Nature. 1965;192:480–3.
13. Crathorne AR, Roberts JJ. Mechanism of the cytotoxic action of alkylating agents in mammalian cells and evidence for the removal of alkylated groups from DNA. Nature. 1966;211:151–3.

14. Loveless A, Cook J, Wheatley P. Recovery from the 'lethal' effects of cross-linking alkylation. Nature. 1965;205:980–3.
15. Brendel M, Ruhland A. Relationships between functionality and genetic toxicology of selected DNA-damaging agents. Mutat Res. 1984;133:51–85.
16. Brookes P. The early history of the biological alkylating agents, 1918–1968. Mutat Res. 1990;233:3–14.
17. Loveless A. Possible relevance of O6-alkylation of deoxyguanosine to mutagenicity and carcinogenicity of nitrosamines and nitrosamides. Nature. 1969;223:206–7.
18. Boritzki TJ, Palmer BD, Coddington JM, Denny WA. Identification of the major lesion from the reaction of an acridine-targeted aniline mustard with DNA as an adenine N1 adduct. Chem Res Toxicol. 1994;7:41–6.
19. Ferguson LR, Denny WA, Boritzki TJ. DNA-directed aniline mustards with high selectivity for adenine or guanine bases: mutagenesis in a variety of *Salmonella typhimurium* strains differing in repair-capability. Mutat Res. 1994;321:27–34.
20. Roberge M, Th'ng J, Hamaguchi J, Bradbury EM. The topoisomerase II inhibitor VM-26 induces marked changes in histone H1 kinase activity, histones H1 and H3 phosphorylation, and chromosome condensation in G2 phase and mitotic BHK cells. J Cell Biol. 1990;111 (Pt 1):1753–62.
21. Adachi Y, Luke M, Laemmli UK. Chromosome assembly in vitro: topoisomerase II is required for condensation. Cell. 1991;64:137–48.
22. Hirano T, Mitchison TJ. Topoisomerase-II does not play a scaffolding role in the organization of mitotic chromosomes assembled in xenopus egg extracts. J Cell Biol. 1993;120:601–12.
23. Liu LF. DNA topoisomerase poisons as antitumor drugs. Annu Rev Biochem. 1989;58:351–75.
24. Wang JC, Caron PR, Kim RA. The role of DNA topoisomerases in recombination and genome stability – a double-edged sword. Cell. 1990;62:403–6.
25. Ferguson LR, Baguley BC. Topoisomerase II enzymes and mutagenicity. Environ Mol Mutagen. 1994;24:245–61.
26. Ralph RK, Judd W, Pommier Y, Kohn KW. DNA topoisomerases. In: Neidle S, Waring M, eds. Molecular aspects of anticancer drug–DNA interactions, vol. 2. London: Macmillan; 1994:1–95.
27. Heck MM, Hittelman WN, Earnshaw WC. Differential expression of DNA topoisomerases I and II during the eukaryotic cell cycle. Proc Natl Acad Sci USA. 1988;85:1086–90.
28. Charron M, Hancock R. DNA topoisomerase-II is required for formation of mitotic chromosomes in Chinese hamster ovary cells – studies using the inhibitor 4′-demethylepipodophyllotoxin 9-(4,6-O-thenylidene-beta-D-glucopyranoside). Biochemistry. 1990;29:9531–7.
29. Lock RB, Ross WE. Inhibition of p34cdc2 kinase activity by etoposide or irradiation as a mechanism of G2 arrest in Chinese hamster ovary cells. Cancer Res. 1990;50:3761–6.
30. Natrajan A, Hecht S. Bleomycins: mechanism of polynucleotide recognition and oxidative degredation. In: Neidle S, Waring M, eds. Molecular aspects of anticancer drug–DNA interactions, vol. 2. London: MacMillan; 1994:197–242.
31. D'Andrea AD, Haseltine WA. Sequence specific cleavage of DNA by the antitumor antibiotics neocarzinostatin and bleomycin. Proc Natl Acad Sci USA. 1978;75:3608–12.
32. Jurlina JL, Lindsay A, Baguley BC, Denny WA. Redox chemistry of the 9-anilinoacridine class of antitumor agent. J Med Chem. 1987;30:473–80.
33. Wendell KL, Wilson L, Jordan MA. Mitotic block in HeLa cells by vinblastine: ultrastructural changes in kinetochore-microtubule attachment and in centrosomes. J Cell Sci. 1993;104(Pt 2):261–74.
34. Jordan MA, Thrower D, Wilson L. Effects of vinblastine, podophyllotoxin and nocodazole on mitotic spindles. Implications for the role of microtubule dynamics in mitosis. J Cell Sci. 1992;102(Pt 3):401–16.
35. Morris SM. The genetic toxicology of 5-fluoropyrimidines and 5-chlorouracil. Mutat Res. 1993;297:39–51.
36. Kunz BA, Kohalmi SE, Kunkel TA, Mathews CK, McIntosh EM, Reidy JA. Deoxyribonucleoside triphosphate levels: A critical factor in the maintenance of genetic stability. Mutat Res. 1994;318:1–64.
37. Fernandes DJ, Catapano CV. Nuclear matrix targets for anticancer agents. Cancer Cells. 1991;3:134–40.
38. Biedler JL, Riehm H. Cellular resistance to actinomycin D in Chinese hamster cells in vitro: cross-resistance, radioautographic and cytogenetic studies. Cancer Res. 1970;30:1174–84.

39. Riordan J, Deuchars K, Kartner N, Alon N, Trent J, Ling V. Amplification of P-glycoprotein genes in multidrug-resistant mammalian cell lines. Nature. 1985;316:817–9.
40. Wilson WR, Harris NM, Ferguson LR. Comparison of the mutagenic and clastogenic activity of amsacrine and other DNA-intercalating drugs in cultured V79 Chinese hamster cells. Cancer Res. 1984;44:4420–31.
41. Alt FW, Kellems RE, Bertino JR, Schimke RT. Selective multiplication of dihydrofolate reductase genes in methotrexate-resistant variants of cultured murine cells. J Biol Chem. 1978;253:1357–70.
42. Yu M, Melera PW. Allelic variation in the dihydrofolate reductase gene at amino acid position 95 contributes to antifolate resistance in chinese hamster cells. Cancer Res. 1993;53:6031–5.
43. Hook EB. Perspectives in mutation epidemiology. 3. Contribution of chromosome abnormalities to human mobidity and mortality and some comments upon surveillance of chromosomal mutation rates. Mutat Res. 1983;114:389–423.
44. Wilcox AJ, Weinberg CR, O'Connor JF, *et al.* Incidence of early loss of pregnancy. N Engl J Med. 1989;319:189–94.
45. National Research Council, ed. Identifying and estimating the genetic impact of chemical mutagens. Washington, D.C.: National Academy Press; 1982.
46. Schwab M, Amler LC. Amplification of cellular oncogenes: a predictor of clinical outcome in human cancer. Genes Chromosomes Cancer. 1990;1:181–93.
47. Hollstein M, Sidransky D, Vogelstein B, Harris CC. p53 mutations in human cancers. Science. 1991;253:49–53.
48. Au WW. Abnormal chromosome repair and risk of developing cancer. Environ Health Perspect. 1993;101 Suppl 3:303–8.
49. Finlay GJ. Genetics, molecular biology and colorectal cancer. Mutat Res. 1993;290:3–12.
50. Dept. of Health, ed. Report on health and social subjects. 35. Guidelines for the testing of chemicals for mutagenicity. London: Her Majesty's Stationary Office; 1989.
51. Maron DM, Ames BN. Revised methods for the *Salmonella* mutagenicity test. Mutat Res. 1983;113:173–215.
52. Russell WL. Reminiscences of a mouse specific-locus test addict. Environ Mol Mutagen. 1989;14 (suppl. 16):16–22.
53. Green S, Auletta A, Fabricant J, *et al.* Current status of bioassays in genetic toxicology – the dominant lethal assay: a report of the USEPA Gene-Tox program. Mutat Res. 1985;154:49–67.
54. Generoso WM, Bishop JB, Gosslee DG, Newell GW, Sheu CJ, von Halle E. Heritable translocation test in mice: a report of the 'GENE-TOX' program. Mutat Res. 1980;76:191–215.
55. Russell LB. The mouse spot test as a predictor of heritable genetic damage and other endpoints. In: de Serres FJ, ed. Chemical mutagens. 1st edn Vol 8. New York: Plenum Press; 1983:95–110.
56. Ward WHJ, Cook PN, Slater AM, Davies DH, Holdgate GA, Green LR. Epidermal growth factor receptor tyrosine kinase – investigation of catalytic mechanism, structure-based searching and discovery of a potent inhibitor. Biochem Pharmacol. 1994;48:659–66.
57. Waters MD, Stack HF. The short-term test activity profile for procarbazine hydrochloride. Mutagenesis. 1988;3:89–94.
58. Anderson D, Bishop JB, Garner RC, Ostrosky-Wegman, Selby PB. Cyclophosphamide: review of its mutagenicity for an assessment of potential germ cell effects. Mutat Res. 1994;[In press].
59. Povirk LF, Austin MJF. Genotoxicity of bleomycin. Mutat Res. 1991;257:127–43.
60. Mosesso P, Palitti F. The genetic toxicology of 6-mercaptopurine. Mutat Res. 1993;296:279–94.
61. McCoy EC, Rosenkranz EJ, Petrullo LA, Rosenkranz HS. Frameshift mutations: relative roles of simple intercalation and of adduct formation. Mutat Res. 1981;90:21–30.
62. Ferguson LR, Denny WA. Frameshift mutagenesis by acridines and other reversibly-binding DNA ligands. Mutagenesis. 1990;5:529–40.
63. Hoshino K, Sato K, Akahane K, *et al.* Significance of the methyl group on the oxazine ring of ofloxacin derivatives in the inhibition of bacterial and mammalian type-II topoisomerases. Antimicrob Agents Chemother. 1991;35:309–12.
64. Levin DE, Hollstein M, Christman MF, Schwiers EA, Ames BN. A new *Salmonella* tester strain (TA102) with A-T base pairs at the site of mutation detects oxidative mutagens. Proc Natl Acad Sci USA. 1982;79:7445–9.

65. Moloney SJ, Wiebkin P, Cummings SW, Prough RA. Metabolic activation of the terminal *N*-methyl group of *N*-isopropyl-alpha-(2-methylhydrazino)-p-toluamide hydrochloride (procarbazine). Carcinogenesis. 1985;6:397–401.
66. Malaveille C, Brun G, Bartsch H. Studies on the efficiency of the Salmonella/rat hepatocyte assay for the detection of carcinogens as mutagens: activation of 1,2-dimethyl-hydrazine and procarbazine into bacterial mutagens. Carcinogenesis. 1983;4:449–55.
67. Ferguson LR, Denny WA. Potential antitumor agents. 30. Mutagenic activity of some 9-anilinoacridines. Relationship between structure, mutagenic potential and antitumour activity. J Med Chem. 1979;22:251–5.
68. Ferguson LR, Denny WA. Potential antitumor agents. 33. Quantitative structure activity relationships of mutagenic activity and antitumour activity of substituted 4′-(9-acridinylamino) methanesulfonanilide derivatives. J Med Chem. 1980;23:269–74.
69. Baguley BC, Ferguson LR. Inverse correlation between bacterial frameshift mutagenicity and yeast mitochondrial effects of antitumour anilinoacridines. Chem Biol Interact. 1985;56:145–55.
70. Anderson RD, Berger NA. Mutagenicity and carcinogenicity of topoisomerase-interactive agents. Mutat Res. 1994;309:109–42.
71. Wurgler FE, Graf U, Frei H, Juon H. Genotoxic activity of the anti-cancer drug methotrexate in somatic cells of Drosophila melanogaster. Mutat Res. 1983;122:321–8.
72. Genther CS, Schoeny RS, Loper JC, Smith CC. Mutagenic studies of folic acid antagonists. Antimicrob Agents Chemother. 1977;12:84–92.
73. DeMarini DM, Doerr CL, Meyer MK, Brock KH, Hozier J, Moore MM. Mutagenicity of m-AMSA and o-AMSA in mammalian cells due to clastogenic mechanism: possible role of topoisomerase. Mutagenesis. 1987;2:349–55.
74. Ferguson LR, Morcombe P, Triggs CM. The size of cytokinesis-blocked micronuclei in human peripheral blood lymphocytes as a measure of aneuploidy induction by Set A compounds in the EEC trial. Mutat Res. 1993;287:101–12.
75. Sanderson BJ, Johnson KJ, Henner WD. Dose-dependent cytotoxic and mutagenic effects of antineoplastic alkylating agents on human lymphoblastoid cells. Environ Mol Mutagen. 1991;17:238–43.
76. Davies MJ, Phillips BJ, Rumsby PC. Molecular analysis of mutations at the tk locus of L5178Y mouse-lymphoma cells induced by ethyl methanesulphonate and mitomycin C. Mutat Res. 1993;290:145–53.
77. de-Boer JG, Glickman BW. Sequence specificity of mutation induced by the anti-tumor drug cisplatin in the CHO aprt gene. Carcinogenesis. 1989;10:1363–7.
78. Ferguson LR, van Zijl P, Baguley BC. Mutagenicity profiles of newer amsacrine analogues with activity against solid tumours; comparison of microbial and mammalian systems. Eur J Cancer Clin Oncol. 1989;25:255–61.
79. DeMarini DM, Doerr CL, Meyer MK, Brock KH, Hozier J, Moore MM. Mutagenicity of m-AMSA and o-AMSA in mammalian cells due to clastogenic mechanism: possible role of topoisomerase. Mutagenesis. 1987;2:349–56.
80. DeMarini DM, Brock KH, Doerr CL, Moore MM. Mutagenicity and clastogenicity of teniposide (VM-26) in L5178Y/TK +/– –3.7.2C mouse lymphoma cells. Mutat Res. 1987;187:141–9.
81. Moore MM, Brock KH, Doerr CL, DeMarini DM. Mutagenicity and clastogenicity of adriamycin in L5178Y/TK+/–.3.7.2C mouse lymphoma cells. Mutat Res. 1987;191:183–8.
82. Ashby J, Tinwell H, Poorman-Allen P, Krehl R, Callander RD, Clive D. Potent clastogenicity of the human carcinogen etoposide to the mouse bone marrow and mouse lymphoma L5178Y cells: comparison to Salmonella responses. Environ Mol Mutagen. 1994;24:51–60.
83. Berger NA, Chatterjee S, Schmotzer JA, Helms SR. Etoposide (VP-16-213)-induced gene alterations – potential contribution to cell death. Proc Natl Acad Sci USA. 1991;88:8740–3.
84. Han YH, Austin MJF, Pommier Y, Povirk LF. Small deletion and insertion mutations induced by the topoisomerase-II inihibitor teniposide in CHO cells and comparison with sites of drug-stimulated DNA cleavage in vitro. J Mol Biol. 1993;229:52–66.
85. Deaven LL, Oka MS, Tobey RA. Cell-cycle-specific chromosome damage following treatment of cultured CHO cells with 4′-[(9-acridinyl)-amino] methanesulphon-m-anisidide-DCl (m-AMSA chloride). J Natl Cancer Inst. 1978;60:1155–9.
86. An J, Hsie AW. Effects of an inhibitor and a mimic of superoxide dismutase on bleomycin mutagenesis in Chinese hamster ovary cells. Mutat Res. 1992;270:167–75.

87. Clive D, Glover P, Applegate M, Hozier J. Molecular aspects of chemical mutagenesis in L5178Y/tk +/– mouse lymphoma cells. Mutagenesis. 1990;5:191–7.
88. Beaula-Helen KD, Subramanyam S. Genotoxic evaluation of Ara-C by multiple parameters. Mutat Res. 1991;263: 185–96.
89. Campbell A. The episomes. Adv Genet. 1962;11:101–46.
90. Campbell A. Genetic structure. In: Hershey AD, ed. The bacteriophage lambda. New York: Cold Spring Harbor;1971:13–44.
91. Dempsey JL, Odagiri Y, Morley AA. In vivo mutations at the H-2 locus in mouse lymphocytes. Mutat Res. 1993;285:45–51.
92. Zotti R, Holt D, Dreimanis M, Morley AA. Mutagenic effects of mitomycin, bleomycin and X-irradiation at the HLA-A locus. In: Fenech M, ed. Natural and man-made toxins in the diet. Adelaide: Australia New Zealand Environmental Mutagen Society; 1994:24.
93. Ferguson LR, Turner PM. Mitotic crossing-over by anticancer drugs in *Saccharomyces cerevisiae*. Mutat Res. 1988;204:239–49.
94. Sarachek A, Henderson L, Wilkens WE. Evaluation of the genotoxic spectrum of cisplatin for Candida albicans. Microbios. 1992;72:183–201.
95. Hannan MA, Nasim A. Mechanisms of cisplatin (cis-diaminodichloroplatinum 11)-induced cytotoxicity and genotoxicity in yeast. Mutat Res. 1984;127:23–30.
96. Mishina Y, Ayusawa D, Seno T, Koyama H. Thymidylate stress induces homologous recombination activity in mammalian cells. Mutat Res. 1991;246:215–20.
97. Sarachek A, Henderson LA, Eddy KB. Genetic destabilization of Candida albicans by hydroxyurea. Microbios. 1991;65:39–61.
98. Rossman TG, Wolosin D. Differential susceptibility to carcinogen-induced amplification of SV40 and dhfr sequences in SV40-transformed human keratinocytes. Mol Carcinog. 1992;6:203–13.
99. Hill AB, Schimke RT. Increased gene amplification in L5178Y mouse lymphoma cells with hydroxyurea-induced chromosomal aberrations. Cancer Res. 1985;45:5050–7.
100. Ferguson LR, Morecombe P. Unpublished data, (this) Laboratory.
101. Natarajan AT, Duivenvoorden WC, Meijers M, Zwanenburg TS. Induction of mitotic aneuploidy using Chinese hamster primary embryonic cells. Test results of 10 chemicals. Mutat Res. 1993;287:47–56.
102. Allen JW, Poorman PA, Backer LC, Gibson JB, Westbrook-Collins B, Moses MJ. Synaptonemal complex damage as a measure of genotoxicity at meiosis. Cell Biol Toxicol. 1988;4:487–94.
103. Brinkley BR, Tousson A, Valdivia MM. The kinetochore of mammalian chromosomes: structure and function in normal mitosis and aneuploidy. Basic Life Sci. 1985;36:243–67.
104. Barbata G, Giglio MC, Granata G, Anzalone A, Carbone P. Clastogenic and aneuploidizing effects of antiblastic busulphan revealed by kinetochore immunofluorescence in CHO cells. Mutat Res. 1991;263:237–42.
105. Rudd NL, Williams SE, Evans M, Hennig UG, Hoar DI. Kinetochore analysis of micronuclei allows insights into the actions of colcemid and mitomycin C. Mutat Res. 1991;261:57–68.
106. Slavotinek A, Perry PE, Sumner AT. Micronuclei in neonatal lymphocytes treated with the topoisomerase-II inhibitors amsacrine and etoposide. Mutat Res. 1993;319:215–22.
107. Whittaker SG, Moser SF, Maloney DH, Piegorsch WW, Resnick MA, Fogel S. The detection of mitotic and meiotic chromosome gain in the yeast Saccharomyces cerevisiae: effects of methyl benzimidazol-2-yl carbamate, methyl methanesulfonate, ethyl methanesulfonate, dimethyl sulfoxide, propionitrile and cyclophosphamide monohydrate. Mutat Res. 1990;242:231–58.
108. Albertini S, Friederich U, Wurgler FE. Reversible inhibition of mammalian tubulin assembly in vitro and effects in Saccharomyces cerevisiae D61.M by mitomycin C. Mutagenesis. 1989;4:39–44.
109. Mayer VW, Goin CJ, Zimmermann FK. Aneuploidy and other genetic effects induced by hydroxyurea in Saccharomyces cerevisiae. Mutat Res. 1986;160:19–26.
110. Kafer E. Botran and bleomycin induce crossing-over, and bleomycin also increases aneuploidy in diploid strains of Aspergillus. Mutat Res. 1990;241:49–66.
111. Sorsa M, Hemminki K, Vainio H. Occupational exposure to anticancer drug – potential and real hazards. Mutat Res. 1985;154:135–49.
112. Sieber SM, Adamson RH. Toxicity of antineoplastic agents in man: Chromosomal aberrations, antifertility effects and carcinogenic potential. Adv Cancer Res. 1975;22:57–155.

113. Russell LB, Hunsicker PR, Cacheiro NL, Rinchik EM. Genetic, cytogenetic, and molecular analyses of mutations induced by melphalan demonstrate high frequencies of heritable deletions and other rearrangements from exposure of postspermatogonial stages of the mouse. Proc Natl Acad Sci USA. 1992;89:6182–6.
114. Rinchik EM, Bangham JW, Hunsicker PR, *et al.* Genetic and molecular analysis of chlorambucil-induced germ-line mutations in the mouse. Proc Natl Acad Sci USA. 1990;87:1416–20.
115. Shelby MD, Bishop JB, Mason JM, Tindall KR. Fertility, reproduction and genetic disease: studies on the reproductive effects of environmental agents on mammalian germ cells. Environ Health Perspect. 1993;100:283–91.
116. Rinchik EM, Flaherty L, Russell LB. High-frequency induction of chromosomal rearrangements in mouse germ cells by the chemotherapeutic agent chlorambucil. Bioessays. 1993;15:831–6.
117. Vogel EW, Zijlstra JA, Nivard MJM. Genetic method for pre-classification of genotoxins into monofunctional or cross-linking agents. Environ Mol Mutagen. 1993;21:319–31.
118. Russell LB, Hunsicker PR, Shelby MD. Melphalan, a second chemical for which specific-locus mutation induction in the mouse is maximum in early spermatids. Mutat Res. 1992;282:151–8.
119. Bentley KS, Working PK. Activity of germ-cell mutagens and nonmutagens in the rat spermatocyte UDS assay. Mutat Res. 1988;203:135–42.
120. Dobrzynska MM, Gajewski AK. Mouse dominant lethal and sperm abnormality studies with combined exposure to X-rays and mitomycin C. Mutat Res. 1994;306:203–9.
121. Hakovirta H, Parvinen M, Lahdetie J. Effects of etoposide on stage-specific DNA synthesis during rat spermatogenesis. Mutat Res. 1993;301:189–93.
122. Sjoblom T, Parvinen M, Lahdetie J. Germ-cell mutagenicity of etoposide – induction of meiotic micronuclei in cultured rat seminiferous tubules. Mutat Res. 1994;323:41–5.
123. Wright SJ, Schatten G. Teniposide, a topoisomerase II inhibitor, prevents chromosome condensation and separation but not decondensation in fertilized surf clam (*Spisula solidissima*) oocytes. Dev Biol. 1990;142:224–32.
124. Generoso WM, Cain WT, Hughes LA, Foxworth LB. A restudy of the efficacy of adriamycin in inducing dominant lethals in mouse spermatogonia stem cells. Mutat Res. 1989;226:61–4.
125. Sudman PD, Rutledge JC, Bishop JB, Generoso WM. Bleomycin: female-specific dominant lethal effects in mice. Mutat Res. 1992;296:143–56.
126. Ehling UH, Kratochvilova J, Lehmacher W, Neuhauser-Klaus A. Mutagenicity testing of vincristine sulfate in germ cells of male mice. Mutat Res. 1988;209:107–13.
127. Sheu CW, Lee JK, Arras CA, Jones RL, Lavappa KS. Detection of vincristine-induced hyperploidy in meiotic II metaphases of male Chinese hamsters. Mutat Res. 1992;280:181–6.
128. Mailhes JB, Aardema MJ, Marchetti F. Investigation of aneuploidy induction in mouse oocytes following exposure to vinblastine-sulfate, pyrimethamine, diethylstilbestrol diphosphate, or chloral hydrate. Environ Mol Mutagen. 1993;22:107–14.
129. Barbin A, Bartsch H. Nucleophilic selectivity as a determinant of carcinogenic potency (TD50) in rodents: a comparison of mono- and bi-functional alkylating agents and vinyl chloride metabolites. Mutat Res. 1989;215:95–107.
130. Allen BC, Crump KS, Shipp AM. Correlation between carcinogenic potency of chemicals in animals and humans. Risk Analysis. 1988;8:531–44.
131. Kaldor MJ, Day NE, Hemminki K. Quantifying the carcinogenicity of antineoplastic drugs. Eur J Cancer Clin Oncol. 1988;24:703–11.
132. Technical Resources I. Seventh Annual Report on Carcinogens. 1st edn. North Carolina: US Dept. of Health and Human Sciences; 1994.
133. Vogel EW, Nivard MJ. International Commission for Protection Against Environmental Mutagens and Carcinogens. The subtlety of alkylating agents in reactions with biological macromolecules. Mutat Res. 1994;305:13–32.
134. Pedersen-Bjergaard J, Philip P. Balanced translocations involving chromosome bands 11q23 and 21q22 are highly characteristic of myelodysplasia and leukemia following therapy with cytostatic agents targeting at DNA-topoisomerase-II. Blood. 1991;78:1147–8.
135. Pedersen-Bjergaard J, Philip P. Two different classes of therapy-related and de-novo acute leukemia? Cancer Cytogenet. 1991;55:119–24.
136. Ratain MJ, Kaminer LS, Bitran JD. Acute nonlymphocytic leukemia following etoposide and cisplatin combination chemotherapy for advanced non-small-cell carcinoma of the lung. Blood. 1987;70:1412–7.

137. Albain KS, LeBeau MM, Ullirsch R. Implication of prior treatment with drug combinations including inhibitors of topoisomerase II in therapy-related monocytic leukemia with a 9;11 translocation. Genes Chromosomes Cancer. 1990;2:53–8.
138. Hawkins MM, Kinnear Wilson LM, Stovall MA. Epipodophyllotoxins, alkylating agents, and radiation and risk of secondary leukemia after childhood cancer. Br Med J. 1992;304:951–8.
139. Sandoval C, Pui CH, Bowman LC, *et al.* Secondary acute myeloid leukemia in children previously treated with alkylating agents, intercalating topoisomerase-II inhibitors, and irradiation. J Clin Oncol. 1993;11:1039–45.
140. Pederson-Bjergaard J, Philip P. Balanced translocations involving bands 11q23 and 21q22 are highly characteristic of myelodysplasia and leukemia following therapy with cytostatic agents targeting at topoisomerase II. Blood. 1992;78:1147–8.
141. Sandoval C, Head DR, Mirro J. The t(9;11)(p21;q23) in pediatric *de novo* and secondary acute myeloblastic leukemia. Leukemia. 1992;6:513–9.
142. Detourmignies L, Castaigne S, Stoppa AM. Therapy-related acute promyelocytic leukemia: a report on sixteen cases. J Clin Oncol. 1992;10:1430–5.
143. Habs M, Schmahl D. Carcinogenicity of bleomycin sulfate and peplomycin sulfate after repeated subcutaneous application to rats. Oncology. 1984;41:114–9.
144. Shirai T, Masuda A, Hirose M, Ikawa E, Ito N. Enhancement of *N*-bis(2-hydroxypropyl)nitrosamine-initiated lung tumor development in rats by bleomycin and *N*-methyl-*N*-nitrosourethane. Cancer Lett. 1984;25:25–31.
145. Gurkalo VK, Volfson NI, Pliss GB. Central mechanism of vinblastine inhibitory effect on experimental carcinogenesis. Exp Pathol. 1987;32:179–86.
146. Csuka O, Szentirmay Z, Sugar J. The effect of promoters on 1,2-dimethylhydrazine-induced colon carcinogenesis. In: Börszönyi M; Day NE, Lapis K, Yamasaki H. IARC Sci Publ. No. 56, Models, mechanisms and etiology of tumour promotion. 1984:129–36.
147. Tsutsui T, Suzuki N, Maizumi H, Barrett JC. Vincristine sulfate-induced cell transformation, mitotic inhibition and aneuploidy in cultured Syrian hamster embryo cells. Carcinogenesis. 1986;7:131–5.
148. Hall EJ. Oncogenic transformation systems involving mammalian cells in vitro to determine the relative risks of different treatment modalities. Strahlentherapie. 1984;160:725–31.
149. Krumdieck CL. Role of folate deficiency in carcinogenesis. In: Butterworth CE, Hutchinson ML, eds. Nutritional factors in the induction and maintenance of malignancy, 1st edn. New York: Academic Press;1983:225–45.
150. Rogers AE, Akhtar R, Zeisel SH. Procarbazine carcinogenicity in methotrexate-treated or lipotrope-deficient male rats. Carcinogenesis. 1990;11:1491–5.
151. Iversen OH. Hydroxyurea enhances methylnitrosourea skin tumorigenesis when given shortly before, but not after, the carcinogen. Carcinogenesis. 1982;3:891–4.
152. Ashby J, Paton D. The influence of chemical structure on the extent and sites of carcinogenesis for 522 rodent carcinogens and 55 different human carcinogen exposures. Mutat Res. 1993;286:3–74.
153. Dunkel VC, Zeiger E, Brusick D, *et al.* Reproducibility of microbial mutagenicity assays: II. Testing of carcinogens and noncarcinogens in Salmonella typhimurium and Escherichia coli. Environ Mutagen. 1985;7(5):1–248.
154. Seino Y, Nagoa M, Yahagi I, Hoshi A, Kawachi T, Sugimura T. Mutagenicity of several classes of antitumor agents to Salmonella typhimurium TA98, TA100, TA92. Cancer Res. 1978;38:2148–56.
155. Hannan MA, al-Dakan AA, Hussain SS, Amer MH. Mutagenicity of cisplatin and carboplatin used alone and in combination with four other anticancer drugs. Toxicology. 1989;55:183–91.
156. Franza Jr BR, Oeschger NS, Oeschger MP, Schein PS. Mutagenic activity of nitrosourea antitumor agents. J Natl Cancer Inst. 1980;65:149–54.
157. Minnich V, Smith ME, Thompson D, Kornfeld S. Detection of mutagenic activity in human urine using mutant strains of Salmonella typhimurium. Cancer. 1976;38:1253–8.
158. Yamada M, Sofuni T, Nohmi T. Preferential induction of AT-TA transversion, but not deletions by chlorambucil at the hisG428 site of Salmonella typhimurium TA102. Mutat Res. 1992;283:29–33.
159. Beck DJ, Fisch JE. Mutagenicity of platinum co-ordination complexes in Salmonella typhimurium. Mutat Res. 1980;77:45–54.

160. Sakamoto Y, Fujikawa K, Nagayabu O, Yamamoto KS, Samejima K. Triple short-term tests with bacteria and Drosophila for assessment of mutagenicity of antineoplastics. J Takeda Res Lab. 1985;44(1/2):96–116.
161. Haworth S, Lawlor T, Mortelmans K, Speck W, Zeiger E. Salmonella mutagenicity test results for 250 chemicals. Environ Mutagen Suppl. 1983;5:3–142.
162. Dunkel VC, Zeiger E, Brusick D, *et al.* Reproducibility of microbial mutagenicity assays: I. Tests with Salmonella typhimurium and Escherichia coli using a standardized protocol. Environ Mutagen. 1984;6(2):1–254.
163. Zeiger E, Anderson B, Haworth S, Lawlor T, Mortelmans K. Salmonella mutagenicity tests: IV. Results from the testing of 300 chemicals. Environ Mol Mutagen. 1988;11(12):1–158.
164. Zeiger E, Anderson B, Haworth S, Lawlor T, Mortelmans K. Salmonella mutagenicity tests: V. Results from the testing of 311 chemicals. Environ Mol Mutagen. 1992;19(21):2–141.
165. Ferguson LR. Unpublished data, this laboratory. 1994.
166. Benedict WF, Baker MS, Haroun L, Choi E, Ames BN. Mutagenicity of cancer chemotherapeutic agents in the Salmonella/microsome test. Cancer Res. 1977;37:2209–13.
167. Babudri N, Pani B, Tamaro M, Monti-bragadin C, Zunino F. Mutagenic and cytotoxic activity of doxorubicin and daunorubicin derivatives on prokaryotic and eukaryotic cells. Br J Cancer. 1984;50:91–6.
168. Au WW, Butler MA, Matney TS, Loo TL. Comparative structure–genotoxicity study of three aminoanthraquinone drugs and doxorubicin. Cancer Res. 1981;41:376–9.
169. Gupta RS, Bromke A, Bryant DW, Gupta R, Singh B, McCalla DR. Etoposide (VP16) and teniposide (VM26): novel anticancer drugs, strongly mutagenic in mammalian but not prokaryotic test systems. Mutagenesis. 1987;2:179–86.
170. Mortelmans K, Haworth S, Lawlor T, Speck W, Tainer B, Zeiger E. Salmonella mutagenicity tests: II. Results from the testing of 270 chemicals. Environ Mutagen Suppl. 1986;8,7:1–119.
171. Zeiger E, Anderson B, Haworth S, Lawlor T, Mortelmans K, Speck W. Salmonella mutagenicity tests: III. Results from the testing of 255 chemicals. Environ Mol Mutagen. 1987;9(9):1–110.
172. Herboid B, Buseimaier W. Induction of point mutations by different chemical mechanisms in the liver microsomal assay. Mutat Res. 1976;40:73–84.
173. Bishop JB, Wassom JS. Toxicological review of busulfan (Myleran). Mutat Res. 1986;168:15–45.
174. Singh B, Gupta RS. Mutagenic responses of thirteen anticancer drugs on mutation induction at multiple genetic loci and on sister-chromatid exchanges in chinese hamster ovary cells. Cancer Res. 1983;43:577–84.
175. Clive D, Johnson KO, Spector JFS, Batson AG, Brown MMM. Validation and characterization of the L5178Y/TK+/– mouse lymphoma mutagen assay system. Mutat Res. 1979;59:61–108.
176. Chibber R, Ord MJ. The mutagenic and carcinogenic properties of three second generation antitumour platinum compounds: a comparison with cisplatin. Eur J Cancer Clin Oncol. 1989;25:27–33.
177. Deen DF, Kendall LE, Marton LJ, Tofilon PJ. Prediction of human tumor cell chemosensitivity using the sister chromatid exchange assay. Cancer Res. 1986;46:1599–602.
178. Bradley MO, Sharkey NA, Kohn KW, Layard MW. Mutagenicity and cytotoxicity of various nitrosoureas in V-79 chinese hamster cells. Cancer Res. 1980;40:2719–25.
179. Mourelatos D, Dozi-Vassiliades J, Granitsas A. Anti-tumor alkylating agents act synergistically with methylxanthines on induction of sister-chromatid exchange in human lymphocytes. Mutat Res. 1982;104:243–7.
180. Dickins M, Wright K, Phillips M, Todd N. Toxicity and mutagenicity of 6 anti-cancer drugs in Chinese hamster V79 cells co-cultured with rat hepatocytes. Mutat Res. 1985;157:189–97.
181. Perry P, Evans HJ. Cytological detection of mutagen-carcinogen exposure by sister chromatid exchange. Nature. 1975;258:121–5.
182. Au W, Sokova OI, Kopnin B, Arrighi FE. Cytogenetic toxicity of cyclophosphamide and its metabolites in vitro. Cytogenet Cell Genet. 1980;26:108–16.
183. Matheson D, Brusick D, Carrano R. Comparison of the relative mutagenic activity for eight antineoplastic drugs in the Ames Salmonella/microsome and TK+/– mouse lymphoma assays. Drug Chemic Toxicol. 1978;1:277–304.

184. Bartoli-Klugmann F, Pani B, Babudri N, Montibragadin C, Tamaro M, Venturini S. In vitro mutagenic activity of 5-(3,3-dimethyl-1-triazeno)-imidazole-4-carboxamide (DTIC) in eukaryotic and prokaryotic cells. Carcinogenesis. 1982;2:467–71.
185. Banerjee A, Benedict WF. Production of sister chromatid exchanges by various cancer chemotherapeutic agents. Cancer Res. 1979;39:797–9.
186. Benedict WF, Banerjee A, Gardner A, Jones PA. Induction of morphological transformation in mouse C3H/10T1/2 clone 8 cells and chromosomal damage in hamster A(T1)C1-3 cells by cancer chemotherapeutic agents. Cancer Res. 1977;37:2202–8.
187. Yajima N, Kondo K, Morita K. Reverse mutation tests in Salmonella typhimurium and chromosomal aberration tests in mammalian cells in culture on fluorinated pyrimidine derivatives. Mutat Res. 1981;88:241–54.
188. Nishi Y, Hasegawa MM, Taketomi M, Ohkawa Y, Inui N. Comparison of 6-thioguanine-resistant mutation and sister chromatid exchanges in Chinese hamster V79 cells with forty chemical and physical agents. Cancer Res. 1984;44:3270–9.
189. Shiraishi Y, Sandberg AA. Effects of various chemical agents on sister chromatid exchanges, chromosome aberrations, and DNA repair in normal and abnormal human lymphoid cell lines. J Natl Cancer Inst. 1979;62:27–35.
190. Suter W, Brennand J, McMillan S, Fox M. Relative mutagenicity of antineoplastic drugs and other alkylating agents in V79 Chinese hamster cells, independence of cytotoxic and mutagenic responses. Mutat Res. 1980;73:171–81.
191. Parkes DJ, Scott D. A quantitative comparison of cytogenetic effects of anti-tumor agents. Cytogenet Cell Genet. 1982;33:27–34.
192. Hittleman WN, Rao PN. Premature chromosome condensation. II. The nature of chromosome gaps produced by alkylating agents and ultraviolet light. Mutat Res. 1974;23:259–66.
193. Tweats DJ, Gatehouse DG. Further debate of testing strategies. Mutagenesis. 1988;3:95–102.
194. Bayer U. The in vivo induction of sister chromatid exchanges in the bone marrow of the chinese hamster. II. *N*-Nitrosodiethylamine (DEN) and *N*-isopropyl-alpha-(2-methylhydrazine)-p-toluamide (Natulan), two carcinogenic compounds with specific mutagenicity problems. Mutat Res. 1978;56:305–9.
195. Amacher DE, Zelljadt I. Mutagenic activity of some clastogenic chemicals at the hypoxanthine guanine phosphoribosyl transferase locus of Chinese hamster ovary cells. Mutat Res. 1984;136:137–45.
196. Clive D, Turner N, Krehl R. Procarbazine is a potent mutagen at the heterozygous thymidine kinase (tk +/–) locus of mouse lymphoma assay. Mutagenesis. 1988;3:83–7.
197. Littlefield LG, Colyer SP, Sayer AM, Dufrain RJ. Sister-chromatid exchanges in human lymphocytes exposed during G0 to four classes of DNA-damaging chemicals. Mutat Res. 1979;67:259–69.
198. Pommier Y, Kerrigan D, Covey JM, Kao-Shan CS, Whang-Peng J. Sister chromatid exchanges, chromosomal aberrations, and cytotoxity produced by antitumor topoisomerase II inhibitors in sensitive (DC3F) and resistant (DC3F/9-OHE) Chinese hamster cells. Cancer Res. 1988;48:512–6.
199. Anderson HC, Kihlman BA. The production of chromosomal alterations in human lymphocytes by drugs known to interfere with the activity of DNA topoisomerase II. I. m-AMSA. Carcinogenesis. 1989;10:123–30.
200. Dillehay LE, Denstman SC, Williams JE. Cell cycle dependence of sister chromatid exchange induction by DNA topoisomerase II inhibitors in Chinese hamster V79 cells. Cancer Res. 1987;47:206–9.
201. Mourelatos D, Dozi-Vassiliades J, Tsigalidou-Balla V, Granitsas A. Enhancement by methylxanthines of sister-chromatid exchange frequency induced by cytostatics in normal and leukemic human lymphocytes. Mutat Res. 1983;121:147–52.
202. Singh B, Gupta RS. Comparison of the mutagenic responses of 12 anticancer drugs at the hypoxanthine-guanine phosphoribosyl transferase and adenosine kinase loci in chinese hamster ovary cells. Environ Mutagen. 1983;5:871–80.
203. Segawa M, Nadamitsu S, Kondo K, Yoshizaki I. Chromosomal aberrations of Don lung cells of chinese hamster after exposure to vinblastine in vitro. Mutat Res. 1979;66:99–102.
204. Morgan WF, Crossen PE. Mitotic spindle inhibitors and sister-chromatid exchange in human chromosomes. Mutat Res. 1980;77:283–6.

205. McGregor DB, Brown A, Cattanch P, *et al.* Responses of the L5178Y tk+/tk– mouse lymphoma cell forward mutation assay: III. 72 coded chemicals. Environ Mol Mutagen. 1988;12:85–154.
206. Amacher DE, Turner GN. The mutagenicity of 5-azacytidine and other inhibitors of replicative DNA synthesis in the L5178Y mouse lymphoma cell. Mutat Res. 1987;176:123–31.
207. Kihlman BA, Andersson HC. Synergistic enhancement of the frequency of chromatid aberrations in cultured human lymphocytes by combinations of inhibitors of DNA repair. Mutat Res. 1985;150:313–25.
208. Aebersold PM. Mutation induction by 5-fluorodeoxyuridine in synchronous Chinese hamster cells. Cancer Res. 1979;39:808–10.
209. Huang P, Siciliano MJ, Plunkett W. Gene deletion, a mechanism of induced mutation by arabinosyl nucleosides. Mutat Res. 1989;210:291–301.
210. Maier P, Schmid W. Ten model mutagens evaluated by the micronucleus test. Mutat Res. 1976;40:325–38.
211. Leonard A, Linden G. Observation of dividing spermatocytes for chromosome aberrations induced in mouse spermatogonia by chemical mutagens. Mutat Res. 1972;16:197–300.
212. Epstein SS, Arnold E, Andrea J, Bass W, Bishop Y. Detection of chemical mutagens by the dominant lethal assay in the mouse. Toxicol Appl Pharmacol. 1972;23:288–325.
213. Bucci LR, Meistrich ML. Effects of busulfan on murine spermatogenesis: cytotoxicity, sterility, sperm abnormalities, and dominant lethal mutations. Mutat Res. 1987;176:259–68.
214. Meistrich ML, Finch M, da Cunha MF, Hacker U, Au WW. Damaging effects of fourteen chemotherapeutic drugs on mouse testis cells. Cancer Res. 1982;42:122–31.
215. Tates AD, Natarajan AT, De Vogel N, Meijers M. A correlative study on the genetic damage induced by chemical mutagens in bone marrow and spermatogonia of mice. III. 1,3-bis-(2-chloroethyl)-3-nitrosurea (BCNU). Mutat Res. 1977;44:87–95.
216. Wiencke JK, Cervenka J, Pauius H. Mutagenic activity of anticancer agent cis-dichlorodiammine platinum-II. Mutat Res. 1979;68:69–77.
217. Suter W, Jaeger I. Comparative evaluation of different pairs of DNA repair-deficient and DNA repair-proficient bacterial tester strains for rapid detection of chemical mutagens and carcinogens. Mutat Res. 1982;97:1–18.
218. Vanparys P, Vermeiren F, Sysmans M, Temmerman R. The micronucleus assay as a test for the detection of aneugenic activity. Mutat Res. 1990;244:95–103.
219. Neal SB, Probst GS. Chemically-induced sister-chromatid exchange in vivo in bone marrow of Chinese hamsters. An evaluation of 24 compounds. Mutat Res. 1983;113:34–43.
220. Jacquet P, Pire P. Morphological and cytogenetic studies of dominant lethality induced by mitomycin C and cyclophosphamide in female germ cells. The use of Robertsonian translocations as a 'marker system' to identify the zygote pronuclei. Mutat Res. 1984;128:181–94.
221. Schlegel R, MacGregor JT. A rapid screen for cumulative chromosomal damage in mice. Accumulation of circulating micronucleated erythrocytes. Mutat Res. 1983;113:481–7.
222. Fox M, Scott D. The genetic toxicology of nitrogen and sulfur mustard. Mutat Res. 1980;75:131–68.
223. Lee IP, Dixon RL. Mutagenicity, carcinogenicity and teratogenicity of procarbazine. Mutat Res. 1978;55:1–14.
224. Liegibel U, Tinwell H, Callander RD, Schmezer P, Ashby J. Clastogenicity to the mouse bone marrow of the mouse germ cell genotoxin streptozotocin. Mutagenesis. 1992;7:471–4.
225. Backer LC, Allen JW, Harrington-Brock K, *et al.* Genotoxicity of inhibitors of DNA topoisomerases-I (camptothecin) and topoisomerases-II (m-AMSA) *in vivo* and *in vitro*. Mutagenesis. 1990;5:541–7.
226. Holmstrom M, Winters V. Micronucleus induction by camptothecin and amsacrine in bone marrow of male and female CD-1 mice. Mutagenesis. 1992;7:189–93.
227. Au WW, Hsu TC. The genotoxic effects of adriamycin in somatic and germinal cells of the mouse. Mutat Res. 1980;79:351–61.
228. Bhuyan BK, Zimmer DM, Mazurek JH, *et al.* Comparative genotoxicity of adriamycin and menogarol, two anthracycline antitumor agents. Cancer Res. 1983;43:5293–7.
229. Meistrich ML, Goldstein LS, Wyrobek AJ. Long-term infertility and dominant lethal mutations in male mice treated with adriamycin. Mutat Res. 1985;152:53–65.
230. Mailhes JB, Marchetti F, Phillips GL, Barnhill DR. Preferential pericentric lesions and aneuploidy induced in mouse oocytes by the topoisomerase II inhibitor etoposide. Teratogen Carcinogen Mutagen. 1994;14:39–51.

231. Sieber SM, Whang-Peng J, Botkin C, Knutsen T. Teratogenic and cytogenetic effects of some plant-derived antitumor agents (vincristine, colchicine, maytansine, VP-16-213 and VM-26) in mice. Teratology. 1978;18:31–48.
232. Poorman-Allen P, Backer LC, Adler I, Westbrook-Collins B, Moses MJ, Allen JW. Bleomycin effects on mouse meiotic chromosomes. Mutagenesis. 1990;5:573–81.
233. Satya-Prakash KL, Liang JC, Hsu TC, Johnson DA. Chromosome aberrations in mouse bone marrow cells following treatment in vivo with vinblastine and Colcemid. Environ Mutagen. 1986;8:273–82.
234. Subramanyam S, Laxinarayana D, Beaula Helen KD. Evaluation of genotoxic potential of vincristine from multiple parameters. Mutat Res. 1984;138:55–62.
235. Hatakeyama Y, Nakajima E, Atai H, Suzuki S. Effects of benzene in a micronucleus test on peripheral blood utilizing acridine orange-coated slides. Mutat Res. 1992;278:193–5
236. Hayashi M. Micronucleus test with mouse peripheral blood erythrocytes by acridine orange supravital staining – the summary report of the fifth collaborative study by CSGMT/JEMS-MMS. Mutat Res. 1992;278:83–98.
237. James DA, Smith DM. Analysis of results from a collaborative study of the dominant lethal assay. Mutat Res. 1982;97:303–14.
238. Albanese R. The cytonucleus test in the rat: a combined metaphase and micronucleus assay. Mutat Res. 1987;182:309–21.
239. Holden HE, Ray VA, Wahrenberg MG, Zelenski JD. Mutagenicity studies with 6-mercaptopurine: 1. Cytogenetic activity in vivo. Mutat Res. 1973;20:257–63.
240. Moreland FM, Sheu CW, Springer JA, Green S. Effects of prolonged chemical treatment with cyclophosphamide and 6-mercaptopurine in the dominant lethal test system. Mutat Res. 1981;90:193–9.
241. Generoso WM, Preston J, Brewen JG. 6-Mercaptopurine, an inducer of cytogenetic and dominant-lethal effects in premeiotic and early meiotic germ cells of male mice. Mutat Res. 1975;28:437–47.
242. Murcia CR, Arroyo Nombela JJ. Cytological aberrations produced by methotrexate in mouse ascites tumours. Mutat Res. 1972;14:405–12.

Index